Complex Clinical Conundrums
in Psychiatry

Kuppuswami Shivakumar
Shabbir Amanullah
Editors

Complex Clinical Conundrums in Psychiatry

From Theory to Clinical Management

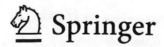

Editors
Kuppuswami Shivakumar
Department of Psychiatry
Northern Ontario School of Medicine
Psychiatry Department
Sudbury, Ontario
Canada

Shabbir Amanullah
Woodstock General Hospital
Woodstock Ontario, University of
Western Ontario
London, Ontario
Canada

ISBN 978-3-319-70310-7   ISBN 978-3-319-70311-4   (eBook)
https://doi.org/10.1007/978-3-319-70311-4

Library of Congress Control Number: 2018942535

Printed on acid-free paper

This Springer imprint is published by the registered company Springer International Publishing AG part of Springer Nature
The registered company address is: Gewerbestrasse 11, 6330 Cham, Switzerland

Dedicated to our parents, wives, and family members for their continuous support.

Preface

In today's world of ever-increasing publications, research papers, opinion leaders, and conferences, one is at loss on what to follow in terms of best practice. The treatment recommendations in guidelines do not work for all patients, and the clinician is left with few options to help the patient. While some access web forums and others call a friend at the university, most are unable to access information that is put together in a concise manner to help navigate challenging cases.

The authors who wrote the book, after years of work as clinicians and researchers in different countries, with the aim of giving their patients the best evidence-based care. However, it became abundantly clear that the evidence available often fell short of getting the desired results for patients in our care. To add to this was the ever-increasing number of publications with recommendations that were at times contrary to one another. This book is made up of several chapters written by leading experts from across the globe, covering a range of topics from conditions in adolescence to those in the elderly.

This book seeks to bridge the gap between theory and clinical application with a view to help clinicians use a combination of evidence, experience, and practical solutions. While the authors advice that one follows the existing guidelines to the best of the clinician's ability, this book offers options based on the experience of the authors from diverse backgrounds with a common interest in patient well being. There are certain conditions where treatment resistance poses a unique challenge and will require the readers to look at emerging best practice and experience; moreover, it is always important to include the patient and where possible the family in decision making.

We are delighted at the support we got from various authors across the globe; despite their busy clinical schedules, they stuck to our deadlines and our comments. We are also grateful to our mentors, colleagues, and graduate students for their editorial support.

Nadina Persaud and her team at Springer have been supportive beyond the call of duty. Thanks to all of them. Finally, there are those who may not respond to the treatments we propose, but this subgroup of nonresponders is the reason for medicine advances. We owe it to them to try our best. We hope you enjoy this book and that it benefits those who need it the most.

Sudbury, ON, Canada   K. Shivakumar
Woodstock, ON, Canada   S. Amanullah
April 2018

Contents

Contributors

Peter Ajueze, MD, MRCPsych(UK), FRCPC Department of Psychiatry, Northern Ontario School of Medicine (NOSM), Sudbury, ON, Canada

Shabbir Amanullah, MD, DPM, FRCPsych(UK), CCT,FRCPC Woodstock General Hospital, Woodstock Ontario University of Western Ontario, London, ON, Canada

University of Western London, Ontario and Dalhousie University Halifax, London, England, UK

Oyedeji Ayonrinde, FRCPsych, MBA Queen's University, Kingston, ON, Canada

Kingston Health Sciences Centre, Hotel Dieu Hospital, Kingston, ON, Canada

Brad D. Booth, MD, FRCPC Integrated Forensic Program, Royal Ottawa Mental Health Centre, Ottawa, ON, Canada

Prabha S. Chandra, MD, FRCPsych, FAMS Department of Psychiatry, National Institute of Mental Health and Neuro Sciences, Bangalore, India

Lynne Drummond National and Trustwide Services for OCD/BDD, SW London and St. George's NHS Trust, London, UK

Bruce Fage, MD Department of Psychiatry, University of Toronto, Toronto, ON, Canada

Sundarnag Ganjekar Department of Psychiatry, National Institute of Mental Health and Neuro Sciences, Bangalore, India

Nisha Nigil Haroon, MD, MSc, Dip NB, CCD, DM Department of Internal Medicine, Northern Ontario School of Medicine (NOSM), Sudbury, ON, Canada

Alkomiet Hasan, MD Department of Psychiatry and Psychotherapy, Klinikum der Universität München, Ludwig-Maximilians Universität München, Munich, Germany

Akiko Kawaguchi, MD, PhD Department of Psychiatry and Cognitive-Behavioral Medicine, Nagoya City University Graduate School of Medical Sciences, Nagoya, Japan

Popuri M. Krishna, MB, BS, DPM, MD, DABPN, FRCPC Department of Psychiatry, Northern Ontario School of Medicine (NOSM), Sudbury, ON, Canada

Tim Lau, MD, FRCP(C), MSc Department of Psychiatry, University of Ottawa, Ottawa, ON, Canada

Jodi Lofchy, MD, FRCPC Psychiatry Emergency Services, Department of Psychiatry, University Health Network, University of Toronto, Toronto, ON, Canada

Michelle D. Mathias, MD, FRCPC Division of Forensic Psychiatry, Department of Psychiatry, University of Ottawa, Ottawa, ON, Canada

M. Nadeem Mazhar, MD, FRCPC Department of Psychiatry, Queen's University, Kingston, ON, Canada

Nirosha J. Murugan, PhD Allen Discovery Center at Tufts; Tufts Center for Regenerative and Developmental Biology, Science and Engineering Complex (SEC), Medford, MA, USA

Vicky P.K.H. Nguyen, MSc, MD, PhD Psychiatry Resident, Northern Ontario School of Medicine, Sudbury, ON, Canada

Ross Norman, PhD PEPP Program, London Health Sciences Centre, Robarts Research Institute and Department of Psychiatry, University of Western Ontario, London, ON, Canada

Najala Orrell, MD Medical student, Schoool of Medicine, Royal College of Surgeons in Ireland, Dublin, Ireland

Lena Palaniyappan, MBBS, FRCPC, PhD PEPP Program, London Health Sciences Centre, Robarts Research Institute and Department of Psychiatry, University of Western Ontario, London, ON, Canada

Soumya Parameshwaran Department of Psychiatry, National Institute of Mental Health and Neuro Sciences, Bangalore, India

Sarah Penfold, MD Department of Psychiatry, Queen's University, Kingston, ON, Canada

Jennifer L. Pikard, MD, MSc Department of Psychiatry, Queen's University, Kingston, ON, Canada

Gautham Pulagam, MD, BSc Schulich School of Medicine, Western University, London, ON, Canada

Adnan Rajeh, MD Victoria Hospital and Children's Hospital of Western Ontario, London, ON, Canada

Arun Ravindran, MB, PhD Department of Psychiatry, University of Toronto, Toronto, ON, Canada

Centre for Addiction and Mental Health, Mood and Anxiety, Toronto, ON, Canada

Nisha Ravindran, MD, FRCPC Department of Psychiatry, University of Toronto, Toronto, ON, Canada

Centre for Addiction and Mental Health, Mood and Anxiety, Toronto, ON, Canada

Alana Rawana, HBSc, MA (Clinical Psychology) Northern Ontario School of Medicine, Thunder Bay, ON, Canada

Andrew Roney National and Trustwide Services for OCD/BDD, SW London and St. George's NHS Trust, London, UK

Nicolas Rouleau, PhD Department of Biomedical Engineering, Initiative for Neural Science, Disease and Engineering (INScide) at Tufts University, Science and Engineering Complex (SEC), Medford, MA, USA

Sarah Russell, MD Department of Psychiatry, University of Ottawa, Ottawa, ON, Canada

Priyadharshini Sabesan, MBBS, MRCPsych Urgent Care and Ambulatory Mental Health, London Health Sciences Centre and University of Western Ontario, London, ON, Canada

Kevin Saroka, BSc, MA, PhD Department of Psychiatry, Northern Ontario School of Medicine (NOSM), Sudbury, ON, Canada

Department of Psychiatry, Health Sciences North, Sudbury, ON, Canada

Kuppuswami Shivakumar, MD, MPH, MRCPsych(UK), FRCPC Department of Psychiatry, Northern Ontario School of Medicine (NOSM), Sudbury, ON, Canada

Ranga Shivakumar, MD, MRCP, FRCPC, ABIM Department of Psychiatry, Northern Ontario School of Medicine (NOSM), Sudbury, ON, Canada

Daya Somasundaram Department of Psychiatry, Faculty of Medicine, University of Jaffna, Jaffna, Sri Lanka

School of Medicine, Faculty of Health Sciences, University of Adelaide, Adelaide, Australia

Sanjeevan Somasunderam Denmark Hill, Camberwell, London, UK

T. Umaharan Post Graduate Institute of Medicine, University of Colombo, Colombo, Sri Lanka

Raj Velamoor, MB, FRCPsych (UK), FRCP (C) Northern Ontario School of Medicine, Laurentian and Lakehead University, Sudbury, ON, Canada

Schulich School of Medicine, Western University, London, ON, Canada

Ramamohan Veluri, MD, DPM, MRCPsych, FRCPC Northern Ontario School of Medicine, Sudbury, ON, Canada

Norio Watanabe, MD, PhD Department of Health Promotion and Human Behavior, Department of Clinical Epidemiology, Graduate School of Public Health, Kyoto University, Kyoto, Japan

Rosalia Sun Young Yoon, MSc, PhD Department of Psychiatry, University of Toronto, Toronto, ON, Canada

Centre for Addiction and Mental Health, Mood and Anxiety, Toronto, ON, Canada

A Complex Case of Major Neurocognitive Disorder: Alzheimer's Disease

Popuri M. Krishna, Kuppuswami Shivakumar, and Shabbir Amanullah

Abbreviations

Aβ42	42-amino acid beta-amyloid
AD	Alzheimer's disease
ADLs	Activities of daily living
APOE	Apolipoprotein E
APP	Amyloid precursor protein
CSF	Cerebrospinal fluid
CT	Computed tomography
DSM	Diagnostic and Statistical Manual
MAPT	Microtubule-associated protein tau
MCI	Minimal cognitive impairment
MRI	Magnetic resonance imaging
NFT	Neurofibrillary tangles
NP	Neuritic plaques
PIB	Pittsburgh compound B
PSEN	Presenilin
SPECT	Single photon emission computed tomography

P.M. Krishna, MB, BS, DPM, MD, DABPN, FRCPC (✉) • K. Shivakumar, MD, MPH, MRCPsych(UK), FRCPC
Department of Psychiatry, Northern Ontario School of Medicine Psychiatry Department, Sudbury, ON, Canada
e-mail: pkrishna@hsnsudbury.ca

S. Amanullah, MD, DPM, FRCPsych(UK), CCT,FRCPC
University of Western Ontario, Woodstock General Hospital University of Western Ontario, Woodstock, ON, Canada

Major Neurocognitive Disorder (MND) is a term that has been incorporated in DSM-5 to replace the term dementia. MND is a clinical syndrome characterized by global cognitive decline from the previous level of functioning as evidenced in loss of one or more cognitive domains (complex attention, executive function, learning and memory, language, perceptomotor or social cognition). Occurring in clear sensorium, this decline interferes with the individual's ability to be independent. MND is a public health issue with significant impact on patients, their families, and the community. Dementia is already an epidemic in developed countries (Murray and Lopez 1997). In more than 50% of cases of Major Neurocognitive Disorders, Alzheimer's disease is the cause (Alzheimer's Association, 2011). The pathology of AD is clearly defined to consist of Neuritic Plaques (NP), Neurofibrillary Tangles (NFT) and subsequent neuronal loss, which is present in a typical distribution in the brains of the afflicted patients. The two most common risk factors for AD are advanced age and family history of dementia.

1.1 Case History

A 52-year-old married female presented with her husband for a geriatric assessment, with concerns about her memory. Over the previous 3 years, her

© Springer International Publishing AG, part of Springer Nature 2018
K. Shivakumar, S. Amanullah (eds.), *Complex Clinical Conundrums in Psychiatry*, https://doi.org/10.1007/978-3-319-70311-4_1

husband noticed that she was repeating the same question, having forgotten that she had asked the same question a number of times previously. This repetition has increased in intensity while waiting for this consult. In the months before the assessment, she started forgetting events. She started misplacing things around the house. In one instance, she forgot where she parked the car and required her husband's help. She frequently forgot her appointments. She did not have any word finding difficulty and was able to recognize people without difficulty. She continued to drive to work, and there were no reports of her losing her way around. She seemed to be more forgetful when she was nervous. She was attending to all her activities of daily living (ADLs). She maintained meaningful employment in the family business – a local shoe store. She was able to handle the customers and the cash register. She did not have any mood changes nor experience incontinence.

Her medical history was positive for lupus, diagnosed about 4 years ago. She also had non-ulcerative dyspepsia. There was no history of diabetes, hypertension, or hypercholesterolemia. She was taking hydroxychloroquine 200 mg P.O. daily. There were no allergies to medication. Her maternal grandmother had a history of Alzheimer's disease at a later age. Her mother died of cancer at 65. Her premorbid personality indicated an outgoing, happy, and jovial person of average intelligence. She liked to sing while at home. She liked cooking and baking.

In her personal history, there is evidence of physical, emotional, and sexual abuse by family members. She completed grade 8 education and later worked as a waitress after moving out of her family home. She got married at 21 and had three children. There is no history of alcohol or substance abuse.

Her physical and neurological examinations were within normal limits. She scored 21/30 on MMSE, but otherwise her mental state examination was normal.

Her CT scan and hematological exam were within normal limits. Her B12 was 229 picograms/ml, TSH 1.10 milli-IU/ L. She was diag-nosed as having Major Neurocognitive Disorder-Alzheimer's Disease. Given the early age of onset, she was referred for further testing for confirmation of diagnosis.

1.2 Genetic Factors Contributing to the Onset of Alzheimer's Disease (AD)

Between 50% and 70% of patients with MND are diagnosed to have the Alzheimer's disease (AD) subtype [26]. A major risk factor for AD is genetic, with 70–80% of cases being hereditary. This is supported by twin studies [7]. AD is a heterogeneous condition involving the interaction of genetic, environmental, and personal factors. Given that the etiology is polygenetic, a predominance of certain gene types may increase the risk of AD, while some genes may be protective [5]. The most well-known gene is the APOE gene. The ε4 allele of APOE gene is a risk factor for AD. Heterozygous ε4 carriers have three times, and homozygous carriers have 15 times the risk of non-ε4 carriers. The APOE ε4 gene is probably involved in the age of onset of the AD [8]. The APOE gene has low penetrance, thus implicating the involvement of other genes involved in the phenotypic expression of AD.

There are two types of expression of AD, familial and sporadic. Among the familial expression, there are two patterns: early-onset and late-onset familial patterns. Late-onset familial AD is the more common form, which is seen in individuals over age 65. Genetic risk decreases with advancing age in some studies [30]. Late-onset familial AD is mediated through several susceptibility genes, including APOE. There are three allelic variations of APOE: ε2, ε3, and ε4. The ε2 allele is relatively rare and may provide protection against the onset of AD. The ε3 allele is most common in the western European population and may be neutral in its effect. However, those individuals who are homozygous for the APOE ε4 allele have the much higher burden of amyloid plaque than those with other genotypes [13].

1.3 Genetic Factors Involved in the Early Onset of Alzheimer's Disease

About 30–40% of early-onset MND-AD has been shown to be due to familial autosomal inheritance pattern. Other genes are probably involved as risk factors (Table 1.1).

The autosomal dominant inheritance pattern of genes shows high penetrance with more severe neuropathological changes. It is also found that the age of onset in these individuals is in the range of 30–50 years. All the genetic forms of MND-AD result in overproduction of the Aβ42 amyloid peptide. The extra chromosome 21 in Down's syndrome with an additional APP gene accelerates the onset of AD by about 30 years earlier than in patients without an extra chromosome 21. PSEN-I mutations are by far the most common gene involved in early-onset AD. The PSEN-II gene is less common and is seen most often in those of German descent living in North America. As noted before, the APOE ε4 gene probably modifies the age of onset of AD by uncertain molecular mechanisms [8]. Other genes may be involved, but their relationship to AD susceptibility or protection is not yet clearly understood (Table 1.2).

1.4 Pathological Effects of the Genetic Factors in an Alzheimer's Disease

The genetic effect of various genes in the pathological process of producing the neurodegenerative changes seen in MND-AD is unclear. The

Table 1.2 Other genes with possible implications in early-onset AD [5]

ACE	MTHFR
CHRNB2	NCSTN
CST3	PRNP
ESRI	GAPDHS
TF	IDE
TFAM	TNF

most common histological changes seen in MND-AD are neuritic plaques (NP) and neurofibrillary tangles (NFT). Other less conspicuous findings are granulovacuolar degeneration, Hirano bodies, and amyloid angiopathy. The neuritic plaques primarily contain amyloid proteins, particularly the Aβ42 peptide in patients with MND-AD. Those individuals who are homozygous for APOE ε4 allele have much higher plaque burden than those who do not. This suggests a pathological effect of APP in persons with MND-AD. APP is cleaved by three secretases: alpha, beta, and gamma. Mutations in PSEN genes lead to an alteration in gamma-secretase, generating higher loads of Aβ42. One hypothesis is that Aβ42 induces an inflammatory response in the brains of patients with MND-AD and promotes oxidative injury to the neurons. The deposit of amyloid in NP may be fairly extensive by the time early symptoms of MND-AD appear [24].

NP are found in the posterior neocortex, especially in the temporal and parietal regions of the brain and, less abundantly, in the frontal regions [2]. Diffuse plaques containing Aβ2 peptide are common in brains without cognitive impairments. In patients with dementia, there is a negligible correlation between NP counts and the degree of cognitive impairment. NP burden does not change even in the progression of symptoms. This is shown by PIB PET imaging studies, where amyloid burden reaches the maximum by the time patients reach the minimal cognitive impairment (MCI) stage in MND-AD.

NFT are primarily intraneuronal. The burden of NFT is better correlated with disease severity than NP count [6]. The NFT formation and neu-

Table 1.1 Genes implicated in early-onset AD [5]

Protein	Chromosome	Inheritance pattern
Amyloid precursor	21	Autosomal dominant
Presenilin I	14	Autosomal dominant
Presenilin II	1	Autosomal dominant
APOE	19	Risk factor

ronal damage progress during MND-AD. The neurotransmitter changes primarily in acetylcholine and other neurotransmitters such as dopamine, serotonin, norepinephrine, and glutamine occur as epiphenomenon due to the disruption of neural pathways. In combination with the inflammatory processes, this leads to neuronal death and disconnections between the neurons by disrupting the dendrites and axons. These changes lead to the cognitive, behavioral, and psychological symptoms in the MND-AD.

NFT are primarily composed of microtubule-associated proteins, tau MAPT [15]. In MND-AD, the tau is excessively phosphorylated. This excessively phosphorylated tau cannot be degraded by the neurons, and it accumulates in the neurons. The genes for different isoforms of tau are located on chromosome 17. It is not clear what induces the hyper-phosphorylation of tau. It is suggested that $A\beta42$ peptide may induce this process. NFT are initially seen around middle age, starting in the transentorhinal area of the brain [6], and then it progresses to entorhinal and hippocampal (CAI) regions. Finally, this progresses to other neocortical association areas. Increased brain volume loss is correlated with the involvement of neocortical regions by NFT.

The hippocampal and medial temporal areas affected are consistent with early anterograde amnestic symptoms in the initial stages of MND-AD. Amyloid angiopathy is commonly found in the brain in patients with MND-AD [14]. However, the presence of amyloid angiopathy does not appear to have a clinical correlate. Other age-related changes in the brain also have a cumulative effect on the pathology of MND-AD.

Loss of memory occurs fairly early with the development of agnosia, apraxia, and aphasia. Patients have gradual deterioration of their functional abilities in the middle stage. In the terminal stages, problems develop with mobility and continence. With good health and good care, patients with MND-AD may live a long time, even in near-vegetative states. Death usually occurs due to frailty resulting from intercurrent infection or other medical causes.

1.5   Continuation of the Case

Four years later, the patient's husband brought her back to the emergency department of the local hospital. Her memory had worsened to the point that she was unable to take care of herself. Her husband and her daughters were providing care along with the support of community services. She was unable to attend to her activities of daily living (ADLs). She had difficulty recognizing familiar people in her life, including her family members. She had difficulty maintaining her sleep. She lost her appetite and dropped 6 pounds in weight. She was often irritable in her mood. Her speech was reduced to simple words, spoken out of context. She was unable to communicate her thoughts coherently. Later, she stopped communicating with her family. Occasionally, she was incontinent of urine.

Over the last 4 years, she was assessed at the tertiary care hospital. She underwent neuropsychological testing after her clinical assessment. Based on the discrepancy of her neuropsychological test scores for her age and the history of sexual abuse, she was diagnosed to have conversion disorder with amnestic symptoms. She was recommended to have psychological counseling and started on a trial of sertraline medication. She was advised to follow up with her primary care physician.

In spite of these interventions, her memory and capacity to function continued to deteriorate. The family was concerned for her safety. They could not leave her at home as she could not live unsupervised. She was deemed incompetent 1 year ago for both personal care and finances, and her husband was appointed substitute decision-maker.

A CT scan and hematological exam done at the second presentation were reported to be normal. She was admitted to the psychiatry unit for further assessment and care planning. A SPECT scan and EEG were performed along with cognitive and functional assessments. The SPECT scan showed a surprisingly abnormal scan for her age of 57 years. She had worse uptake in parietal areas in comparison to the frontal areas. There were decreased uptake in temporal areas, more so on the left side, and only mild decreased uptake in occipital areas. There was a normal uptake in the basal ganglia. Her EEG was abnormal, with slow background activity. There was a persistent mixture of delta and theta wave activity. These findings were consistent with advanced Alzheimer's disease. Her MMSE was 3/30, compared to 21/30 4 years earlier. She showed severe functional impairment. She needed assistance with her ADLs. She was diagnosed to have a major neurocognitive disorder of early-onset Alzheimer's disease, moderate in severity. She was started on galantamine 4 mg P.O. twice daily, gradually to be increased up to a maximum of 24 mg daily. Her antidepressant medication was stopped. Her husband wanted to provide care at home with community supports. Thus, she was discharged back to her home.

1.6 Natural History of Alzheimer's Disease?

It has been shown that the pathological process of MND-AD begins several years before the onset of clinical and functional changes of the individuals with MND-AD [3]. It is possible to have imaging studies for amyloid deposition by Pittsburgh compound B (PIB), PET, and SPECT studies [21]. The natural history of Alzheimer's dementia has been well-described. Time from diagnosis to death in the tertiary centers is on the order of 10–12 years. The median time from onset of symptoms to death is around 3–5 years [20]. Most patients exhibit slow progression. In Cache County Study, a quarter of the patients showed limited progression from milder stages of MND-AD, even after 3–5 years of onset [18]. The presence of psychosis and extrapyramidal symptoms is associated with faster progression, along with the presence of

hypertension, diabetes, hyperlipidemia, and atrial fibrillation.

1.7 Investigations Used to Establish the Diagnosis?

After completing a comprehensive history and physical exam, most cases of MND-AD are diagnosed clinically. Obtaining baseline labs and electrocardiograms is the first step in the investigation. Less than 1% of the dementias are truly reversible, even with intervention. Less than 10% of patients with dementia may show a reversible cause by the laboratory investigations [11]. Additional lab evaluation workup can be done if other risk factors are identified in the patient's history. Lumbar puncture (LP) and electroencephalograph (EEG) are done in patients where diagnosis is unclear. The American Academy of Neurology recommends either computed tomography (CT) or magnetic resonance imaging (MRI) [19]. Other methods of assessment include PET, SPECT, genetic testing, and brain biopsy. Some examples are given below (Figs. 1.1, 1.2, and 1.3).

MND-AD like the case presented: typical posterior temporoparietal predominant hypometabolism with hypometabolism more prominent in the left hemisphere and lesser involvement of the frontal lobes. Behavioral bifrontal (could be asymmetric) predominant FTD with little or no posterior temporoparietal hypometabolism.

F18-fluorodeoxyglucose positron emission tomography (FDG-PET) in patients with autopsy-confirmed Alzheimer's disease (AD, rows 3 and 4) frontotemporal degeneration with ubiquitin inclusions (FTD, rows 5 and 6). Scan data are displayed using three-dimensional stereotactic surface projection (3D–SSP) maps from six perspectives, illustrated in a reference image of the brain surface (row 1). These reference images show regions of the brain typically most affected in AD in shades of orange and most affected in FTD in blue, purple, and aqua. Local cerebral metabolic rates for glucose (LCMRGlc) relative to the pons are displayed

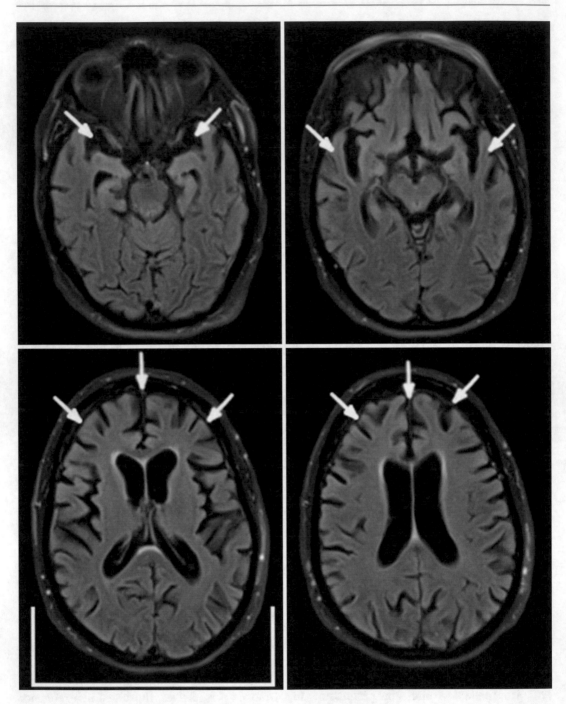

Fig. 1.1 Typical brain magnetic resonance imaging (MRI) findings in a patient with autopsy-confirmed frontotemporal degeneration with TDP-43-positive inclusions. The MRI obtained when the patient had only mild symptoms shows the characteristic focal pattern of atrophy (arrows). There is symmetric widening of sulci and shrinkage of gyri in the anterior temporal regions (top row) and in the bilateral frontal cortex (bottom row). These regional changes are easy to overlook and best recognized when compared in the same scan with the size of sulci in posterior regions of the cerebral cortex (bracket)

MORPHOMETRY RESULTS

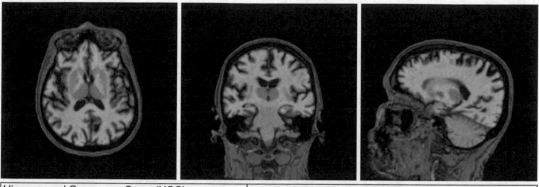

Hippocampal Occupancy Score (HOC)		0.62	
Brain Structure	Volume (cm³)	% of ICV (5%-95% Normative Percentile)	Normative Percentile
Hippocampi	5.00	0.31 (0.38-0.52)	< 1
Lateral Ventricles	30.03	1.84 (1.09-3.87)	40
Inferior Lateral Ventricles	3.09	0.19 (0.08-0.21)	91

AGE-MATCHED REFERENCE CHARTS

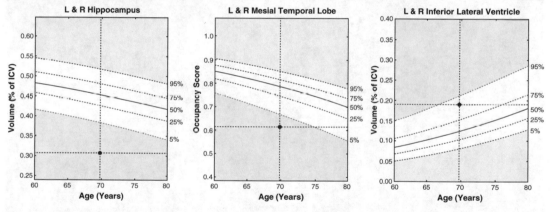

Fig. 1.2 Typical MND-AD qMRI NeuroQuant and MRI selection of horizontal slices – CACIR 06379. Illustrate selective hippocampal atrophy in MND-AD (Figure provided Courtesy of Norman L. Foster, MD; Richard D. King, MD, PhD; and Yao He, Center for Alzheimer's Care, Imaging and Research, University of Utah)

using a color scale shown below the images with the hotter colors representing higher rates of glucose metabolism (rows 2, 3, and 5). Statistical maps also can be constructed with z-scores of metabolic rates for each patient (rows 4 and 6) compared to 27 cognitively normal elderly individuals (row 2) using the same color scale. The patient with AD had symptoms similar to the case presented in the text and shows typical posterior temporoparietal hypometabolism, with hypometabolism more prominent in the left hemisphere corresponding to the patient's prominent language deficits, whereas a patient with FTD with behavioral symptoms shows bifrontal and left anterior temporal predominant hypometabolism (Fig. 1.4)

Amyloid PET imaging of Alzheimer's disease neuritic plaque pathology with AV-45 (florbetapir) in two elderly individuals with dementia in the Alzheimer's Disease Neuroimaging Initiative (ADNI). Scan data are displayed using 3D–SSP as in Fig. 1.4. Semiquantitative values of tracer binding in the brain surface relative to the cerebellum are shown in standard uptake value ratios (SUVr). Average values in 168 ADNI elderly control subjects (row 2) only show expected nonspecific binding in white matter tracts in the brainstem and corpus callosum. This same pat-

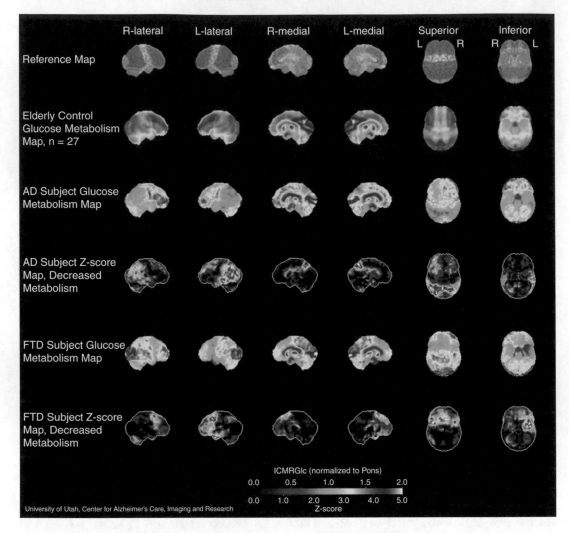

Fig. 1.3 FDG-PET: typical single-case stereotactic surface projection image presentation

tern is seen in the patient in row 3, who has a negative scan. The patient in row 4 shows the typical diffuse pattern of increased binding seen in Alzheimer's disease dementia. In this patient, the visual cortex is the only cerebral cortical region spared. Note that the distribution of amyloid plaque is not limited to regions of the brain that are typically hypometabolic on FDG-PET and that binding is minimal in the cerebellum of all cases, including those with Alzheimer's disease dementia (Fig. 1.1).

(Figure) provided Courtesy of Norman L. Foster, MD; Richard D. King, MD, PhD; and Yao He, Center for Alzheimer's Care, Imaging and Research, University of Utah).

1.8 Making a Diagnosis of MND-AD

In general, making a diagnosis of MND is a two-step process. In the first step, determine if there is a dementia process. Second, proceed with the inquiry of the type of MND. The most common clinical conditions to be ruled out are cognitive changes due to depression or chronic delirium. Secondary medical conditions such as normal pressure hydrocephalus (a triad of dementia, ataxia, and urinary incontinence) and hypothyroidism should be ruled out. Confirm if the criteria for MND are fulfilled (Table 1.3 and 1.4)

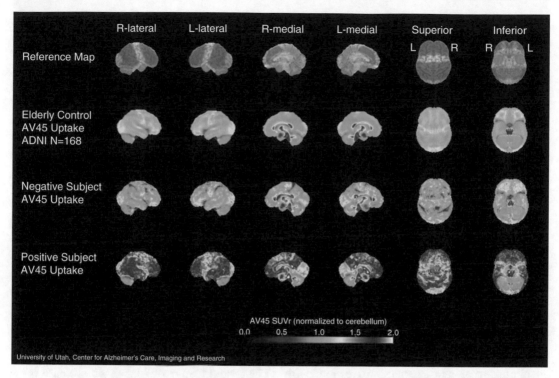

Fig. 1.4 Positive AV-45 amyloid case typical single-case SSP image (Figure provided Courtesy of Norman L. Foster, MD; Richard D. King, MD, PhD; and Yao He, Center for Alzheimer's Care, Imaging and Research, University of Utah)

Table 1.3 Cognitive domains and relevant neuropsychological tests

Cognitive domain	Neuropsychological test
Complex attention	Trail Making Test A, Digit Span
Learning and memory	California Learning and Memory Wechsler's Memory Scale
Perceptual motor	Finger-tapping test
Language	Boston Naming, verbal fluency
Executive function	Wisconsin Card Sorting, Trail Making Test B
Social cognition	Thematic Apperception Test

Table 1.4 Differences between mild neurocognitive disorder, major neurocognitive disorder, and major neurocognitive disorder due to Alzheimer's disease

Mild neurocognitive disorder	Major neurocognitive disorder	Major neurocognitive disorder due to Alzheimer's disease
Modest decline in one or more cognitive domains	Significant decline in 1 or > cognitive domains	Significant decline in 1 or > cognitive domains
Person is concerned of the change	Usually, family are concerned of the change	Usually, family are concerned of the change
Cognitive deficits do not interfere with ADL or IADLs	Significant interference of ADL or IADLs	Significant interference of ADL or IADLs
Cognitive deficits are not due to delirium or other mental disorders	Cognitive deficits are not due to delirium or other mental disorders	Cognitive deficits are not due to delirium or other mental disorders
Progression is variable 5–10% may convert to Alzheimer's disease	Variable depending on the type	Insidious onset and gradual progression over years

Most cases of MND are due to Alzheimer's disease. The next most common cause is a mixture of vascular and Alzheimer's disease (reference for epidemiological studies latest). Vascular dementia and DLB are the next most common causes. FTD is more common in earlier ages of onset (30–64 years) and decreases as age advances. It is rarely seen after 70 years of age. In one community study in the UK [27], frontotemporal dementia (FTD) was 15.7% and Alzheimer's dementia (AD) was 25% in people with dementia between the ages of 30 and 64 years.

With available clinical investigations, the Alzheimer's dementia is classified as probable, possible, and definite.

According to McKhann's criteria, the diagnostic certainty of AD has three levels: definite, probable, and possible. A definite diagnosis can only be done by brain biopsy. A probable diagnosis is done when the dementia syndrome has insidious onset and gradual progression, with cognitive deficits in multiple domains and at least basic cognitive testing (MMSE). When these criteria are not completely met (e.g., a fluctuating course, sudden onset), then a diagnosis of possible AD should be made [23].

About a week later, the patient was brought back to the hospital as she was becoming more aggressive with family members. The family was unable to manage her at home. Her husband was not able to sleep and was feeling helpless. She was admitted to the medical unit to rule out acute medical conditions and to make an appropriate care plan. Galantamine, which had been initiated earlier, was continued.

In the hospital, she was started on (SSRIs) escitalopram 10 mg P.O. daily along with risperidone, 0.25 mg twice daily. Her medical investigations were negative. Her agitation increased, and she was given frequent doses of haloperidol for management of her agitation. Three weeks later, she was noted to be walking around naked and sexually disinhibited in the hospital. She also had decreased sleep and was found to talk loudly when awake. She was euphoric in her mood. She was wandering into other patients' rooms. Occasionally, she was irritable and impulsive in her behavior. She was noted to be talking to herself. The nursing staff was unable to redirect her behavior. She needed assistance with all her ADL care.

Her risperidone was gradually increased and escitalopram was discontinued; memantine was added with the family consent, and they visited often. They declined genetic testing for the patient owing to cost. Her daughters also refused genetic testing for themselves. The poor prognosis was discussed with the family. There were no advanced directives from the patient. The family decided to keep her comfortable and safe, agreeing to long-term care in a supported environment.

1.9 The Cognitive and Behavioral Symptoms in MND-AD

The central feature of Alzheimer's disease is the gradual progression of multiple neurocognitive dysfunctions, initially starting as difficulties in new learning and recent memory. Amnestic patients often repeat themselves in conversation, ask the same question repeatedly, or forget recent conservations. Family members often ignore symptoms as these are misinterpreted as "normal aging." Symptoms are typically present before family members bring the patient for medical attention. The loss of ability to carry on activities such as shopping, driving, handling money, or doing chores around the house is more frequently the reasons than forgetfulness for such presentations. Sometimes getting lost while driving or accidents while driving may bring the patient medical attention. Neuropsychiatric symptoms are more likely to bring the patient for evaluation than forgetfulness.

Deficits in frontal executive function are noted in the difficulty in planning the meal for dinner, organizing the kitchen, or following a recipe. Other changes include difficulty in recognition of people (agnosia), difficulty in cutting the vegetables or difficulty in dressing (apraxia), and difficulty in naming or finding the right word to speak (aphasia). Other cognitive deficits include difficulties in reading (dyslexia) or writing (dysgraphia) and difficulties in doing simple calculations (acalculia). In moderate to severe stages, patients may have right/left disorientation.

Behavioral symptoms are often due to delusions, hallucinations, or mood changes. Common mood changes are anxiety, depression, irritability, anger, and elation. Other behavioral symptoms are apathy, hyperactivity, and aggression. Sometimes the behavioral changes occur due to the personality changes.

In some patients, changes in biological functions such as sleeping, eating, and sexual disinhibition occur in all stages of AD. Other physical symptoms such as swallowing, continence, and gait difficulties occur as the disease progresses.

As the dementia progresses, difficulties in day-to-day functioning and behavioral symptoms become more common. Misidentification syndromes occur commonly. The patient may complain that someone else has been in the house. Sometimes they identify the family members as someone else in the disguise of other family members (Capgras syndrome). Sometimes they misidentify their own image in the mirror as someone else.

1.10   General Principles of Management of a Patient with Alzheimer's Disease

Management of Alzheimer's disease follows the general four pillars of dementia care. The first pillar is to modify the aspect of the disease. Only a few therapies such as choline esterase inhibitors are available at this time. The approved medications are donepezil, rivastigmine, and galantamine. The second pillar is to manage the symptoms of AD. These are the cognitive, neuropsychiatric, and functional symptoms.

The third pillar is to provide supportive care for the patient with AD. The final and fourth pillar is to support the caregivers for the dementia care. These interventions should be evidence-based approaches.

1.11   Effects of MND-AD on the Family Caregivers

Prolonged activity of providing care for a family member with Alzheimer's disease will frequently lead to chronic stress in one or several members of that family. The caregiver's burden is the subjective perception of that burden of providing care. This stress may interfere with physical, social, emotional, and financial functioning of the family care providers. Several scales can subjectively or objectively measure the caregiver's burden. The Caregiver Self-Assessment Questionnaire is a 16-item scale that can be answered yes/no. This can be used in an office setting for rapid screening of caregiver burden. Anxiety and depressive symptoms are common, while some families express pride in providing care for their loved ones. Successful family caregivers are flexible in adjusting the expectations of themselves and the older adult. The primary caregiver at home needs occasional breaks, respite, backup, and services to support them [12].

Sometimes interpersonal difficulties arise when siblings attempt to divide the responsibilities of caregivers. Families face the realities of loss and grief during the process of caregiving. Sleep quality can be affected significantly in caregivers. The Pittsburgh Sleep Quality Index can measure this more reliably [10]. Primary care physicians must be aware of these factors in the family when they are planning the care for MND-AD patients. Physical symptoms such as hypertension, diabetes, and coronary artery diseases are also higher in the family care providers than the general population [29]. Premature death is associated with spousal caregiver strain [28].

1.12   Legal and Ethical Encounters when Managing a Patient with MND-AD

As the major neurocognitive disorder of MND-AD has a prolonged course of 8–10 years, families face various legal and ethical issues during its course. Retrospectively, in the early stages after the diagnosis, the family is better served when an open discussion occurs with the family members, including the patient and their primary care physician [9]. Advanced directives are sought and recorded by the family members. Prior wishes of the patient are respected throughout the course of MND-AD. It is wise for the family to discuss the patient's wishes in a sensitive manner. This discussion may include end-of-life issues as well.

Capacity assessment in regard to driving will be encountered in moderate stages of MND-AD. Given the possibility that the patient may lose their ability to take reasonable decisions toward their personal treatment, care choices, and ability to manage her finances, a power of attorney might be chosen by the patient. Ideally, such advanced directives and the power of attorney papers are kept with the patient's lawyer and documented with their physician. Patients sometimes may make advanced directives to participate in the research [16].

In most of the cases, the patient presents to the physicians in moderately advanced stages of MND-AD. There may not be any documentation of their advanced directives, including their resuscitation status. In these situations, appropriate substitute decision-makers for the patient need to be identified and documented to make decisions on behalf of the patient [4]. In those situations where there is no responsible substitute decision-maker from the family, an official of the government or court-appointed guardian needs to be appointed. The management of the patient's care should proceed in collaboration with the substitute decision-maker. Several clinical dilemmas occur in taking the treatment, care decisions, and end-of-life issues during the management of the patient as the disease progresses toward the terminal stages. Patients and their families' wishes must be respected throughout the course of MND-AD. Several of these issues related to capacity are discussed by Hope et al. [17].

In terms of the case presented here, the ethical questions mainly pertain to genetic testing as a method of establishing the cause of her major neurocognitive disorder. Genetic testing, though available to rule out some known familial variants, may not be conclusive. Also, the lack of ready availability in the local hospitals and cost must be considered along with the family's wishes. Once the genetic variant is identified to be of a familial variety correlated with early-onset MND-AD, the family must understand the implications for themselves. Such testing must be performed only if pretest and posttest counseling and support are available for the family members. Finally, the definitive diagnosis of MND-AD in this case can only be made by brain biopsy, either antemortem or postmortem. The family's wishes either for personal or academic reasons must be sought in all such diagnostic dilemmas [24]. Invasive procedures such as a lumbar puncture for CSF analysis can be discussed with the family to improve diagnostic accuracy. CSF can be analyzed for proteins. Total tau (T-tau) in combination with neurofilament light (NFL) has potential for biomarkers for prediction of MND-AD [22].

Ethical issues will arise around the sexual behaviors noted in moderate and severe stages of dementia. In North American and Scandinavian countries, physician-assisted deaths are seriously considered in advanced stages of the disease. These are complicated with several controversies, and careful decisions must be taken within the legal realities of those countries.

Conclusion

As the world's population continues to age, the prevalence of major neurocognitive disorders will increase. Molecular genetics is furthering our understanding both in early diagnosis and research in new pharmacological interventions. Despite this, families and communities will likely experience more caregiver burden. Future planning and management of persons with Alzheimer's disease are fraught with several ethical and legal issues.

Disclosure Statement "The authors have nothing to disclose."

References

1. The Alzheimer Disease and Frontotemporal Dementia Mutation Database. Available online www.molgen.ua.ac.be/ADmutations, provides up-to-date information on various genes involved in AD.
2. Arnold SE, Hyman BT, Flory J, Damasio AR, Van Hoesen GW. The topographical and neuroanatomical distribution of neurofibrillary tangles and neuritic plaques in the cerebral cortex of patients with Alzheimer's disease. Cereb Cortex. 1991;1(1):103–16.
3. Blennow K, de Leon MJ, Zetterberg H. Alzheimer's disease. Lancet. 2006;368(9533):387–403.
4. Berger JT, DeRenzo EG, Schwartz J. Surrogate decision making: reconciling ethical theory and clinical practice surrogate decision making. Ann Intern Med. 2008;149(1):48–53.
5. Bertram L, Lill CM, Tanzi RE. The genetics of Alzheimer disease: back to the future. Neuron. 2010;68(2):270–81.
6. Braak H, Braak E. Neuropathological stageing of Alzheimer-related changes. Acta Neuropathol. 1991;82(4):239–59.
7. Breitner JC, Murphy EA, Folstein MF, Magruder-Habib K. Twin studies of Alzheimer's disease: an approach to etiology and prevention. Neurobiol Aging. 1990;11(6):641–8.
8. Breitner JCS, Wyse BW, Anthony JC, Welsh-Bohmer KA, Steffens DC, Norton MC, et al. APOE-ε4 count predicts age when prevalence of AD increases, then declines the cache county study. Neurology. 1999;53(2):321.
9. Burlá C, Pessini L, Siqueira JE, Nunes R. Aging and Alzheimer's disease: reflections on the loss of autonomy and the challenges of care. Revista Bioética. 2014;22(1):85–93.
10. Buysse DJ, Reynolds CF, Monk TH, Berman SR, Kupfer DJ. The Pittsburgh sleep quality index: a new instrument for psychiatric practice and research. Psychiatry Res. 1989;28(2):193–213.
11. Clarfield AM. The decreasing prevalence of reversible dementias: an updated meta-analysis. Arch Intern Med. 2003;163(18):2219–29.
12. Derence K. Dementia-specific respite: the key to effective caregiver support. N C Med J. 2005;66(1):48–51.
13. Drzezga A, Grimmer T, Henriksen G, Mühlau M, Perneczky R, Miederer I, et al. Effect of APOE genotype on amyloid plaque load and gray matter volume in Alzheimer disease. Neurology. 2009;72(17):1487–94.
14. Greenberg SM, Vonsattel JP, Segal AZ, Chiu RI, Clatworthy AE, Liao A, et al. Association of apolipoprotein E ε2 and vasculopathy in cerebral amyloid angiopathy. Neurology. 1998;50(4):961–5.
15. Iqbal etal. Mechanisms of tau-induced neuro-degeneration. Acta Neuropathol. 2009;118:53–69.
16. Jongsma K, van de Vathorst S. Advance directives in dementia research: the opinions and arguments of clinical researchers– an empirical study. Research ethics. 2015;11(1):4–14.
17. Hope T, Savulescu J, Hendrick J. Medical ethics and law: the core curriculum. London: Churchill Livingstone/Elsevier; 2003.
18. Jellinger KA, Paulus W, Wrocklage C, Litvan I. Effects of closed traumatic brain injury and genetic factors on the development of Alzheimer's disease. Eur J Neurol. 2001;8(6):707–10.
19. Knopman DS, DeKosky ST, Cummings JL, Chui H, Corey–Bloom J, Relkin N, et al. Practice parameter: diagnosis of dementia (an evidence-based review) Report of the quality standards subcommittee of the american academy of neurology. Neurology. 2001;56(9):1143–53.
20. Larson EB, Shadlen MF, Wang L, McCormick WC, Bowen JD, Teri L, Kukull WA. Survival after initial diagnosis of Alzheimer disease. Ann Intern Med. 2004;140(7):501–9.
21. Lockhart A. Imaging Alzheimer's disease pathology: one target, many ligands. Drug Discov Today. 2006;11(23):1093–9.
22. Mattsson N, Insel PS, Palmqvist S, Portelius E, Zetterberg H, Weiner M, et al. Cerebrospinal fluid tau, neurogranin, and neurofilament light in Alzheimer's disease. EMBO Mol Med. 2016;8(10):1184–96.
23. McKhann G, Drachman D, Folstein M, Katzman R, Price D, Stadlan EM. Clinical diagnosis of Alzheimer's disease report of the NINCDS-ADRDA work group* under the auspices of department of health and human services task force on Alzheimer's disease. Neurology. 1984;34(7):939.
24. Montine TJ, Phelps CH, Beach TG, Bigio EH, Cairns NJ, Dickson DW, et al. National institute on aging–Alzheimer's association guidelines for the neuropathologic assessment of Alzheimer's disease: a practical approach. Acta Neuropathol. 2012;123(1):1–11.
25. Murray CJ, Lopez AD. Alternative projections of mortality and disability by cause 1990–2020: Global burden of disease study. Lancet. 1997;349(9064):1498–504.
26. Ranginwala NA, Hynan LS, Weiner MF, White CL. Clinical criteria for the diagnosis of Alzheimer disease: still good after all these years. Am J Geriatr Psychiatry. 2008;16(5):384–8.
27. Ratnavalli E, Brayne C, Dawson K, Hodges JR. The prevalence of frontotemporal dementia. Neurology. 2002;58(11):1615–21.
28. Schulz R, Beach SR. Caregiving as a risk factor for mortality: the caregiver health effects study. JAMA. 1999;282(23):2215–9.
29. Schulz R, Martire LM. Family caregiving of persons with dementia: prevalence, health effects, and support strategies. Am J Geriatr Psychiatry. 2004;12(3):240–9.
30. Silverman JM, Smith CJ, Marin DB, Mohs RC, Propper CB. Familial patterns of risk in very late-onset Alzheimer disease. Arch Gen Psychiatry. 2003;60(2):190–7.

A Complex Case of Delirium: From Theory to Clinical Management

2

Tim Lau and Sarah Russell

2.1 Case Presentation: Part I

Mr. D is a 78-year-old retired physician who was diagnosed with Parkinson's disease 7 years ago. He was taking Sinemet 100/250 two tablets TID and entacapone 200 mg TID to manage his motor symptoms which consisted of a resting tremor, rigidity, and shuffling gait. His Parkinson's medication was managed by his family physician under the guidance of his neurologist.

Three years ago, he was started on divalproic acid 500 mg BID after it was discovered he was experiencing absence seizures. His dose and level had been stable and his seizures diminished in frequency.

He had been doing very well, going out with his wife several times a week to see movies and to the theater. Although he had a pronounced tremor, he enjoyed going for walks and playing Scrabble with his wife. His ability to form new memories at the time was intact.

He was found to have a large basal cell carcinoma on his scalp which was removed by surgical excision under local anesthetic. He developed a cellulitis and subsequently required hospitalization after he became acutely confused over the course of 2 days. His wife noted that he started having visual hallucinations and became convinced that people were trying to hurt him. A CAM screening was positive for delirium, and his severity using the CAM-S scores was 9 out of a possible 19. His mini mental status exam score was 7/30.

While hospitalized he became combative. The internal medicine service where he was admitted diagnosed him with dementia of unclear etiology, possibly Alzheimer's disease or Parkinson's disease dementia. It was suspected that his symptoms were related to a superimposed delirium in someone with a decreased cognitive reserve. He was treated with cephalexin without any change improvement in his confusion. His entacapone was discontinued. His Sinemet was reduced. Despite these interventions, his delirium worsened. A further medical workup was unremarkable. His white count normalized, and his bloodwork remained otherwise unremarkable. A CT scan of his head was read as nil acute. His chest X-ray, abdominal X-ray, and urine cultures were unremarkable during his admission.

Mr. D was frequently somnolent in a hospital gown during the day, having a clear day-night reversal. He was unable to walk safely but kept trying to get up. He was put into a wheelchair with a safety belt to prevent rising. He subsequently became even more agitated. His agitation was severe at times as evidenced by extreme aggression during care. He received regular low doses of Haldol to manage his behaviors, but this seemed only to worsen his agitation and had little effect on his psychotic symptoms.

T. Lau, MD, FRCP(C), MSc (✉) • S. Russell, MD
Department of Psychiatry, University of Ottawa,
Ottawa, ON, Canada
e-mail: tim.lau@theroyal.ca

© Springer International Publishing AG, part of Springer Nature 2018
K. Shivakumar, S. Amanullah (eds.), *Complex Clinical Conundrums in Psychiatry*,
https://doi.org/10.1007/978-3-319-70311-4_2

Trazodone was also added to help both with sleep and provide some sedation during the day. It seemed inevitable that he would require admission to a long-term care facility, but his care needs at the time exceeded what a nursing home could provide. The question of a Lewy body dementia was raised despite him having the motor symptoms of Parkinson's for more than 1 year.

After 4 weeks, there was no improvement in his fluctuating level of consciousness, his agitation, and his psychosis. He was transferred to a geriatric psychiatry unit. The severity of his delirium was measured using the CAM-S. He scored 19 out a possible 19. His MMSE was 5/30. He was given adequate hydration, and a regular bowel pattern was ensured over the course of the first week.

We gradually reduced the dose of the antipsychotic that he was regularly getting and stopped all PRN antipsychotics and benzodiazepines which internal medicine had been using to manage his behavior. We further examined his medications to see if there was something that could be discontinued. We tried holding his Sinemet without any real change in his motor symptoms or his agitation. Next we tried to remove the trazodone which had been added in an effort to calm him. There was not a noticeable effect when it was stopped. Later divalproic acid was stopped. A remarkable improvement was seen when divalproic acid was discontinued. Over the course of 3 days, his sleep normalized and his confusion improved. His wife was able to spend more time with him and was able to comfort him. Two weeks after his divalproic acid was discontinued, he was walking again, was able to feed himself, and was much clearer cognitively. His MMSE at that time was 25/30. His Sinemet but not his entacapone was restarted to help with his mobility. He continued to improve and was able to regain the full function he had prior to having his basal cell carcinoma resected. He returned home with his wife and continues to enjoy going to the theater, exercising, and playing Scrabble. His MMSE when he returned home was 27/30.

2.2   What Is Delirium?

Delirium is an acute-onset confusional state that is characterized by a loss of function, fluctuating consciousness, disturbances in attention, and disorganization. The presentation can be extremely variable person to person but typically is associated with other cognitive deficits; changes in arousal; perceptual disturbances including hallucinations, delusions, and paranoia; and an altered sleep-wake cycle. Disturbances in affect can be seen with depression, irritability, and fear [1, 2].

Delirium can also be classified into hypoactive and hyperactive delirium. Hypoactive delirium is more common in the elderly with symptoms of sedation and psychomotor retardation with slowed physical movements and verbal response. By contrast, hyperactive delirium is characterized by increased activity, agitation, and hypervigilance. Mixed picture states also exist with both hypoactive and hyperactive symptoms seen.

Delirium is not a disease but a clinical diagnosis based upon a collection of symptoms. The *Diagnostic and Statistical Manual of Mental Disorders*, Fifth Edition (DSM-5), has the following diagnostic criteria:

1. Disturbance in attention (i.e., reduced ability to direct, focus, sustain, and shift attention) and awareness.
2. Change in cognition (e.g., memory deficit, disorientation, language disturbance, perceptual disturbance) that is not better accounted for by a preexisting, established, or evolving dementia.
3. The disturbance develops over a short period (usually hours to days) and tends to fluctuate during the course of the day.
4. There is evidence from the history, physical examination, or laboratory findings that the disturbance is caused by a direct physiologic consequence of a general medical condition, an intoxicating substance, medication use, or more than one cause.

The DSM-5 includes several specifiers related to delirium including substance intoxication delirium, substance withdrawal delirium, and medication-induced delirium. This highlights how important it is to identify and examine substance- and medication-induced causes of delirium. These causes often have a clear treatment plan. There are also a specifier regarding length of diagnosis, acute vs. persistent, and a specifier looking at activity level, hyperactive, hypoactive, and mixed level of activity [1].

The International Statistical Classification of Diseases and Related Health Problems (**ICD**) is a medical classification system put out by the World Health Organization. The latest iteration, the ICD-10, has the following diagnostic criteria [3]:

2.3   FO5 Delirium, Not Induced by Alcohol and Other Psychoactive Substances

A. Clouding of consciousness, i.e., reduced clarity of awareness of the environment, with reduced ability to focus, sustain, or shift attention.
B. Disturbance of cognition, manifest by both:
    1. Impairment of immediate recall and recent memory, with relatively intact remote memory
    2. Disorientation in time, place, or person
C. At least one of the following psychomotor disturbances:
    1. Rapid, unpredictable shifts from hypoactivity to hyperactivity
    2. Increased reaction time
    3. Increased or decreased flow of speech
    4. Enhanced startle reaction
D. Disturbance of sleep or the sleep-wake cycle, manifest by at least one of the following:
    1. Insomnia, which in severe cases may involve total sleep loss, with or without daytime drowsiness, or reversal of the sleep-wake cycle
    2. Nocturnal worsening of symptoms
    3. Disturbing dreams and nightmares which may continue as hallucinations or illusions after awakening
E. Rapid onset and fluctuations of the symptoms over the course of the day.

F. Objective evidence from history, physical and neurological examination, or laboratory tests of an underlying cerebral or systemic disease (other than psychoactive substance-related) that can be presumed to be responsible for the clinical manifestations in AD.

2.4   Prevalence of Delirium

Overall prevalence of delirium is low in the community, with an estimated rate of 1–2% [1]. Delirium is very commonly seen in hospital and nursing home settings. It's estimated that 6–56% of hospitalized patients will experience delirium at one point during their admission [2]. In special populations, this number rises even higher. A study that looked strictly at ICU patients found rates of delirium in 44.4%. In patients who were mechanically ventilated, this number rose to 62.5% [4]. Hip fractures are also commonly associated with delirium. A study involving patients aged 65 and over with a hip fracture found that 58% of patients had delirium preoperatively and 42% had delirium postoperatively [5]. Higher rates of delirium are also seen in stroke patients, postoperative patients, and patients approaching end-of-life [2].

2.5   Typical Course of Delirium

Delirium was long thought to be an acute, reversible condition with return to function once the reversible cause has been treated. However, clinical experience shows us that delirium often persists and is associated with decreased functional status. Delirium is also associated with increased mortality with a 1-year mortality of 35–40% and is considered a life-threatening emergency [2]. In ICU settings, it's associated with increased length of ICU admission and total hospital days, increased time spent on mechanical ventilation, and increased institutionalization. It's the most common complications of hospitalized elderly. Long-term outcomes show increased risk of functional disability and cognitive impairment and increased risk of dementia with delirium independent of previous dementia status [6, 7].

2.6   Causes of Delirium

The pathophysiology of delirium is poorly understood but several theories exist. It develops when
noxious stimuli are imposed on vulnerable brain
structures. Precipitating causes are vast and
include infection, metabolic disturbances, and
medications. Cholinergic deficiency is one theory
based on the fact that anticholinergic medications
are frequently the cause of delirium. In addition,
the cholinergic system is thought to be a key
mediator in attention which is heavily affected in
delirium. Dopamine is also listed as a potential
contributor based on the propensity of psychotic
symptoms in delirium and symptom reduction
with use of antipsychotic medications which
block dopamine in the brain. Further support for
this theory is that Parkinson's medications are
also known to precipitate delirium. Other neurotransmitters that are thought to be involved in
delirium include glutamate, gaba-aminobutyric
acid, 5-HT (5-hydroxytryptamine), and norepinephrine. Inflammation, aberrant stress response,
and neuronal injury are also thought to contribute
[2, 8, 9].

The workup for causes of delirium is broad.
The emphasis has shifted in recent years to
looking at medications first, both started and
stopped, as well as drug interactions. This may
be because both the prognosis is more favorable
if the confusion is drug induced and the intervention more obvious and successful. Even
with this in mind, the causes of delirium are
broad and can include almost any organic etiology. Several mnemonics exist to help provide a
systematic approach to remembering the different causes of delirium. I WATCH DEATH looks
at common causes of delirium, whereas
WHHHHIMPS looks at potentially deadly
causes [10].

I WATCH DEATH	
Infection	Urinary tract infection, pneumonia, cellulitis, wound infection, endocarditis, septicemia, osteomyelitis, gastroenteritis, septic arthritis, HIV, syphilis
Withdrawal	Alcohol, benzodiazepine, opioid, typical neuroleptics, barbiturates, and anticholinergics
Acute metabolic	Metabolic acidosis and alkalosis, renal failure, hepatic failure, electrolyte disturbances(ca, mg, Ph, K, Na), hyper- and hypoglycemia, pancreatitis
Trauma	Head injury (subdural or subarachnoid hemorrhage), pain, burns, postoperative, fracture, concealed bleed, urinary retention, fecal impaction, electrocution
Central nervous system	Seizures, status epilepticus, infection (abscesses, encephalitis, meningitis), stroke, tumor, arteriovenous malformation, CNS vasculitis
Hypoxia	Cardiac and pulmonary failure, COPD, severe anemia, carbon monoxide poisoning, shock/hypotension, pulmonary embolism
Deficiencies	B12, folate, malnutrition, dehydration, thiamine, niacin, hypovitaminosis
Endocrinopathies/ environment	Hyperparathyroidism, hypoparathyroidism, hypothyroidism, hyperthyroidism, adrenal, hypothermia, hyperthermia
Acute vascular	Hypertensive emergencies, stroke, intracerebral bleed, myocardial infarction, sagittal vein thrombosis
Toxins or drugs	Medications, pesticides, solvents (gasoline, kerosene, turpentine), drugs of abuse, industrial poisons, cyanide
Heavy metals	Lead, arsenic, mercury

WHHHIMPS—life-threatening causes of delirium	
	Treatment
Wernicke's encephalopathy	Thiamine 500 mg IV TID for 2 days and then 200IM or IV daily for several days)
Withdrawal	Depends on substance from which they are withdrawing, for alcohol withdrawal—Benzodiazepines, monitored setting, protocol such as CIWA also exist
Hypertensive crisis	Slow reduction in blood pressure

WHHHIMPS—life-threatening causes of delirium	
Hypoperfusion/ hypoxia of the brain	Treat underlying cause, oxygen
Hypoglycemia	Glucagon IM/SC 0.5–1 mg if no IV access, if IV access then 25grams of 50% glucose IV. Monitoring may require glucose drip
Hyper–/hypothermia	Treatment depends on severity; resuscitation and air support may be necessary. Cooling and rewarming techniques based on clinical situation
Intracranial process/ infection	Antibiotics for infection, surgical vs. nonsurgical management of elevated intracranial pressure
Metabolic/meningitis poisons	Depends on poison (e.g., flumazenil for benzodiazepine overdose, naloxone for opioid), antibiotics/antivirals for meningitis
Status epilepticus	Supportive management, benzodiazepines, and an antiepileptic medication for longer-term control (e.g., fosphenytoin)

Medications are a very common cause of delirium. Many classes of medications can contribute to or cause delirium. Frequent offenders are Parkinson's medications and anticholinergic medications such as diphenhydramine and dimenhydrinate. Steroids and opioid pain medications are other common offenders [11].

A mnemonic exists for identifying frequent medications that cause delirium called ACUTE CHANGE in MS [10].

Drug class (10)	Examples
Antibiotics	Cefepime, penicillin, metronidazole, sulfonamide
Cardiac drugs	Antiarrhythmics, digoxin, antihypertensives
Urinary incontinence drugs	Oxybutynin, tolterodine, solifenacin, darifenacin
Theophyilline	Theophylline
Ethanol	Ethanol
Corticosteroids	Prednisone, prednisolone, dexamethasone
H2 blockers	Ranitidine, famotidine
Antiparkinsonian drugs	Carbidopa-levodopa, amantadine, pramipexole, bromocriptine, ropinirole
Narcotics	Morphine, hydromorphone, meperidine, codeine, methadone
Non-prescription	Antihistamines, antiemetic medications, medication containing alcohol, mandrake, henbane, jimsonweed, atropa belladonna extract
Geriatric psychiatric drugs	TCAs, lithium, antipsychotics
ENT drugs	Betahistine
Insomnia drug	Zopiclone, eszopiclone

Drug class (10)	Examples
NSAIDS	Ibuprofen, celecoxib, naproxen, indomethacin
Muscle relaxants	Baclofen, cyclobenzaprine
Seizure medicines	Barbiturates, valproic acid

2.7   Risk Factors for Delirium

There are many modifiable and non-modifiable risk factors for delirium. The non-modifiable risk factors include older age, preexisting cognitive impairment such as dementia, previous episodes of delirium, history of stroke, and male sex and hepatic and renal failure. Other risk factors include choice of medications; opioids, benzodiazepines, and anticonvulsants are all associated with increased risk of delirium. Pain, new pressure ulcers, sleep disturbance, emotional distress, malnutrition, constipation, immobilization, physical restraints, and depression can increase the risk. Sensory impairment such as uncorrected impaired vision and hearing deficits also increases the risk. In patients with cancer, brain cancer/metastases, malnutrition constipation, and decreased PPS (palliative performance scale) were all associated with increased risk of delirium [2, 4, 9, 11, 12].

2.8   Diagnosis of Delirium

Several tools exist to help diagnose delirium. The CAM (Confusion Assessment Method) is one of the most commonly used tools. It looks at four separate features: (A) acute onset and fluctuating course, (B) inattention, (C) disorganized thinking, and (D) altered level of consciousness. In order to make a diagnosis of delirium, both A and B need to be present and one of C or D. The CAM also exists in format for ICU use called CAM-ICU. The CAM-S can be used to monitor the severity of delirium. The MMSE (mini mental status exam) is another cognitive tool frequently used to follow the course of delirium. It tests orientation, memory, attention, delayed recall, language, and visual-spatial skills. The MoCA (Montreal Cognitive Assessment) is another bedside tool that tests cognition across several domains. Asking a patient to recite the months of the year backward is another method to quickly assess attention with no equipment necessary [13–16].

2.9   Mimetics of Delirium

Overlapping symptoms that occur among delirium, dementia, depression, and psychosis can make a diagnosis of delirium challenging. Dementia increases an individual's risk for delirium. Dementia is a usually irreversible condition which results in progressive changes in memory, personality, and executive function. The onset of dementia is often subacute, and progression is usually gradual or stepwise in nature. Level of consciousness is generally normal. Changes are seen in mood and sleep. Agitation, delusions, and hallucinations can occur. Lewy body dementia can be especially difficult to differentiate, as fluctuating consciousness and hallucinations can commonly occur. Depression is characterized by changes in mood and interest with a subacute onset, variable duration, and propensity recurrence. The level of consciousness and orientation is generally preserved. Similarly, patients with psychosis usually present with predominant symptoms of hallucinations and delusions, and typically orientation is maintained. Finally, catatonia may have symptoms that overlap with delirium including the apparent confusion associated with catatonic excitement, stupor as well as mutism, and extreme negativism [17]. Key

features that characterize delirium include acute onset, fluctuating attention and consciousness, and abrupt cognitive changes [1, 9, 18].

2.10   Treatment of Delirium

Finding the cause, if possible, is the first goal of treatment for delirium. Once a cause is determined, hope of reversibility improves; however, oftentimes no precipitating cause is found even after a battery of tests.

Initial workup often includes CBC, electrolytes (Na, Cl, K) and extended electrolytes (Ca, Ph, Mg), urea, creatinine, glucose, liver function tests, TSH, B12, folate, urinalysis and urine culture, and chest X-ray. CT of the head is also frequently done.

In addition to trying to reverse the cause, the main components of delirium management include supportive therapy and pharmacologic management. Supportive therapy includes trying to facilitate an environment that is stable, quiet, and well-lit during the day. Additionally, facilitating a normalized sleep cycle and allowing family members to be present are interventions that are now recognized to be extremely helpful. Reorientation techniques or memory cues such as calendars, clocks, and family photos may also be helpful. Finally, maintaining adequate fluid intake and minimizing the use of Foley catheters and restraints are important [18].

Pharmacologic management includes the removal of medications that may be contributing to confusion if possible. Common culprits include benzodiazepines, opioids, and anticonvulsants. These medications may need to be gradually discontinued. It is important to keep in mind that the effect of medications that cause cognitive impairment may be additive, particularly in the case of anticholinergic medication. In patients where alcohol withdrawal is suspected, thiamine can be beneficial. As a recent Cochrane review suggests, cholinesterase inhibitors and melatonin have not proven to be effective treatments for delirium [19].

Depending on the behaviors that accompany the delirium, medications may be required to promote the safety and well-being of patients and staff. Low-dose antipsychotics are the most commonly used medications for this indication. Haldol has historically been the most commonly used antipsychotic for use in delirium. Doses of Haldol used in the management of delirium are generally much lower than those used for antipsychotic purposes or in acute agitation. Typically, doses of 2–5 mg are used in divided doses. Side effects of Haldol include QTc prolongation, extrapyramidal symptoms, and akathisia. When used intravenously, there is greater risk for QTc prolongation but less so for EPS. Other medications used include second-generation antipsychotic such as risperidone, quetiapine, and olanzapine. Second-generation antipsychotics have similar efficacy to Haldol in the management of delirium. These medications have greater propensity for metabolic side effects, orthostatic hypotension, and sedation, and they can all increase the QTc as well. All antipsychotics are associated with increased risk of death in the elderly, and informed consent should be obtained and documented prior to the use of these medications [18, 20].

Benzodiazepines often are used for withdrawal states but otherwise can make delirium worse and should be avoided.

2.11   Non-pharmacologic Strategies in the Management of Delirium

Intervention	Examples of strategies
Family involvement	Allow family members to visit frequently and often
Remove lines if possible	This includes IV and Foley tubes
Re-orient	Clocks and calendars in the room
Correct day-night reversal	Leave lights on during the day
Nutrition	Ensure adequate PO intake
Decrease environmental stimuli	Try to reduce noise, evaluate need for noisy monitors
Mobility	Mobilize out of bed early if possible

Intervention	Examples of strategies
Review medication list	Try to reduce or stop medications associated with delirium if safe to do so
Correct sensory impairment	Glasses and hearing aids should be brought in and be available at the bedside

2.12   Case Presentation: Part II

As evidenced by the case discussed above, delirium may have psychosis as a feature. The diagnosis of delirium in this case is complicated by the patient's previous diagnosis of Parkinson's disease and the concurrent presence of medications that are known to induce confusion and psychosis. It is important to note that Parkinson's disease has moved from being conceptualized as a motor disease to being a disease of three areas: motor, cognitive, and emotions/behavior. Lewy body dementia, which is characterized by visual hallucinations, fluctuations, and parkinsonism, is widely thought to be on a continuum with Parkinson's disease dementia. When the patient in the case developed hallucinations, it could have theoretically been a symptom of Parkinson's disease or an adverse side effect of his Parkinson's medications. Currently, when psychosis is present in Parkinson's disease, the recommendations advise removing all Parkinson's medications, sparing Sinemet for the last. In this case, these strategies were tried and patient's confusion persisted. Ultimately, discontinuation of divalproic acid resulted in the patient's clinical improvement.

Supportive therapy in this case included transferring the patient to a geriatric psychiatry unit that specializes in trying to create a more stable, quiet environment.

2.13   Key Points

1. Delirium is a severe illness with many negative consequences.
2. Although potentially reversible, it is very rarely completely recoverable.

3. The most effective approach is prevention, including caution with medications, focusing on frail patients as the most important population of interest (less frail patients are more likely to recover).
4. In the presence of delirium, your most important job is to identify and address treatable causes.
5. When using medications to manage behavior, use very low-dose neuroleptics, so the underlying causes can be addressed.
6. Always use environmental modifications including involving families.

Disclosure Statement "The authors have nothing to disclose."

References

1. Association AP. Diagnostic and statistical manual of mental disorders, 5th edition (DSM-5). 5th ed. Washington, DC: American Psychiatric Publishing; 2013. ISBN: 9780890425558
2. Inouye SK. Delirium in older persons. N Engl J Med. 2006;354(11):1157–65.
3. [cited 2017 Feb 11]. Available from: http://apps.who.int/classifications/icd10/browse/2014/en#F05.1.
4. Limpawattana P, Panitchote A, Tangvoraphonkchai K, Suebsoh N, Eamma W, Chanthonglarng B, et al. Delirium in critical care: a study of incidence, prevalence, and associated factors in the tertiary care hospital of older Thai adults. Aging Ment Health. 2016;20(1):74–80.
5. Freter S, Dunbar M, Koller K, MacKnight C, Rockwood K. Risk of pre-and post-operative delirium and the delirium elderly at risk (DEAR) tool in hip fracture patients. Can Geriatr J. 2015;18(4):212–6.
6. Witlox J, Eurelings LS, de Jonghe JF, Kalisvaart KJ, Eikelenboom P, van Gool WA. Delirium in elderly patients and the risk of postdischarge mortality, institutionalization, and dementia: a meta-analysis. JAMA. 2010;304(4):443–51.
7. Salluh JI, Wang H, Schneider EB, Nagaraja N, Yenokyan G, Damluji A, et al. Outcome of delirium in critically ill patients: systematic review and meta-analysis. BMJ. 2015;350:h2538.
8. Cerejeira J, Nogueira V, Luís P, Vaz-Serra A, Mukaetova-Ladinska EB. The cholinergic system and inflammation: common pathways in delirium pathophysiology. J Am Geriatr Soc. 2012;60(4):669–75.
9. Gower LE, Gatewood MO, Kang CS. Emergency department management of delirium in the elderly. West J Emerg Med. 2012;13(2):194–201.
10. Caplan JP, Stern TA. Mnemonics in a nutshell: 32 aids to psychiatric diagnosis. Curr Psychiatr Ther. 2008;7(10):27–33.
11. Alagiakrishnan K, Wiens CA. An approach to drug induced delirium in the elderly. Postgrad Med J. 2004;80(945):388–93.
12. Şenel G, Uysal N, Oguz G, Kaya M, Kadioullari N, Koçak N, et al. Delirium frequency and risk factors among patients with cancer in palliative care unit – Dec 31, 2015. American Journal of Hospice and Palliative Medicine®. 2015 Dec 31 [cited 2017 Feb 11]. Available from: https://doi.org/10.1177/1049909115624703 doi: https://doi.org/10.1177/1049909115624703.
13. Han JH, Zimmerman EE, Cutler N, Schnelle J, Morandi A, Dittus RS, et al. Delirium in older emergency department patients: recognition, risk factors, and psychomotor subtypes. Acad Emerg Med. 2009;16(3):193–200.
14. Han JH, Wilson A, Graves AJ, Shintani A, Schnelle JF, Dittus RS, et al. Validation of the confusion assessment method for the intensive care unit in older emergency department patients. Acad Emerg Med. 2014;21(2):180–7.
15. Inouye SK, Kosar CM, Tommet D, Schmitt EM, Puelle MR, Saczynski JS, et al. The CAM-S: development and validation of a new scoring system for delirium severity in 2 cohorts. Ann Intern Med. 2014;160(8):526–33.
16. Meagher J, Leonard M, Donoghue L, O'Regan N, Timmons S, Exton C, et al. Months backward test: a review of its use in clinical studies. World J Psychiatry. 2015;5(3):305–14.
17. Malone M, Lau T. Hidden in plain sight: recognizing catatonia amidst its medical complications. Univ Ott J Med. 2015;5(2):22–5.
18. Popeo DM. Delirium in older adults. Mt Sinai J Med. 2011;78(4):571–82.
19. Siddiqi N, Harrison JK, Clegg A, Teale EA, Young J, Taylor J, et al. Interventions for preventing delirium in hospitalized non-ICU patients. Cochrane Database Syst Rev. 2016; (3):CD005563.
20. Fong TG, Tulebaev SR, Inouye SK. Delirium in elderly adults: diagnosis, prevention and treatment. Nat Rev Neurol. 2009;5(4):210–20.

Geriatric Psychopharmacology: A Complex Case of Psychosis Complicated by Neuroleptic Malignant Syndrome (NMS) and Metabolic Syndrome (MetS)

3

Raj Velamoor and Gautham Pulagam

Abbreviations

ALT	Alanine transaminase
AMPK	Adenosine monophosphate-activated protein kinase
AST	Aspartate transaminase
BUN	Blood urea nitrogen
CPK	Creatine phosphokinase
CVD	Cardiovascular disease
CYP	Cytochrome P 450
GABA	Gamma-amniobutyric acid
HDL	High-density lipoprotein
LDL	Low-density lipoprotein
LFT	Liver function test
MetS	Metabolic syndrome
NMS	Neuroleptic malignant syndrome
PPAR α	Peroxisome proliferator-activated receptor alpha
SSRI	Selective serotonin reuptake inhibitors
START	Screening Tool to Alert doctors to Right Treatment
STOPP	Screening Tool of Older Person's Prescriptions
TNFα	Tumor necrosis factor alpha

R. Velamoor, MB, FRCPsych (UK), FRCP (C)
Northern Ontario School of Medicine, Laurentian and Lakehead University, Sudbury, ON, Canada

Schulich School of Medicine, Western University, London, ON, Canada

G. Pulagam, MD, BSc (✉)
Schulich School of Medicine, Western University, London, ON, Canada
e-mail: mbasaguilar@northwell.edu

3.1 Introduction

Geriatric mental health care has assumed great clinical importance as our aging population has been consistently increasing over the last six decades. According to the US Census Bureau, the growth of elderly people over the age of 65 has gone up from 7% in 1940 to nearly 13% in 2010 [1]. Geriatric pharmacology is a delicate and complex subject that has been gaining importance over the last few years. Given the likelihood of multiple comorbidities and prescribers in this population, individuals on prescription and over-the-counter non-prescription medications have increased disproportionately [2]. A survey done in the USA found that 87% of the population over the age of 65 used at least one prescription medication, while 36% used at least five or more prescription medications. In the same survey, it was found that approximately 38% of the respondents used over-the-counter medications [3]. The incidence of adverse effects in individuals over the age of 65 has been increasing. Hence, physicians are often faced with the challenge of striking the

© Springer International Publishing AG, part of Springer Nature 2018
K. Shivakumar, S. Amanullah (eds.), *Complex Clinical Conundrums in Psychiatry*,
https://doi.org/10.1007/978-3-319-70311-4_3

right balance between the dose of medications prescribed and their possible side effects. The benefits should outweigh the risks in this calculation.

With the improvement in the standard of living and accessibility to mental health care, the number of older individuals seeking treatment for psychiatric disorders has also increased. The likelihood of older individuals over the age of 70 being admitted to a hospital for management of adverse drug reactions from psychotropic drugs is 3.5 times higher than in young individuals [4]. This has led to a greater interest in the research and publication of material in geriatric psychopharmacology. This chapter reviews the age-related changes in the pharmacokinetic and pharmacodynamic functions, commonly used psychotropic drugs, as well as the negative influence of multiple comorbidities and polypharmacy on the health of the elderly.

3.2   Case Presentation

The importance of pharmacodynamic and kinetic effects in the elderly is illustrated through the following case vignette:

A 77-year-old male was brought to the ER after striking out at his wife following an argument. Upon further questioning, his wife stated that he had been getting increasingly agitated, forgetful, and dependent on her for activities of daily living like self-care, transportation, and managing finances. His past medical history was significant for hypertension, diabetes, osteoarthritis, depression, and coronary artery disease. His medications included captopril, metformin, fluoxetine, acetaminophen, and aspirin. His wife stated that she had been giving him ginkgo biloba, as she was told that it improves memory. The patient had a one pack/day smoking history for 30 years but quit 6 months ago. He did not drink alcohol or use illicit drugs.

His blood pressure in the ER was 136/86, heart rate 90/min, temperature 37.2 °C (99° F), and respiration rate 14/min. Examination revealed a disheveled man with dry mucus membranes and a S3 murmur. The rest of the physical examination was unremarkable. Mental status exam revealed an agitated and confused elderly gentleman. His labs revealed the following:

Serum chemistry	Reference range	
Serum sodium	140 mEq/L	136–146 mEq/L
Serum potassium	4.5 mEq/L	3.5–5.0 mEq/L
Chloride	108 mEq/L	95–105 mEq/L
Bicarbonate	28 mEq/L	22–28 mEq/L
BUN	35 mg/dL	7–18 mg/dL
Creatinine	1.4 mg/dL	0.6–1.2 mg/dL
Calcium	9.5 mg/dL	8.4–10.2 mg/dL
Blood glucose	148 mg/dL	70–110 mg/dL

Liver function test (LFT)		
Total bilirubin	1.8 mg/dL	0.1–1 mg/dL
Direct bilirubin	0.4 mg/dL	0.0–0.3 mg/dL
Alkaline phosphatase	120 U/L	30–100 U/L
AST	65 U/L	40–80 U/L
ALT	75 U/L	40–80 U/L

The patient was started on IV fluids. As he was restless and pulling out the tubes, he was administered haloperidol 5 mg intramuscularly. 24 h later he appeared confused and diaphoretic. He developed cogwheel rigidity, which did not respond to benztropine 2 mg IM. His vitals revealed a blood pressure of 162/98, heart rate of 110/min, respiratory rate of 22/min, and temperature of 38.6 °C (101.5 °F). CT of the brain ruled out any intracranial pathology. His metabolic panel revealed:

		Reference range
Serum sodium	145 mEq/L	136–146 mEq/L
Serum potassium	5 mEq/L	3.5–5 mEq/L
Chloride	110 mEq/L	95–105 mEq/L
Bicarbonate	30 mEq/L	22–28 mEq/L
BUN	38 mEq/L	7–18 mEq/L
Creatinine	1.6 mg/dL	0.6–1.2 mg/dL
Calcium	9.5 mg/dL	8.4–10.2 mg/dL
Blood glucose	160 mg/dL	70–110 mg/dL
Creatine kinase	710 U/L	25–90 U/L

Within a time span of 24 h, the patient had developed a high fever, heart rate (above 25% of baseline), and respiratory rate (above 50% of baseline) along with a significant change in blood pressure (systolic BP above 25% baseline). A rapid increase in BUN and creatine also signified worsening renal function. Furthermore, his creatine kinase was nearly eight times the normal value. A diagnosis of neuroleptic malignant syndrome was suspected, and neurology was consulted. He was transferred to a medical floor for further investigations and management.

3.2.1 Pharmacokinetics

Aging leads to a loss of functional units along with dysregulation of various processes in the body. This can often lead to inadequate homeostasis as the pharmacokinetics and pharmacodynamics of the psychotropic drugs in the body are altered [5]. The pharmacokinetic implications of a drug include its absorption, distribution, metabolism, and elimination. So far, studies on geriatric pharmacology have not provided any conclusive evidence that the physiological changes in older individuals that affect drug absorption would necessarily lead to a higher incidence of adverse side effects [5, 6]. However, the remaining components of pharmacokinetics seem to play a role in increased drug sensitivity. Aging results in reduction of first-pass metabolism due to reduced blood flow to the liver and also decreased liver mass. This increases the bioavailability of drugs undergoing first-pass metabolism [7]. Polar, hydrophilic drugs have a small volume of distribution, which increases the drug serum levels in older individuals. The content of body water drops around 10–15% until the age of 80 [8]. So, the volume of distribution of hydrophilic drugs will result in a higher plasma concentration in elderly individuals as compared to younger individuals. On the other hand nonpolar, hydrophobic drugs have a higher volume of distribution, thus prolonging the half-life of the drug [9]. Renal clearance also plays a key role in the drug toxicity in the elderly. Glomerular filtration rate linearly decreases by age 40 and by age 60; this decline is exponential [10]. This physiological loss of renal function decreases the rate of elimination, especially for medications like lithium that are primarily excreted through the kidneys. Recent studies have shown that a decline in renal function can also affect drug metabolism in the liver, thus enhancing the drug toxicity in the body [11]. The integrity of the liver and kidneys is therefore vital to the tolerance of drugs prescribed.

Aging also causes a loss of cell integrity, especially between the tight junctions in the blood-brain barrier [12]. This leads to an increased access of the brain to certain medications like antipsychotics and antidepressants. Changes in central pharmacokinetics such as increased sensitivity to drugs and decreased dopamine levels make the elderly more susceptible to antipsychotics. It is predicted that a young patient would experience extrapyramidal effects when antipsychotics occupy over 80% of the dopamine D2 receptors in the brain. However, this threshold is lowered in the elderly as symptoms manifest when there is even less than 80% occupancy of D2 receptors. This threshold might also be much lower in patients with behavioral and psychological symptoms [13].

All the above changes in the physiological and biochemical mechanisms, as well as impairment of the liver and renal functions, behoove the clinician to be vigilant and judicious in their prescribing habits.

3.2.2 Pharmacodynamics

Pharmacodynamics refers to the effects of a drug on the body. The effect of a drug depends on the number of receptors in the target organ, signal transduction, and counter-regulatory processes that maintain a functional equilibrium. A decrease in all these factors is postulated to cause a decline in the dopaminergic system. There is an overall decline in the number of dopamine D2 receptors in the striatum [7]. Postmortem studies have shown that aging causes a decrease in the number of dopaminergic binding sites in the basal ganglia by at least 10% per decade [14]. A few other age-related changes include a decrease in the number of synapses, counter-regulatory measures, and also a decline in brain weight [8, 15]. These pharmacodynamic changes increase the sensitivity of drugs in the elderly.

Age-related pharmacodynamic changes also include a decrease in the cholinergic receptors [7]. This combined with reduced homeostasis makes them susceptible to anticholinergic effects [16, 17]. These side effects can be quite disabling and may include peripheral effects such as urinary retention, dry mouth, constipation, blurred vision, and increased frequency of falls and risk of infection. Central cerebral effects may include memory impairment, confusion, agitation, anxiety, and even severe cognitive impairment with increased risk of Alzheimer's dementia. Among the antipsychotics, olanzapine has the greatest binding affinity to M1 receptors and is thus known to have a higher risk of causing anticholinergic side effects. Risperidone in comparison causes relatively less anticholinergic side effects [18]. An increase in sedation secondary to CNS medications can be explained by a decrease in GABAminergic receptors resulting in a higher plasma drug concentration [19]. These central and peripheral anticholinergic effects can result in an overall decrease in the activities of daily living [20].

3.2.3 Polypharmacy

In addition to the age-related changes, another variable that profoundly affects the tolerance and safety of medication use is polypharmacy. Multiple prescribers prescribe multiple medications in a system of care that is often not coordinated. The prevalence of multiple medication use among patients with schizophrenia and other psychotic disorders is between 3% and 71% [21]. This polypharmacy has been associated with an increased incidence of adverse side effects. Some of the most common adverse effects associated with combination antipsychotic therapy include increased sedation, anticholinergic side effects, hyperprolactinemia, and an overall increase in metabolic and cardiovascular risk. Polypharmacy also increases the risk of drug interactions. For example, it is reported that nearly 50% of geriatric patients suffer from varying forms of depression for which many are prescribed selective serotonin reuptake inhibitors (SSRI) [22]. Fluoxetine and paroxetine are potent inhibitors of CYP2D6 isoenzymes, and these medications are often concomitantly used with antipsychotics for treatment of depressive psychosis or for the treatment of negative symptoms of schizophrenia [23, 24]. In vitro studies have shown that such combinations can cause a remarkable increase in plasma concentrations of drugs.

First-generation antipsychotics like haloperidol and fluphenazine when combined with fluoxetine could possibly lead to increase in incidence of CNS adverse effects, including but not limited to NMS [22]. Fluoxetine also interferes with the elimination of second-generation antipsychotics like clozapine and olanzapine by inhibiting CYP3A4 and CYP2D6 isoenzymes. The same study also mentions that fluoxetine increases the concentration of clozapine by twofold and fluvoxamine, another SSRI, increases it by nearly five- to tenfold. This results in an increased incidence of adverse effects like agranulocytosis and metabolic syndrome. Since SSRIs inhibit CYP isoenzymes, it can also cause drug interactions with some of the most common medications used in the geriatric population such as beta-blockers, digoxin, oral anticoagulants, and also other psychotropic drugs.

3.3 Neuroleptic Malignant Syndrome (NMS)

3.3.1 Neuroleptic Malignant Syndrome (NMS)

Neuroleptic malignant syndrome is a rare but potentially lethal form of drug-induced hyperthermia. First described in 1960 by Delay et al., the overall incidence of NMS ranges between 0.02% and 3.23% [25]. NMS affects patients of all ages, while men have a higher reported incidence than women. This may be because young adult males may be receiving higher doses of neuroleptics. The four principal symptoms of NMS are hyperthermia, rigidity, mental status changes, and autonomic dysfunction. This is usually characterized by rigidity unresponsive to anticholinergic medications, hyperthermia of unknown cause, diaphoresis, dysphagia, changes in level of consciousness ranging from confusion to coma, and elevated creatine phosphokinase (CPK) levels [25]. Studies suggest that the symptoms of NMS might progress in a predictable manner. It has been observed that mental status changes and muscle rigidity precede hyperthermia and autonomic dysregulation [26, 27]. The presentation and course of NMS can be variable. NMS usually develops within 4 weeks of starting an antipsychotic treatment, while two-thirds of cases develop within the first week [25, 26]. Caroff and Mann reported that 16% of patients developed signs of NMS within 24 h of administration of antipsychotics, with 66% within the first week and 96% within the 4 weeks of antipsychotic therapy [28]. In some individuals, NMS also develops after having taken the same dose of antipsychotic medication for several months.

3.3.2 Pathophysiology

Central dopaminergic systems are involved in temperature regulation, muscle tone, and movement. Blockade of these systems offers the most compelling evidence for causation of NMS. Neuroleptic-induced dopamine blockade in the nigrostriatal pathway is said to cause rigidity, and blockade in the hypothalamus may explain the impairment of the autonomic as well as central thermoregulation. Alteration of dopamine neurotransmission in the brain stem reticular activating system may be responsible for the alterations in consciousness like mutism, coma, and other disturbances in arousal. Other cofactors may include imbalance of norepinephrine, GABA, and serotonin systems. Dysregulated sympathoadrenal hyperactivity has also been postulated as a likely explanation in the etiology of NMS [29]. The hypermetabolic state is possibly a result of excess noradrenaline relative to dopamine when individuals are on dopamine antagonist therapy. Recent studies in pharmacogenetics implicate a role for genetic predisposition as well in the causation of NMS [30].

3.3.3 Diagnosis

The four principal symptoms of NMS are hyperthermia, rigidity, mental status changes, and autonomic impairment. NMS is generally characterized by the presence of rigidity and hyperthermia following antipsychotic administration, as well as other symptoms which may include profuse sweating, tremor, incontinence, mental status changes, changes in heart rate and blood pressure, leukocytosis, and CPK elevation. The medical workup is usually negative.

There is however a lack of general agreement among experts about the significance of these items. This impedes research and clinical management of patients. While classical full-blown forms are recognized, diagnosed, and treated, partial or milder forms may be missed. This heterogeneity in presentation, course, and response to treatment warrants development of specific criteria that can be applied uniformly across varying clinical presentations with confidence. An international multispecialty expert panel (including psychiatrists, neurologists, emergency medicine specialists, and anesthesiologists) converged to establish critical values and offer guidance regarding the relative importance of individual diagnostic elements [27]. The table below represents the findings of the panel of experts based on a formal consensus procedure (Table 3.1).

The consensus study criteria have been validated recently in a study accepted for publication [31]. The latest edition of DSM 5 makes reference to the abovementioned consensus diagnostic criteria in the general clinical review of NMS under the heading of diagnostic features [32]. This will hopefully advance research in the field, as well as the clinical management of patients with NMS.

The criteria of negative medical workup are critically important in the elderly in view of the presence of concomitant medical disorders and morbidities. Laboratory abnormalities in NMS generally include elevated creatine kinase levels as stated above, leukocytosis, metabolic acidosis, elevated catecholamines, and electrolyte changes [25, 33]. A prospective study revealed that patients with NMS have a low serum iron level by as much as 10 µmol/l or lower in 96% of the cases analyzed [34]. This suggests that iron deficiency may possibly have a role in NMS as a risk factor.

Table 3.1 Neuroleptic malignant syndrome diagnostic criteria: expert panel consensus

Diagnostic criterion	Priority score
Exposure to dopamine antagonist, or dopamine agonist withdrawal, within past 72 h	20
Hyperthermia (>100.4 °F or 38.0 °C on at least 2 occasions, measured orally)	18
Rigidity	17
Mental status alteration (reduced or fluctuating level of consciousness)	13
Creatine kinase elevation (at least four times the upper limit of normal)	10
Sympathetic nervous system lability, defined as at least two of the following: Blood pressure elevation (systolic or diastolic ≥25% above baseline) Blood pressure fluctuation (≥20 mmHg diastolic change or ≥25 mm hg systolic change within 24 h) Diaphoresis Urinary incontinence	10
Hypermetabolism, defined as heart rate increase (≥25% above baseline) and respiratory rate increase (≥50% above baseline)	5
Negative workup for infectious, toxic, metabolic, or neurological causes	7
Total	100

Reproduced with permission from "An international consensus study of neuroleptic malignant syndrome diagnostic criteria using the Delphi method"

3.3.4 Differential Diagnoses

NMS is a diagnosis of exclusion; it is therefore important to rule out various medical and neurological conditions that may mimic this condition. Sewell and Jeste, in their 1992 study of 34 hospitalized patients with suspected NMS, found that 24 of those patients had NMS, while the symptoms of the remaining 10 patients were more likely attributable to other acute medical conditions. A stroke, especially involving the brain stem and basal ganglia, can simulate NMS. Recent studies have indicated that elderly patients undergoing treatment with second-generation antipsychotics are at an increased risk of stroke [35]. Another important condition to consider while diagnosing NMS is parkinsonism-hyperthermia syndrome seen in patients with Parkinson's disease and other disorders of the basal ganglia [36]. These patients can develop rebound parkinsonian symptoms resembling NMS such as hyperthermia and rigidity due to abrupt withdrawal of dopamine agonist treatment. This, according to Caroff et al., is analogous to inhibiting dopamine activity with antipsychotics. Another possible differential diagnosis to consider is neuroleptic sensitivity syndrome in patients with Lewy body dementia. In these patients, any exacerbation of psychotic symptoms is often managed with multiple antipsychotics. Over a period of time, repeated use of these antipsychotics can sensitize the patients to neurological side effects of medications [37, 38]. Like NMS, neuroleptic sensitivity syndrome if not managed could be fatal as the patient can rapidly deteriorate with increased confusion, rigidity, fixed flexion posture, and dehydration. It is important to note that anticholinergic agents do not reverse these symptoms and might actually make it worse [39]. Heatstroke and serotonin syndrome are also confused with NMS as the clinical presentations may be similar. However, there are important differences. Patients with heatstroke present with hyperthermia but with a dry skin and loss of muscle tone. Hyperthermia in NMS on the other hand is usually associated with muscle rigidity and diaphoresis [37]. The use of polypharmacy in geriatric patients, especially a combination of SSRIs and other medications, can cause the serotonin syndrome. Although they present with hyperthermia and autonomic changes as seen in NMS, they also manifest gastrointestinal symptoms, myoclonus and hyperreflexia, which are not characteristic of NMS [25].

Given the common prevalence of the use of anticholinergic agents, the elderly are also susceptible to atropinic poisoning, which presents with hyperthermia and mental status changes along with autonomic signs similar to NMS [37, 40]. Some of the other disorders to consider and exclude for the differential diagnosis of NMS in the elderly include infectious causes like meningitis, encephalitis, brain abscess or sepsis, toxic effects from salicylate poisoning and substance abuse, and endocrine causes like thyrotoxicosis and pheochromocytoma [29, 41].

3.3.5 Risk Factors

NMS can occur across the life span in children, adults, as well as the elderly. However, geriatric patients are more susceptible due to their comorbidities and other risk factors associated with age. These may include polypharmacy, dehydration, malnutrition, rapid or parenteral administration of antipsychotics, ethanol intoxication, and adjunctive use of anticholinergic medications and lithium. Alzheimer's dementia and, especially, Lewy body dementia are predisposing factors for NMS [28, 42]. Certain conditions such as organic brain syndrome and mood disorders, as well as agitation and exhaustion, can cause vulnerability to NMS [43].

3.3.6 Management

The most important aspect of treatment is prevention. This includes taking necessary precautions to reduce possible risk factors, early recognition of suspected cases, and prompt discontinuation of the offending agent. Specific treatment should always be based empirically on the duration and severity of the symptoms. For mild cases, treatment should mainly be conservative. Supportive management should start with fluid replacement, correction of electrolyte and acid-base imbalance, reduction of body temperature by active cooling measures, and monitoring of cardiac, respiratory, and renal functions [25, 38]. Woodbury and Woodbury suggested that benzodiazepines and anticholinergic agents can be used for catatonia and extrapyramidal symptoms [44]. A trial of lorazepam 0.5–1 mg IM q4–6 hourly has been found to be quite effective as an initial approach. Several case studies have reported the complete resolution of NMS symptoms with high divided doses of benzodiazepines [45, 46]. A similar case report by Francis and Yacoub showed a resolution of muscle rigidity and fever within 24–72 h after the initiation of lorazepam [47]. However, one needs to be cautious about respiratory depression due to benzodiazepine use, especially in the elderly.

Severe cases may warrant dopamine agonist drugs to correct the hypodopaminergic state. In patients with muscle rigidity and a body temperature ranging between 38.3 and 40.0 °C, treatment with a dopamine agonist should be considered. Treatment should start with bromocriptine 2.5 mg every 8 h or amantadine 100 mg every 8 h [25]. This dosage may be continued over the next 10 days and gradually tapered thereafter.

If the body temperature is greater than 40 °C, IV dantrolene 2 mg–3 mg/kg body weight should be considered. Dantrolene is a muscle relaxant and hydantoin derivative and acts centrally by blocking specific receptors responsible for calcium release in the skeletal muscles. This in turn decreases the excitation-contraction mechanism of the muscles, reducing spasticity [48]. It is especially indicated in NMS patients with refractory hyperthermia. It lowers the temperature by reducing muscle rigidity, muscle metabolism, and heat generation [38]. Once the symptoms are controlled, the medication can be switched to oral dantrolene 1 mg/kg every 6 h for another 10 days and then gradually tapered off.

Bromocriptine and dantrolene significantly reduce the mortality rate in patients with severe hyperthermia caused by cardiorespiratory failure, myoglobinuric renal failure, arrhythmias, seizures, etc. A combination of bromocriptine and dantrolene, however, has not proven to be superior to either one or the other drug used alone [38]. Once the patients are initiated on either a dopamine agonist or dantrolene, physicians should monitor for the most common side effects associated with these drugs. Both these drugs can cause drowsiness, dizziness, and overall weakness along with some nausea and headaches [49]. Dantrolene can be toxic to the liver. In patients with NMS who are refractory to pharmacotherapy, ECT may be considered. ECT is the treatment of choice for patients in whom the hypermetabolic state has resolved but without the resolution of catatonia [38].

Following a drug-free clearance period of at least 2 weeks following the complete resolution of NMS symptoms, treatment of ongoing psychosis may be attempted. This may be done by rechallenging the patient with a neuroleptic class of drug other than the one that caused the episode. A low-dose atypical antipsychotic like aripiprazole, a partial dopamine antagonist and agonist, may be considered. Alternative medications (if still sensitive to neuroleptics) may include mood stabilizers (low-dose lamotrigine, divalproex, or lithium) and cautious use of benzodiazepines. Serial monitoring of creatine kinase levels may be helpful in warning us of further episodes of NMS. Education of the patient and family, as well as the importance of thorough documentation, cannot be overemphasized.

3.3.7 Case Progression

Two weeks after the resolution of NMS, the patient was initiated on olanzapine, an atypical antipsychotic at 5 mg bedtime for agitation and labile mood secondary to dementia. The dose was titrated up over the next few months to 15 mg daily. In addition, he was continued on captopril, metformin, aspirin, acetaminophen, and fluoxetine for his other comorbidities. The patient missed two follow-up appointments with the psychiatrist and did not see his primary care physician. Five months after starting therapy with olanzapine, the patient returned with his wife. She stated that although he remained confused, there had been an improvement in his mental status with very few episodes of agitation. However, she was concerned about his physical health as he was experiencing shortness of breath and a noticeable increase in weight. He had gained 20 lbs. in weight unintentionally since his last visit, and his blood pressure had increased to 160/105. His labs revealed:

		Reference range
Creatinine	1.5 mg/dL	0.6–1.2 mg/dL
High-density lipoprotein	28 mg/dL	30–70 mg/dL
Low-density lipoprotein	140 mg/dL	< 160 mg/dL
Triglycerides	220 mg/dL	101–150 mg/dL
Hemoglobin A1c	8.2%	< 6%

Based on ATP III guidelines, a diagnosis of olanzapine-induced metabolic syndrome was made.

3.4 Metabolic Syndrome

3.4.1 Metabolic Syndrome

Atypical antipsychotics have become the mainstay in the management of psychosis, in both the young and elderly patients. They are preferred over the older typical antipsychotics like haloperidol, as they are known to cause fewer extrapyramidal symptoms. However, these antipsychotics are associated with a few side effects of their own, of which metabolic syndrome is most concerning. Referred to as syndrome X when it was first described in 1988 by Reaven, it has since been mainly associated with atypical antipsychotics [21, 50]. Metabolic syndrome (MetS) is a culmination of metabolic disturbances, which include weight gain, hypertriglyceridemia, increased insulin, blood glucose, and low-density lipoprotein cholesterol levels. The current definitions used for MetS are proposed by the Adult Treatment Panel III (ATP III), American Heart Association (ATP III A), and the International Diabetes Federation (IDF) [51] (Fig. 3.1).

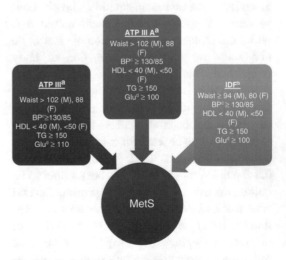

Fig. 3.1 Definitions for metabolic syndrome. [a]Diagnosis if three of five criteria are met. [b]Diagnosis if waist plus another two criteria are met. [c]Or if treated with antihypertensive medication. [d]Or if treated with hypoglycemic agent or insulin. Waist (cm); *HDL (mg/dL)* high-density lipoprotein, *TG (mg/dL)* triglycerides, *Glu (mg/dL)* glucose, *M* male, *F* female

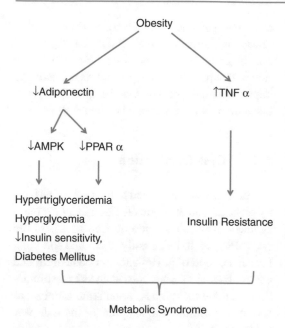

Fig. 3.2 The pathophysiology of metabolic syndrome. *AMPK* Adenosine monophosphate-activated protein kinase, *PPAR α* Peroxisome proliferator-activated receptor alpha, *TNFα* Tumor necrosis factor alpha

3.4.2   Pathophysiology

Adipose tissue plays a key role as the regulator of many endocrine functions in the body. Adipocytes produce many biologically active molecules known as adipokines such as adiponectin, leptin, and tumor necrosis factor α (TNFα) [52]. Dysregulation of these adipokines is directly linked to metabolic disturbances. Adiponectin is known for its antidiabetic activity by increasing insulin sensitivity. Studies have shown that hypoadiponectemia is independently associated with MetS [52, 53]. Adiponectin stimulates adenosine monophosphate-activated protein kinase phosphorylation and also the activation of peroxisome proliferator-activated receptor alpha (PPAR α), which directly regulate glucose metabolism [54]. Obesity and accumulation of visceral fat reduce the expression of adiponectin, which further decreases AMPK and PPAR α activity [54, 55]. This in turn leads to hyperglycemia, insulin resistance, diabetes mellitus, and hypertriglyceridemia. In contrast to adiponectin, high TNFα levels are directly linked to insulin resistance [56] (Fig. 3.2).

Weight gain is a common side effect of most atypical antipsychotics. These medications bind multiple neurotransmitters including histaminergic, serotonergic, dopaminergic, and cholinergic receptors at varying degrees. Blocking of histamine H1 receptors by atypical antipsychotics is found to cause metabolic disturbances [57]. These receptors are implicated in weight regulation through H1 receptor-linked activation of hypothalamic AMPK [58]. Similarly, atypical antipsychotics also block 5-HT2C receptors, which cause further weight gain [59]. In addition, blockade of muscarinic M3 receptors and 5-HT1A receptors causes desensitization of the pancreatic beta cells leading to insulin dysregulation. Impaired glucose uptake can be attributed to antagonism of 5HT2A receptors [57]. Certain antipsychotics are also implicated in impairing the effect of insulin on adipocytes, causing lipid accumulation and dyslipidemia [60].

3.4.3   Risk Factors

The prevalence of MetS is twice as high in patients suffering from a mental illness when compared to the general population. In a study of patients with schizophrenia and bipolar disorder, they were found to have glucose dysregulation and diabetes even before they were treated with any antipsychotic medications [61]. A pattern of insulin resistance is also suspected in these patients. Weight gain is another important risk factor, perhaps the most bothersome for some patients. Studies have shown that clozapine and olanzapine are associated with the most significant weight gain, especially within the first 6 months of initiating atypical antipsychotic therapy. In their review, Newcomer and Haupt found that patients on olanzapine reported a mean weight gain of 6 kg, while it was over 10 kg for patients on a dose higher than 12.5 mg. Studies have also shown that the risk of both short- and long-term weight gain is highest for clozapine, while it was reported to be the lowest for patients taking ziprasidone [62]. Individual case studies have also shown a marked increase in blood glucose levels in patients treated with clozapine and olanzapine [61]. Approximately two-thirds of all the studies done to identify the role of antipsychotics in MetS found that drugs such as olanzapine were also associated with an increased risk for diabetes. A meta-analysis on published cases regarding new onset of diabetes showed that the incidence of new-onset diabetes was 45% within the first 3 months of antipsychotic treatment [63].

3.4.4   Management

While clozapine and olanzapine are associated with the highest incidence of metabolic syndrome, it is relatively less to none with ziprasidone and aripiprazole [64]. If the patient has considerable risk factors for metabolic syndrome, a low initial dose of either ziprasidone or aripiprazole may be considered. Optimal medical monitoring and management of the elderly on psychotropic medications are of paramount importance. However, elderly patients with mental illnesses often do not receive optimal attention for their medical concerns like cardiovascular or metabolic illness [63]. Once antipsychotic therapy is initiated, it is important to regularly monitor the patient so as to keep track of any metabolic changes. The psychiatrist or the primary care physician should get a baseline fasting glucose level along with lipid profile, BMI, and EKG before initiating the antipsychotic therapy. If the patients begin to exhibit abnormal glucose levels, they should be referred for medical management promptly. Similarly, these patients should be closely monitored for diabetic ketoacidosis (DKA), especially the more vulnerable elderly population. The mortality risk from DKA increases from 2% in the general population to 20% in the elderly [65]. Metformin therapy along with lifestyle modifications like diet regulation and exercise has shown to significantly improve the quality of life in patients with metabolic syndrome [66].

Collaboration between psychiatry and primary care is critically essential in the psychiatric and medical management of the elderly. Effective communication between the primary care physician and the psychiatrist is key to good outcome [67]. This will not only improve the quality of monitoring of the patient but also help in early detection and management of metabolic abnormalities. Educating the patient, their family members, and also other health-care providers involved in the care of that patient will help to optimize treatment, improve compliance, and facilitate prompt discontinuation of unnecessary medications [68].

3.4.5   Case Disposition

The patient was discharged to the care of his family physician on aripiprazole 2 mg daily for management of psychosis and quetiapine 25–50 mg orally PRN up to twice daily to be used sparingly for severe agitation. Reliance on behavioral and environmental interventions such as low stimulation, calming techniques, orientation training, as well as counseling and support for his wife was emphasized.

3.5   Discussion and Conclusions

3.5.1   Discussion

Comorbid medical conditions, pharmacokinetic and pharmacodynamic changes of aging, drug interactions associated with polypharmacy, and compliance issues to medications are some of the most common and interlinked factors that affect the response to medications in geriatric patients. Medications are prescribed to manage many psychiatric disorders. The most common disorders are new-onset psychosis later in life, dementia-related syndromes with psychosis, delirium- or drug-induced psychosis, and primary psychiatric disorders especially depression [69]. Dementia is the greatest risk factor for the development of psychotic symptoms in geriatric patients [43]. According to the Lewy Body Dementia Association, more than 50% of the patients with Lewy body dementia treated with antipsychotics may also develop NMS.

In the case of our 77-year-old patient, there was an interplay of all the above mentioned (age-related) factors. Pharmacokinetic and pharmacodynamic changes along with polypharmacy could have led to an increase in plasma haloperidol to toxic levels triggering an episode of NMS. Specifically as haloperidol is mainly biotransformed in the liver, pharmacokinetic changes could have caused the increase in plasma haloperidol levels [70]. As hepatic mass and blood flow to the liver decrease with age, haloperidol is not metabolized at the same rate as in a young patient. In a comparison study, it was reported that plasma levels of haloperidol were twice as high in older patients for the same oral dose as in younger patients with schizophrenia. Reduced haloperidol, a metabolite of haloperidol, has also been reported to be five times higher in elderly patients [71]. Abnormal liver enzyme levels in this patient prior to admission would confirm hepatic dysfunction, which can decrease the rate of drug metabolism. However, impaired haloperidol metabolism alone may not induce a toxic increase in blood level. An additional factor that may occur with aging is an increase in peripheral fat stores in the body, which causes an increase in the bioavailability of lipophilic drugs like haloperidol [70]. Even though these changes in peripheral pharmacokinetics play a role in increased drug sensitivity in older individuals, explanation for the full panoply of adverse effects to antipsychotics is not fully understood [13].

As in this case, antipsychotic therapy increases the risk for metabolic syndrome in older patients. Olanzapine is well known to be the offending agent in weight gain. Patients who are on two or more second-generation antipsychotics are more likely to have a higher BMI than patients on antipsychotic monotherapy [21]. Similarly, these patients have a poorer metabolic health. They are found to have significantly higher rates of lipid markers of insulin resistance and metabolic syndrome. All the symptoms that define metabolic syndrome such as hyperglycemia, hypertension, increase in triglycerides and overall adiposity are also significant risk factors for cardiovascular disease.

3.5.2   Recommendations

3.5.2.1   Collaborative Care Management

The interface between psychiatry and primary care is becoming critically important in delivering timely and efficient care to the elderly. Despite access to mental health, only 20% of patients seek help from a mental health-care specialist, as they prefer to see their primary care physician [67]. Unfortunately, patients who seek help from a mental health-care provider have limited access to medical care. This in turn has increased the mortality rate in these patients. As many as 70 randomized control trials have confirmed that collaboration between psychiatry and family medicine, especially for common psychiatric conditions like depression, anxiety, schizophrenia, etc., is more effective and efficient than conventional models of care that operate in isolation. In another exhaustive review of the evidence base for collaborative mental health care in the primary care setting, it was concluded that collaboration makes intuitive sense and is supported by promising results, especially for management of depressive disorders [72]. Both psychiatry and family medicine should monitor the patients regularly for extrapyramidal side effects, tardive dyskinesia, anticholinergic toxicity, and metabolic changes following the initiation of an antipsychotic. Patients should be screened for hyperglycemia, hyperlipidemia, and any weight changes to forestall the development of a metabolic syndrome. If the patient exhibits symptoms, the primary care physician should educate the patient about this condition and recommend lifestyle changes. If indicated, symptomatic treatment with hypoglycemic agents and lipid lowering drugs may be prescribed [65]. The patient should also be carefully monitored for any electrolyte or EKG abnormalities as well as screened for orthostatic hypotension and risk of falls. We should always be vigilant for occurrence of adverse drug reactions as a result of polypharmacy.

3.5.2.2   Criteria and Guidelines

Physicians may consult Beers Criteria for the list of medications that are contraindicated, relatively contraindicated, or avoided in conjunction with other medical conditions before prescribing a new psychotropic drug to geriatric patients. Since its inception in 1991, the Beers Criteria for Potentially Inappropriate Medication Use in Older Adults has been constantly updated with the recommended list of medications that are deemed appropriate and inappropriate in the elderly population over the age of 65 [73]. Other screening tools such as Screening Tool of Older Person's Prescriptions (STOPP) and Screening Tool to Alert doctors to Right Treatment (START) are helpful in decreasing the incidence of hospitalization due to inappropriate medications in the elderly population [74].

3.5.2.3 Management of Risk Factors

Both NMS and metabolic syndrome are prevented by attending to risk factors. As the risk for NMS increases with certain factors including the administration of high-potency neuroleptics such as haloperidol, rapid increase in dosage, parenteral administration, dehydration and high ambient temperature, multiple medications, withdrawal of parkinsonian medications, and medical comorbidities especially in the elderly, great care and caution should be exercised in their prevention and management. The Adult Treatment Panel Guidelines are helpful in the prevention and management of metabolic syndrome and other medical conditions. They report that a decrease in cholesterol levels by 10% will result in a 30% reduction in cardiovascular disease risk. Similarly, lowering blood pressure by 4–6% will decrease the CVD risk by 15%, and this risk is lowered to 35–55% if the BMI is maintained below 25 [75]. Increasing intake of fiber, reducing fat and cholesterol consumption, smoking cessation, and an overall increase in physical activity can significantly lower the risk of cardiovascular disease.

3.5.2.4 Drugs of Choice and Dosage

When initiating the patient on a psychotropic drug, the initial dosage should be low. Two cross-sectional prescription surveys conducted in Pittsburg and Tokyo, respectively, demonstrated that older patients received 50–75% of the mean daily dose of antipsychotics prescribed to young patients to avoid adverse side effects [13]. The Expert Consensus Guidelines recommends risperidone 1.25 mg –3.25 mg/day as the first line of treatment for late onset schizophrenia. If aripiprazole is considered as the second line of treatment, a dose 15–30 mg/day is recommended [76–78]. Ziprasidone (20–40 mg bid) may be

another option. It is prudent to always order an EKG prior to prescribing antipsychotic or antidepressant medications to rule out QT and other abnormalities. When considering an antidepressant, citalopram and sertraline may be preferred over fluoxetine due to their low CYP inhibitory effects. Atypical antipsychotics may be added as useful adjuncts in the management of anxiety and mood disorders. For the management of acute agitation, the suggested initiation dose for haloperidol is between 0.25 and 0.5 mg per day and a maintenance dose of 0.25–4 mg per day [4]. If quetiapine is used for agitation, PRN doses of 25–50 mg, 2–3 times daily, may be considered. If olanzapine is prescribed for agitation or mood stability, the dosage should be as low as 2–5 mg to start with and titrated up gradually to a total of 15 mg daily. With both quetiapine and olanzapine, we should be mindful of their propensity to cause weight gain.

Conclusion

Geriatric psychopharmacology is a complex and intricate science that informs physicians about the unique pharmacokinetic and pharmacodynamic considerations relevant to the use of psychotropic medications in the elderly. This enables the prescribing of the right type of drug, in the right dosage, for the appropriate psychiatric condition. Polypharmacy in medically compromised and physiologically challenged older individuals can lead to disabling and life-threatening toxic effects. Rare but serious conditions like neuroleptic malignant syndrome can follow from indiscriminate use of antipsychotics in the treatment of psychosis. This can be avoided by awareness of the condition and prevention of the risk factors. Morbidity and mortality in NMS can be significantly reduced by early recognition and prompt management.

Psychotropic medications can also cause the metabolic syndrome in the elderly. This can cause type 2 diabetes with critical elevations in weight, sugar, cholesterol, and lipid levels. This can be prevented by careful selection of drugs, avoidance of unnecessary medications and polypharmacy, monitoring of dosage and side effects, active surveillance of the biochemical parameters, and education of patients regarding lifestyle issues of diet, exercise, and nutrition. Providing integrated patient-centered care in a culture of collaboration with primary care providers, allied health-care professionals, and mental health-care specialists working harmoniously can lead to very positive health outcomes.

Disclosure Statement "The authors have nothing to disclose."

References

1. Ortman JM, Velkoff VA, Hogan H. An aging nation: the older population in the United States. US Census Bur Econ Stat Adm US Dep Commer. 2014;1964:1–28.
2. Mintzer J, Burns A. Anticholinergic side-effects of drugs in elderly people. J R Soc Med. 2000;93(9):457–62.
3. Rochon PA. Drug prescribing for older adults. In: Post TW, editor. UpToDate. Waltham, MA: UpToDate; 2016. Accessed 26 July 2016.
4. Lindsey PL. Psychotropic medication use among older adults: what all nurses need to know. J Gerontol Nurs. 2011;35(9):28–38.
5. Mangoni AA, Jackson SHD. Age-related changes in pharmacokinetics and pharmacodynamics: basic principles and practical applications. Br J Clin Pharmacol. 2004;57(1):6–14.
6. Cohen JL. Pharmacokinetic changes in aging. Am J Med. 1986;80(5 SUPPL. 1):31–8.
7. Catterson ML, Preskorn SH, Martin RL. Pharmacodynamic and pharmacokinetic considerations in geriatric psychopharmacology.pdf. Psychiatr Clin North Am. 1997;20(1):205–18.
8. Turnheim K. Drug therapy in the elderly. Exp Gerontol. 2004;39(11):1731–8.
9. Fülöp T, Wórum I, Csongor J, Fóris G, Leövey A. Body composition in elderly people: I. determination of body composition by multiisotope method and the elimination kinetics of these isotopes in healthy elderly subjects. Gerontology. 1985;31(1):6–14.
10. Bennett WM. Geriatric pharmacokinetics and the kidney. Am J Kidney Dis. 1990;16:283–8.
11. Yuan R, Venitz J. Effect of chronic renal failure on the disposition of highly hepatically metabolized drugs. Int J Clin Pharmacol Ther. 2000;38(5):245–53.
12. Davson H, Segal MB. Physiology of the CSF and blood-brain-barriers. Diabetes Care. 1995;33(Suppl 1):S11–61.
13. Uchida H, Mamo D, Mulsant B, Pollock B, Kapur S. Increased antipsychotic sensitivity in elderly patients. J Clin Psychiatry. 2009;70(3):397–405.
14. McGeer PL, McGeer EG, Suzuki JS. Aging and extra-pyramidal function. Arch Neurol. 1977;34(1):33–5.
15. Katzman R. Human nervous system. Compr Physiol. 1995;12:325–44.
16. Kompoliti K, Goetz C. Neuropharmacology in the elderly. Neurol Clin. 1998;16:599–610.
17. Turnheim K. Drug dosage in the elderly. Is it rational? Drugs Aging. 1998;13(5):357–79.
18. Richelson E. Preclinical pharmacology of neuroleptics: focus on new generation compounds. J Clin Psychiatry. 1996;57:4–11.
19. DeVane LC, Pollock BG. Pharmacokinetic considerations of antidepressant use in the elderly. J Clin Psychiatry. 1999;60(suppl 12):38–44.
20. Tune LE. Anticholinergic effects of medication in elderly patients. J Clin Psychiatry. 2001;62(SUPPL. 22):11–4.
21. Correll CU, Frederickson AM, Kane JM, Manu P. Does antipsychotic polypharmacy increase the risk for metabolic syndrome? Schizophr Res. 2007;89(1–3):91–100.
22. Spina E, Scordo MG. Clinically significant drug interactions with antidepressants in the elderly. Drugs Aging. 2002;19(4):299–320.
23. Evins AE, Goff DC. Adjunctive antidepressant drug therapies in the treatment of negative symptoms of schizophrenia. CNS Drugs. 1996;6(2):130–47.
24. Avenoso A, Spina E, Campo G, Facciola G, Ferlito M, Zuccaro P, et al. Interaction between fluoxetine and haloperidol: pharmacokinetic and clinical implications. Pharmacol Res. 1997;35(4):335–9.
25. Velamoor VR. Neuroleptic malignant syndrome. Recognition, prevention and management. Drug Saf. 1998;19(1):73–82.
26. Velamoor VR, Norman RM, Caroff SN, Mann SC, Sullivan KA, Antelo E. Progression of symptoms in neuroleptic malignant syndrome. J Nerv Ment Dis. 1994;182(3):168–73.
27. Gurrera RJ, Caroff SN, Cohen A, Carroll BT, DeRoos F, Francis A, et al. An international consensus study of neuroleptic malignant syndrome diagnostic criteria. J Clin Psychiatry. 2011;72(9):1222–8.
28. Caroff SN, Mann SC. Neuroleptic malignant syndrome. Med Clin North Am. 1993;77(1):185–202.
29. Gurrera RJ. Sympathoadrenal hyperactivity and the etiology of neuroleptic malignant syndrome. Am J Psychiatry. 1999;156(2):169–80.
30. Kawanishi C. Genetic predisposition to neuroleptic malignant syndrome: implications for antipsychotic therapy. Am J Pharmacogenomics. 2003;3(2):89–95.
31. Gurrera RJ, Mortillaro G, Velamoor VR, Caroff SN. A Validation study of the international consensus diagnostic criteria for neuroleptic malignant syndrome. J Clin Psychopharmacol. 2017;37(1):67–71.
32. American Psychiatric Association. Diagnostic and statistical manual of mental disorders: DSM V. In: American Psychiatric Association. Washington; 2013. p. 709–11.
33. Strawn JR, Keck PE, Caroff SN. Neuroleptic malignant syndrome. Am J Psychiatry. 2007;164(6):870–6.

34. Rosebush PI, Mazurek MF. Serum iron and neuroleptic malignant syndrome. Lancet. 1991; 338(8760):149–51.
35. Hall RCW, Appleby B, Hall RCW. Atypical neuroleptic malignant syndrome presenting as fever of unknown origin in the elderly. South Med J. 2005;98(1):114–7.
36. Mizuno Y, Takubo H, Mizuta E, Kuno S. Malignant syndrome in Parkinson's disease: concept and review of the literature. Parkinsonism Relat Disord. 2003;9(SUPPL. 1):3–9.
37. Caroff SN, Cambell CE, Sullivan KA. Neuroleptic malignant syndrome in elderly patients. Expert Rev Neurother. 2007;7(4):423–31.
38. Velamoor VR, Swamy G, Parmar R, Williamson P, Caroff S. Management of suspected neuroleptic malignant syndrome. Can J Psychiatr. 1995;40:545–50.
39. Hall RCW, Hall RCW, Chapman M. Neuroleptic malignant syndrome in the elderly: diagnostic criteria, incidence, risk factors, pathophysiology, and treatment. Clin Geriatr. 2006;14(5):39–46.
40. Granner MA, Wooten GF. Neuroleptic malignant syndrome or parkinsonism hyperpyrexia syndrome. Semin Neurol. 1991;11(3):228–35.
41. Gurrera RJ, Romero JA. Sympathoadrenomedullary activity in the neuroleptic malignant syndrome. Biol Psychiatry. 1992;32(4):334–43.
42. Sewell DDJD. Distinguishing neuroleptic malignant syndrome (NMS) from NMS-like acute medical illnesses: a study of 34 cases. J Neuropsychiatry Clin Neurosci. 1992;4(3):265–9.
43. Seitz DP, Gill SS. Neuroleptic malignant syndrome complicating antipsychotic treatment of delirium or agitation in medical and surgical patients: case reports and a review of the literature. Psychosomatics. 2009;50(1):8–15.
44. Woodbury M, Woodbury M. Neuroleptic-induced catatonia as a stage in the progression toward neuroleptic malignant syndrome. J Am Acad Child Adolesc Psychiatry. 1992;31(6):1161–4.
45. Francis A, Chandragiri S, Rizvi S, Koch M, Petrides GI. Lorazepam a treatment for neuroleptic malignant syndrome? CNS Spectr. 2000;5(7):54–7.
46. Khaldarov V. Benzodiazepines for treatment of neuroleptic malignant syndrome. Hosp Physician. 2011;6:51–5.
47. Yacoub A, Francis A. Neuroleptic malignant syndrome induced by atypical neuroleptics and responsive to lorazepam. Neuropsychiatr Dis Treat. 2006;2(2):235–40.
48. Krause T, Gerbershagen MU, Fiege M, Weisshorn R, Wappler F. Dantrolene--a review of its pharmacology, therapeutic use and new developments. Anaesthesia. 2004;59(4):364–73.
49. Ward A, Chaffman M, Sorkin E, Dantrolene A. Review of its pharmacodynamic and pharmacokinetic properties and therapeutic use in malignant hyperthermia, the neuroleptic malignant syndrome and an update of its use in muscle spasticity. Drugs. 1986;32(2):130–68.

50. Saddichha S, Manjunatha N, Ameen S, Akhtar S. Metabolic syndrome in first episode schizophrenia – a randomized double-blind controlled, short-term prospective study. Schizophr Res. 2008;101(1–3):266–72.
51. De Hert MA, Van Winkel R, Van Eyck D, Hanssens L, Wampers M, Scheen A, et al. Prevalence of the metabolic syndrome in patients with schizophrenia treated with antipsychotic medication. Schizophr Res. 2006;83(1):87–93.
52. Furukawa S, Fujita T, Shumabukuro M, Iwaki M, Yamada Y, Makajima Y, et al. Increased oxidative stress in obesity and its impact on metabolic syndrome. J Clin Invest. 2004;114(12):1752–61.
53. Kadowaki T, Yamauchi T, Kubota N, Hara K, Ueki K, Tobe K. Adiponectin and adiponectin receptors in insulin resistance, diabetes, and the metabolic syndrome. J Clin Invest. 2006;116(7):1784–92.
54. Clarke SD. Polyunsaturated fatty acid regulation of gene transcription: a molecular mechanism to improve the metabolic syndrome. J Nutr. 2001;131(4):1129–32.
55. Kola B. Role of AMP-activated protein kinase in the control of appetite. J Neuroendocrinol. 2008;20(7):942–51.
56. Bai YM, Chen TT, Yang WS, Chi YC, Lin CC, Liou YJ, et al. Association of adiponectin and metabolic syndrome among patients taking atypical antipsychotics for schizophrenia: a cohort study. Schizophr Res. 2009;111(1–3):1–8.
57. Nasrallah HA. Atypical antipsychotic-induced metabolic side effects: insights from receptor-binding profiles. Mol Psychiatry. 2008;13(1):27–35.
58. Kim SF, Huang AS, Snowman AM, Teuscher C, Snyder SH. Antipsychotic drug-induced weight gain mediated by histamine H1 receptor-linked activation of hypothalamic AMP-kinase. Proc Natl Acad Sci U S A. 2007;104(9):3456–9.
59. Reynolds GP, Hill MJ, Kirk SL. The 5-HT2C receptor and antipsychoticinduced weight gain - mechanisms and genetics. J Psychopharmacol. 2006;20(4 Suppl):15–8.
60. Vestri HS, Maianu L, Moellering DR, Garvey WT. Atypical antipsychotic drugs directly impair insulin action in adipocytes: effects on glucose transport, lipogenesis, and antilipolysis. Neuropsychopharmacology. 2007;32(4):765–72.
61. Lieberman JA. Metabolic changes associated with antipsychotic use. Prim Care Comp J Clin Psychiatry. 2004;6(Suppl 2):8–13.
62. Newcomer JW, Haupt DW. The metabolic effects of antipsychotic medications. Can J Psychiatr. 2006;51(8):480–91.
63. Newcomer J. Antipsychotic medications: metabolic and cardiovascular risk. J Clin Psychiatry. 2007;68 Suppl 4(suppl 4):8–13.
64. American Diabetes Association. Consensus development conference on antipsychotic drugs and obesity and diabetes. Diabetes Care. 2004;27:596–601.
65. Newcomer JW. Metabolic risk during antipsychotic treatment. Clin Ther. 2004;26(12):1936–46.

66. De Hert M, Schreurs V, Sweers K, Van Eyck D, Hanssens L, Šinko S, et al. Typical and atypical antipsychotics differentially affect long-term incidence rates of the metabolic syndrome in first-episode patients with schizophrenia: a retrospective chart review. Schizophr Res. 2008;101(1–3):295–303.

67. Unützer J, Harbin H, Schoenbaum M, Druss BG. The collaborative care model: an approach for integrating physical and mental health care in medicaid health homes (Internet). 2013 (cited 26 July 2016). Available from: http://www.chcs.org/media/HH_IRC_Collaborative_Care_Model_052113_2.pdf

68. Stahl SM. The metabolic syndrome: psychopharmacologists should weigh the evidence for weighing the patient. J Clin Psychiatry. 2002;63:1094–5.

69. Brendel RW, Stern TA. Psychotic symptoms in the elderly. Prim Care Comp J Clin Psychiatry. 2005;7(5):238–41.

70. Kudo S, Ishizaki T. Pharmacokinetics of haloperidol. Clin Pharmacokinet. 1999;37(6):435–56.

71. Chang WH, Jann MW, Chiang TS, Lin HN, WH H, Chien CP. Plasma haloperidol and reduced haloperidol concentrations in a geriatric population. Neuropsychobiology. 1996;33(1):12–6.

72. Velamoor R, State SA. Collaborative mental health care: the evolving narrative in primary care. In: State SA, Vingilis E, editors. Applied research and evaluation in community mental health services: an update

of key research domains. 1st ed. Quebec: McGill-Queen's University Press; 2011. p. 160–81.

73. American Geriatrics Society 2015 Beers Criteria Update Expert Panel. American Geriatrics Society 2015 updated beers criteria for potentially inappropriate medication use in older adults. J Am Geriatr Soc. 2015;63(11):2227–46.

74. Gallagher P, Ryan C, Byrne S, Kennedy J, O'Mahony DSTOPP. (screening tool of older Person's prescriptions) and START (screening tool to alert doctors to right treatment). Consensus validation. Int J Clin Pharmacol Ther. 2008;46(2):72–83.

75. National Cholesterol Education Program. (NCEP) expert panel. Third report of the National Cholesterol Education Program (NCEP) expert panel on detection, evaluation, and treatment of high blood cholesterol in adults (adult treatment panel III) final report. Circulation. 2002;106(25):3143–421.

76. Alexopoulos GS, Streim J, Docherty JP. Using antipsychotic agents in older patients. J Clin Psychiatry. 2004;65:5–99. discussion 100

77. Hutchison LC, O'Brien C. Changes in pharmacokinetics and pharmacodynamics in the elderly patient. Prim Care Companion J Clin Psychiatry. 2008;7(1):47–58.

78. Tsan JY, Stock EM, Gonzalez JM, Greenawalt DS, Zeber JE, Rouf E, et al. Mortality and guideline-concordant care for older patients with schizophrenia: a retrospective longitudinal study. BMC Med. 2012;10:147.

A Complex Case of Obsessive-Compulsive Disorder (OCD)

Lynne Drummond and Andrew Roney

4.1 Case History

Joyce is a 32-year-old single woman with two children. Her problems had started 10 years ago during her pregnancy with her oldest child. Her symptoms consisted of fear of contamination by dirt and germs. Although realising her worries were "out of proportion", she was concerned that she may lead to one of her children becoming seriously ill. Consequently she was extremely careful and meticulous in her everyday life. She also exhibited a number of compulsions including extensive handwashing, bathing and house-cleaning compulsions. Handwashing would occur anything between 50–100 times a day and would be performed until she "felt clean". Bathing would take up to 2 hours, and she ensured she washed her entire body "properly". Indeed, more recently she had been adding antiseptic to her bath which had resulted in a widespread skin rash. In addition, she cleaned the kitchen on a daily basis using a dilute bleach solution for 2–3 hours per day. Despite this, she still would rewash kitchen items several times when preparing food for the children.

Joyce had visited her GP on several occasions over the last 10 years but had not always told her the complete story. More recently however the headmistress of her children's school had asked to see her as they were concerned that the children were very cautious in certain outside activities and seemed unduly worried about getting "dirty". This time on visiting the GP, she told her the complete story and broke down in tears as she was concerned she may be "passing the OCD on to her children".

The GP listened to her story and prescribed her the selective serotonin reuptake-inhibiting drug, fluoxetine. This was to be taken initially in a dose of 20 mg a day, increasing by 20 mg at weekly intervals up to a dose of 60 mg a day. In addition, she was referred for some psychological therapy.

The medication did not seem to have any effect on Joyce's symptoms. She was seen by the Psychological Therapy Service who started her on some individual treatment involving graded exposure and self-imposed response prevention (ERP). Unfortunately, however, unlike most people with OCD, Joyce did not seem to be responding to this regime. Her GP became concerned about her lack of progress, and she was referred to secondary care services in her local hospital.

Whilst under the psychiatric services, she underwent a physical examination, blood tests and an electrocardiogram. A comprehensive history was taken at consultation in which she disclosed the true extent of the impact her OCD was

L. Drummond (✉) • A. Roney
National and Trustwide Services for OCD/BDD,
SW London and St. George's NHS Trust,
London, UK
e-mail: lynnemd@sgul.ac.uk; andrew.roney@nhs.net

© Springer International Publishing AG, part of Springer Nature 2018
K. Shivakumar, S. Amanullah (eds.), *Complex Clinical Conundrums in Psychiatry*,
https://doi.org/10.1007/978-3-319-70311-4_4

having on her daily life and her children. Overall, she was in good health, although she had severe eczema over her body. Her children were assessed by the local children's team, and Joyce and the children were to attend family meetings to encourage the children to engage in normal childhood activities.

It was decided to switch her medication from fluoxetine to sertraline. Fluoxetine has a long half-life, and so this transition needs to be done carefully. The fluoxetine was reduced by 20 mg every week. After her dose of fluoxetine had been reduced to 20 mg a day, sertraline was introduced initially at a dose of 50 mg a day. This was then titrated up to 200 mg a day which is the recognised effective dose for OCD.

Once the sertraline was at 200 mg, further ERP treatment was started. Gradually Joyce found her condition improving and her mood lifting. She engaged well in ERP treatment even though she found the exposure exercises demanding. After she had, with the therapist's help, devised a hierarchy of feared situations concerning her obsessive fear, she would perform an exposure exercise 1 week with the therapist without performing any of her compulsive behaviours. Following on from the session with the therapist, she would practise the same exposure episodes three times a day at home. Whereas initially her anxiety would be high and would last for 2–3 hours, once she had practised the behaviour, she found that the anxiety began to reduce and did not last as long. From time to time, she would find herself performing her handwashing compulsions. She had been advised that, if this did occur, she should "recontaminate" herself with her exposure programme. Because everyone washes their hands, it is important to ensure that the person with OCD is taught a new way to wash their hands different to that of their compulsions. In Joyce's case, she was always washing her hands under running water, using antibacterial liquid soap and being meticulous about every area. Instead of this she was asked to only wash her hands immediately before meals and cooking, and after using the toilet. She was to place the plug in the handbasin and wash with normal soap for no longer than 30 sec (or the time it took her to sing "happy birthday to you" in her head). There was to be no washing of the taps afterwards and no washing further up her arms than to her wrists. Similarly she was to bath using soap only and was to take no longer than 5 min. The timing was done by setting her mobile phone and leaving it outside the bathroom door. If she had not "completely" bathed at 5 min, she was to get out of the bath and to "take the risk" of leaving part of herself unwashed. She was allowed no more than 1 bath a day.

4.2   Psychopharmacological Management of OCD

First-line psychopharmacological treatment of OCD involves drugs which act on the serotonin system. Clomipramine, a tricyclic antidepressant, was the first drug which was reported to have a beneficial effect on OCD [1]. Further observations led to the development of the serotonin theory for the genesis for OCD. Although clomipramine is an effective drug for the treatment of OCD, its side effects are burdensome, and it should rarely be used as a first-line treatment these days [2]. The selective serotonin reuptake-inhibiting drugs (SSRIs) are much better tolerated with far fewer side effects than clomipramine. The dosages of SSRI needed to treat OCD are generally higher than those used to treat depression [3]. Although it has previously been thought that the speed of response of OCD to SSRIs was much slower than that seen in depression, a recent meta-analysis demonstrated that most patients showed a significant reduction in symptoms after 2 weeks of treatment and that this improvement then continued over the following weeks [4]. Accumulated beneficial effects of SSRIs or clomipramine can continue up to 2 years [5]. The serotonin reuptake-inhibiting drugs which have been shown to be useful in OCD are shown in Table 4.1.

All patients receiving a high-dose SSRI of any type should receive an annual ECG.

Table 4.1 SSRIs used in OCD

Drug	Maximum daily adult dosage for OCD (mg)	Occasionally prescribed maximal daily dosage (mg)	Notes
Sertraline	200	400	
Fluoxetine	60	120	Has a longer half-life than other SSRIs
Paroxetine	60	100	
Fluvoxamine	300	450	One of the older SSRIs and may have more side effects
Citalopram	40		Although evidence suggested citalopram was effective in OCD in dosages of 60 mg, fears of QT prolongation mean that doses >40 mg (>20 mg in those aged over 60 years) can no longer be prescribed in many countries
Escitalopram	20		Although evidence suggested escitalopram was effective in OCD in dosages of 40 mg, fears of QT prolongation mean that doses >40 mg can no longer be prescribed in many countries
Clomipramine	250		Should not be prescribed in higher doses due to toxicity, including cardiotoxicity

If a patient does not respond to an SSRI at maximal dosage for 3 months, it is worthwhile switching to an alternative drug. This is shown by the case history above. Joyce failed to respond to fluoxetine but responded much better to sertraline.

SSRIs have been shown to be efficacious in treating OCD in multiple studies [2, 6].

4.3 Psychological Treatment of OCD

The psychological treatment of choice for OCD is prolonged graded exposure in real life to the feared situation combined with self-imposed response (or ritual) prevention (ERP). This treatment was first demonstrated to be effective by Marks et al. [7]. An early study of this therapy by Foa and Goldstein suggested that 66% of patients treated as inpatients were greatly clinically improved using ERP [8].

In more recent years there have been attempts to replace ERP with more cognitive treatments. However, ERP has stood this test of time. Cognitive behaviour therapy (CBT) has been used but with no clear evidence that it has any advantage over ERP [9, review in [10–12]. ERP as treatment of choice is supported by multiple studies – McLean et al. [13] demon-strated significantly better results in the use of ERP over CBT, and Drummond [14, 15] suggests that for severe, chronic OCD patients, ERP should be treatment of choice but CBT may be of use for specific difficulties. A meta-analysis of studies examining the use of ERP and CBT in OCD concluded that ERP is the first-line psychotherapeutic treatment for OCD but use of cognitive therapy at the same time to target specific symptom-related problems could improve tolerance and adherence to treatment [16].

Approximately half of patients treated with serotonin reuptake inhibition for obsessive-compulsive disorder do not respond fully and continue to experience distressing symptoms [17, 18]. Thus augmentation strategies will often need to be considered using either pharmacological or psychological approaches.

Augmentation with the use of psychological therapy with SSRIs has shown to be of benefit with up to 70% of patients showing a response [19–21]. Many studies are now of patients under-going combination therapy with the use of ERP along side pharmacological treatments [20, 22, 23]. A systematic review and network meta-analysis by Skapinakis et al. concluded that combination treatment was efficacious and likely better than monotherapy in the treatment of patients with a severe illness presentation [2].

4.4   Treatment of Refractory OCD

If a person with OCD has tried good-quality ERP treatment from a therapist experienced in delivering the therapy and they have failed to respond to this in addition to two trials of SSRI treatment or clomipramine in recommended dosages for at least 3 months each, then they can be considered treatment refractory.

There are two main approaches to treatment refractory OCD which are:

- Addition of a low-dose dopamine-blocking agent to the SSRI or clomipramine
- Trial of above usual SSRI dosages (not clomipramine due to toxicity).

It is preferable to use the term "dopamine blocker" rather than "antipsychotic" as the dosage used in augmenting serotonin reuptake-inhibiting drugs in OCD is far lower than that used in psychotic disorders. Dopamine blockers act on the basal ganglia and reduce the effect of dopamine in these areas. It has long been recognised that certain abnormalities of the basal ganglia and their connections can result in obsessions and compulsions. Examples include some movement disorders including chorea, and it also worth noting that sometimes the medicines used to treat Parkinson's disease can result in obsessions and compulsions.

Side effects with dopamine blockers at low doses are much less frequently seen than with the much higher doses used for schizophrenia. Most of the dopamine blockers also have the ability to cause prolongation of the QT interval and are another reason why at least annual ECG monitoring is worthwhile in OCD. Aripiprazole is and exception, and is not recognised to have an effect on the QT interval. Some of the drugs used in OCD are listed below in Table 4.2.

In general, studies of the use of dopamine blockers for OCD are small, and thus the evidence of their efficacy is patchy. Overall, there is probably more positive evidence for risperidone than the others.

In total about 1/3 of people who have not responded to an SSRI or clomipramine will experience improvement with the addition of a dopamine blocker [18]. A large study also found that the addition of psychological therapy for OCD which comprises a form of treatment known as cognitive behaviour therapy (CBT) was more effective than adding in a dopamine blocker. [24].

The use of above normal dosages of SSRIs has been mentioned above. Again there are relatively few studies with small numbers. A retrospective study by Pampaloni et al. [25] demonstrated that this was generally well tolerated and effective. A more recent study has examined patients on high doses of sertraline and demonstrated that despite dosages up to 400 mg sertraline a day, all patients had blood levels within therapeutic range. This suggested that patients refractory to SSRIs may

Table 4.2 Antipsychotics used in OCD

Drug name	Usual dose for OCD	Common side effects	Notes
Risperidone	0.5 mg up to 1–2 mg if helpful	Drowsiness. Dizziness. Can occasionally cause weight gain	This is the atypical drug with the greatest number of studies to demonstrate its effectiveness in OCD
Aripiprazole	2.5–5 mg	Can cause an increase in activity and even anxiety. Drowsiness is less common. Can cause loss of appetite.	Does not have any effect on the heart
Olanzapine	2.5–5 mg	Drowsiness. Dizziness. Weight gain is common	Weight gain is common with olanzapine and is therefore not advisable for those who are overweight
Quetiapine	25 mg	Drowsiness. Dizziness. Difficulty sleeping. Increased appetite and weight gain	Weight gain is generally less than with olanzapine

either have abnormalities in absorbing the drug or they may metabolise it rapidly [26].

Other agents have also been examined, but again the numbers in studies are too small to come to definitive conclusions. These have included some studies on serotonin- and norepinephrine-inhibiting drugs, drugs which act on pleasure centres in the brain such as morphine derivatives and mood-stabilising agents. Recently there has been increasing interest in the possible adjunctive use of drugs acting on the glutaminergic system in OCD. So far all of these studies are small and the results speculative.

Disclosure Statement "The authors have nothing to disclose".

References

1. Thoren P, Åsberg M, Cronholm B, Jörnestedt L, Träskman L. Clomipramine treatment of obsessive-compulsive disorder: I. A controlled clinical trial. Arch Gen Psychiatry. 1980;37(11):1281–5.
2. Skapinakis P, Caldwell DM, Hollingworth W, Bryden P, Fineberg NA, Salkovskis P, Welton NJ, Baxter H, Kessler D, Churchill R, Lewis G. Pharmacological and psychotherapeutic interventions for management of obsessive-compulsive disorder in adults: a systematic review and network meta-analysis. The Lancet Psychiatry. 2016;3(8):730–9.
3. Bloch MH, McGuire J, Landeros-Weisenberger A, Leckman JF, Pittenger C. Meta-analysis of the dose-response relationship of SSRI in obsessive-compulsive disorder. Mol Psychiatry. 2010;15(8):850–5.
4. Issari Y, Jakubovski E, Bartley CA, Pittenger C, Bloch MH. Early onset of response with selective serotonin reuptake inhibitors in obsessive-compulsive disorder: a meta-analysis. J Clin Psychiatry. 2016;77(5):605–11.
5. Fineberg NA, Pampaloni I, Pallanti S, Ipser J, Stein DJ. Sustained response versus relapse: the pharmacotherapeutic goal for obsessive–compulsive disorder. Int Clin Psychopharmacol. 2007;22(6):313–22.
6. Soomro GM, Altman DG, Rajagopal S, Oakley Browne M. Selective serotonin re-uptake inhibitors (SSRIs) versus placebo for obsessive compulsive disorder (OCD). Cochrane Database of Systematic Reviews 2008;1: DOI:10.1002/14651858.CD001765.pub3.
7. Marks IM, Hodgson R, Rachman S. Treatment of chronic OCD two years after in vivo exposure. Brit J Psychiat. 1975;127:349–64.
8. Foa EB, Goldstein AJ. Continuous exposure and complete response prevention in the treatment of obsessive-compulsive neurosis. Behav Ther. 1978;9:821–9.
9. Ougrin D. Efficacy of exposure versus cognitive therapy in anxiety disorders: systematic review and meta-analysis. BMC Psychiatry. 2011;11(1):1.
10. Tyagi H, Drummond LM, Fineberg NA. Treatment for obsessive compulsive disorder. Curr Psychiatr Rev. 2010;6(1):46–55.
11. Whittal ML, Thordarson DS, McLean PD. Treatment of obsessive–compulsive disorder: cognitive behavior therapy vs. exposure and response prevention. Behav Res Ther. 2005;43(12):1559–76.
12. Cottraux J, Note I, Yao SN, Lafont S, Note B, Mollard E, Bouvard M, Sauteraud A, Bourgeois M, Dartigues JFA. Randomized controlled trial of cognitive therapy versus intensive behavior therapy in obsessive compulsive disorder. Psychother Psychosom. 2001;70(6):288–97.
13. McLean PD, Whittal ML, Thordarson DS, Taylor S, Söchting I, Koch WJ, Paterson R, Anderson KW. Cognitive versus behavior therapy in the group treatment of obsessive-compulsive disorder. J Consult Clin Psychol. 2001;69(2):205.
14. Drummond LM. The treatment of severe, chronic, resistant obsessive-compulsive disorder. An evaluation of an in-patient programme using behavioural psychotherapy in combination with other treatments. Br J Psychiatry. 1993;163(2):223–9.
15. Drummond LM. CBT for adults: a practical guide for clinicians. London: Royal College of Psychiatrists; 2014. p. 93–111.
16. McKay D, Sookman D, Neziroglu F, Wilhelm S, Stein DJ, Kyrios M, Matthews K, Veale D, Accreditation Task Force of The Canadian Institute for Obsessive Compulsive Disorders. Efficacy of cognitive-behavioral therapy for obsessive-compulsive disorder. Psychiatry Res. 2015;227(1):104–13.
17. Erzegovesi S, Cavallini MC, Cavedini P, Diaferia G, Locatelli M, Bellodi L. Clinical predictors of drug response in obsessive-compulsive disorder. J Clin Psychopharmacol. 2001;21(5):488–92.
18. Bloch MH, Landeros-Weisenberger A, Kelmendi B, Coric V, Bracken MB, Leckman JFA. Systematic review: antipsychotic augmentation with treatment refractory obsessive-compulsive disorder. Mol Psychiatry. 2006;11(7):622–32.
19. Foa EB, Liebowitz MR, Kozak MJ, Davies S, Campeas R, Franklin ME, Huppert JD, Kjernisted K, Rowan V, Schmidt AB, Simpson HB. Randomized, placebo-controlled trial of exposure and ritual prevention, clomipramine, and their combination in the treatment of obsessive-compulsive disorder. Am J Psychiatr. 2005;162(1):151–61.
20. Simpson HB, Foa EB, Liebowitz MR, Ledley DR, Huppert JD, Cahill S, Vermes D, Schmidt AB, Hembree E, Franklin M, Campeas RA. Randomized, controlled trial of cognitive-behavioral therapy for augmenting pharmacotherapy in obsessive-compulsive disorder. Am J Psychiatr. 2008;165(5):621–30.
21. Wheaton MG, Schwartz MR, Pascucci O, Simpson HB. Cognitive-behavior therapy outcomes for

obsessive-compulsive disorder: exposure and response prevention. Psychiatr Ann. 2015;45(6):303–7.

22. Boschen MJ, Drummond LM, Pillay A, Morton K. Predicting outcome of treatment for severe, treatment resistant OCD in inpatient and community settings. J Behav Ther Exp Psychiatry. 2010;41(2):90–5.

23. Boschen MJ, Drummond LM. Community treatment of severe, refractory obsessive-compulsive disorder. Behav Res Ther. 2012;50(3):203–9.

24. Simpson HB, Foa EB, Liebowitz MR, Huppert JD, Cahill S, Maher MJ, McLean CP, Bender J, Marcus SM, Williams MT, Weaver J. Cognitive-behavioral therapy vs risperidone for augmenting serotonin reuptake inhibitors in obsessive-compulsive disorder: a randomized clinical trial. JAMA Psychiat. 2013;70(11):1190–9.

25. Pampaloni I, Sivakumaran T, Hawley CJ, Al Allaq A, Farrow J, Nelson S, Fineberg NA. High-dose selective serotonin reuptake inhibitors in OCD: a systematic retrospective case notes survey. J Psychopharmacol. 2010;24(10):1439–45.

26. Vaughan, R, O'Donnell, C and Drummond, L.M. Blood Levels of Treatment Resistant Obsessive-Compulsive Disorder Patients Prescribed Supra-normal Dosages of Sertraline Faculties of Child & Adolescent Psychiatry and General Adult Psychiatry. Annual Conference 2016 06–07 October 2016. The ICC, Birmingham.

Clinical Conundrum: A Complex Case of Postpartum Depression

Prabha S. Chandra, Sundarnag Ganjekar, and Soumya Parameshwaran

5.1   Objectives

1. To use a biopsychosocial approach in the evaluation and understanding of postpartum depression (PPD)
2. To consider the role of medical comorbidity in the etiology and course of PPD
3. To discuss social and cultural issues such as income, gender disadvantage, trauma, and violence in PPD
4. To highlight the role of personality factors as a contributing factor in PPD and in mother-infant attachment issues due to PPD
5. To discuss the current evidence related to pharmacological management of PPD especially in the context of breastfeeding
6. To discuss the current evidence on psychological management of PPD and the role of the partner and family

The Case

Ms. V was a 29-year-old lady who was brought to the emergency room 3 weeks after delivering a healthy female infant by cesarean section. During the first week postpartum, she had difficulty in

P.S. Chandra, MD, FRCPsych, FAMS (✉)
S. Ganjekar • S. Parameshwaran
Department of Psychiatry, National Institute of
Mental Health and Neuro Sciences,
Bangalore, India
e-mail: chandra@nimhans.ac.in

breastfeeding and reported feeling helpless and inadequate as she had less milk. These feelings gradually increased, and she was often found crying and trying to feed the infant repeatedly. When the infant cried, she would get extremely anxious. She felt she was not a good mother as she did not have enough milk to satisfy the needs of her infant. By the third week postpartum, the family noticed that she had stopped taking care of the infant and would avoid being with her. She appeared depressed and expressed her wish to give away her daughter for adoption. She reported feelings of helplessness and expressed suicidal thoughts. On the day that she was brought to the emergency room, she had tried to take her own life by hanging. During the evaluation at the emergency room, her eyes were downcast; she was weeping and appeared depressed. She said she heard a voice in her head telling her that she was the worst mother in the world and she had no right to live.

Her medical history revealed hypothyroidism prior to and during pregnancy for which she had been on 50mcg of thyroxine supplementation. However, she had stopped thyroxine supplementation during her last few weeks of pregnancy.

Clinical Issues and Challenges

- What is the prevalence of PPD?
- What are the psychosocial, obstetric, and biological risk factors for PPD?
- Which medical conditions can complicate the clinical picture of PPD?

© Springer International Publishing AG, part of Springer Nature 2018
K. Shivakumar, S. Amanullah (eds.), *Complex Clinical Conundrums in Psychiatry*,
https://doi.org/10.1007/978-3-319-70311-4_5

Table 5.1 Prevalence of PPD in different time frames of the postpartum period—a comparison between developed and developing countries using EPDS [2]

	Duration of postpartum	Prevalence of PPD (%)
Developed countries	<4 weeks	5.5–34.4
	4–8 weeks	2.6–35
	8 weeks–6 months	2.9–25.5
	6–12 months	6–29
Developing countries	<4 weeks	12.9–50.7
	4–8 weeks	4.9–50.8
	8 weeks–6 months	8.2–38.2
	6–12 months	21–33.2

5.2 Prevalence of PPD

Postpartum depression is usually a nonpsychotic depressive episode which is mild to severe in nature, seen during the first 12 months following childbirth [1]. There are variations in the reported prevalence of PPD across various countries and across various studies. The difference in rates is due to two factors: (1) assessment tools used and (2) time frame of postpartum period [2]. Self-reported tools, diagnostic clinical interviews, or both have been used to measure the prevalence of PPD [2]. The Edinburgh Postnatal Depression Scale (EPDS) is the most commonly used self-reported instrument [2]. Table 5.1 shows a comparison of the prevalence of PPD in developed and developing countries using EPDS. A systematic review of the prevalence of PPD in high-income countries has shown a prevalence rate of around 10% [3]. The prevalence of PPD is higher in middle- and low-income countries as compared to high-income countries (see Table 5.1) [4]. Two systematic reviews have shown that in middle- and low-income countries, one in five women may experience PPD within the first year after childbirth [5, 6].

5.3 Risk Factors for PPD (Fig. 5.1)

5.3.1 Sociodemographic Factors

Maternal Age Studies exploring the significance of lower maternal age as a risk factor for PPD

have been inconclusive. While some studies have shown that lower maternal age is a risk factor for PPD, there have been other subsequent studies that have shown no correlation or a reverse correlation between the two [2, 7–11].

Economic Status Social and economic status can be indicators of the risk of PPD. Poor educational backgrounds, low income or unemployment, and being unmarried are all factors that increase the risk of PPD [12]. This is especially true in low-income settings where financial strain is a significant risk factor for PPD [13–15]. Irrespective of the economic status, however, a lack of social support for the mother is a significant risk factor for PPD [2].

Partner Violence Partner violence has been consistently found to be a strong predictor of PPD irrespective of economic status [16–18].

5.3.2 Obstetric Factors

Several studies have investigated the association of PPD with factors such as unwanted or unplanned pregnancies and pregnancy-related complications such as emergency cesarean section, physical illness in the newborn, and absence of breastfeeding. While the findings have been inconsistent for pregnancy-related complications [20, 21], a few studies have found a significant relationship between unplanned pregnancy and postpartum depression [19].

5.3.2.1 Cesarean Section

Studies conducted in the past found that women who undergo an emergency cesarean section are more at risk of developing PPD compared to women who undergo spontaneous vaginal delivery or forceps delivery [22, 23]. However, recent studies haven't replicated these findings [19, 21, 24], so the association is inconclusive.

Medical Illness in the Newborn When a newborn has a medical illness or a neonatal intensive care unit admission, there is an increased risk of the mother developing PPD [25, 26].

Fig. 5.1 Risk factors for postpartum depression

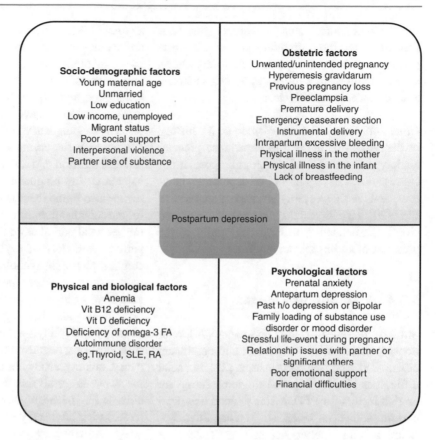

Breastfeeding Absence of breastfeeding in the postpartum period was believed to be a risk factor for developing PPD [19, 23], but studies have been inconclusive on the correlation between breastfeeding and PPD [21].

Though the presence of these obstetric factors might potentially put the mother at risk of developing PPD, no definite association can be made based on these studies [2].

5.3.3   Physical and Biological Factors

Nutrition A mother's nutritional requirements increase during pregnancy and the postpartum period. This is due to the increased maternal metabolic needs specific to reproduction and fetal and infant growth. Nutritional deficiencies can be a risk factor for PPD. For instance, iron-deficiency anemia, which is common in women from developing countries, can lead to generalized fatigue, reduced energy levels, loss of interest, and

depressed affect [27]. It is also associated with stress and cognitive impairment [30]. Low levels of 25-hydroxy vitamin D are associated with higher scores on the EPDS [28]. Also, a deficiency of omega-3 polyunsaturated fatty acids during the postpartum period has been found to be a risk factor for postpartum depression [29]. There is also a possible association between reduced serum zinc concentration and the severity of the mother's depressive symptoms [31].

Autoimmune Disorders Among the other medical conditions that can present as behavioral symptoms during the postpartum period are autoimmune disorders. Autoimmune thyroiditis (Hashimoto's disease) can present as postpartum depression and postpartum psychosis. On rare occasions, autoimmune hyperthyroid state (Graves' disease) can present as postpartum delirium [32]. The presence of thyroid peroxidase (TPO) antibodies during gestation maybe used as a biomarker for postpartum depression

[33]. Other autoimmune disorders that can worsen during the postpartum period with postpartum depression are systemic lupus erythematosus, rheumatoid arthritis, systemic sclerosis, and keratoconjunctivitis sicca.

Other Biological Factors Women with a history of depression or those who experience prenatal anxiety are at risk of developing postpartum depression. A family history of depression, however, does not necessarily predispose mothers to PPD [20]. Hypothyroidism has been shown to be closely associated with PPD, especially in the presence of antithyroid antibodies.

5.3.4 Psychological Factors

Stressful life events during pregnancy [34], relationship issues with the partner and significant others [35], poor support systems [21], financial difficulties [13–15, 36], and single parenting are all risk factors for PPD. A study found that postpartum mothers experience higher cognitive dysfunction and higher scores on scales for depression, anxiety and stress [39]. Relationship problems and poor partner support in the postpartum period is not only a risk factor for depression in mothers but also in fathers [40] and poor mother-infant attachment may be an early indicator for PPD [41].

5.3.5 Suicide During Pregnancy

Suicide and suicidal attempts are relatively less common during pregnancy as compared to the general population. Suicidal ideations are more common than suicidal attempts and completed suicide, with prevalence ranging from 5% to 14% during pregnancy and postpartum [37, 38, 42]. Mothers who have suicidal thoughts and suicidal ideation during pregnancy are at risk of developing postpartum depression [43]. A prospective study of pregnant women from urban India in their early pregnancy (<20 weeks) reported a prevalence of suicidality in 7.6%, with suicidal plans in 2.4% and 1.7% having made suicidal

attempts [44]. In the same study, authors found that women at young age; belonging to a middle socioeconomic strata; having poor perceived support, depressive symptoms, and a past history of suicidality; and experiencing domestic violence were predicted to have suicidal ideation during the current pregnancy [44].A systematic review of suicide in the perinatal period has found that suicidal ideation and attempts are more likely to happen during pregnancy than postpartum. The review also found that the use of violent methods for the suicide attempt was more common during the perinatal period as compared to non-perinatal periods. A history of psychiatric illness, family conflict, physical/psychological violence, loneliness, a situation where the father has rejected the paternity, gender inequality, racial discrimination, inadequate housing, nulliparity, premenstrual irritability, perceived pregnancy complications, negative attitude toward the pregnancy, anxiety about the birth, and poor coping mechanisms are all risk factors for perinatal suicide. It has been emphasized that suicidal ideation during pregnancy should be taken very seriously and must be systematically assessed by mental health professionals [45].

The Case

Ms. V was admitted into the mother-baby inpatient unit and was started on treatment. On more detailed evaluation, Ms. V spoke of a difficult childhood where she was criticized by her parents for not being as good-looking as her siblings and for being the third female child. She said that she was constantly compared with others and belittled for not being smart enough. As she grew into adolescence, she reported having mood swings and being unable to sustain friendships. She felt rejected and lacked any relationships of confidence. She reported feeling depressed and spoke of an episode where she cut herself after a breakup when she was 15 years old. However, she was good at school and later graduated to earn her college degree. She worked as a data entry operator for a year. Her parents pressurized her to get married soon, but she faced several rejections from potential partners and finally agreed to marry someone that her parents chose for her. Her husband was less educated than her and did not hold a steady job.

After her marriage, Ms. V moved away from the city to a rural area where she had little support and barely any friends. She lived with her husband, and his parents and sisters lived nearby. Her husband would drink often and get verbally and physically abusive, accusing her of being lazy and not being good enough for him. She got minimal support from her in-laws who were also critical of her. She was discouraged from going out to work, which added to her sense of isolation and loneliness. Money was a problem, and her husband had several large debts. Ms. V would often lose her temper and was found to be irritable and weepy. On two occasions she had left home after a misunderstanding with her husband.

She had wanted to hold off pregnancy for a few years after marriage, but the couple did not use any contraception, and soon she found herself pregnant. She was unhappy throughout her pregnancy. She reported having no feelings toward her unborn baby and did not prepare for its arrival. On several occasions she hoped for a miscarriage. During pregnancy a hypothyroid state was detected, and she was started on 50mcg of thyroid supplementation. Her TSH was 10.09μIU/ml, and her T3 = 50 ng/dL and T4 = 4.09 μgm/dL were on the lower end of the clinical range.

In addition to this, her in-laws who were from a traditional Indian family wanted her to have a male child. Ms. V reported feeling angry and resentful about this as well. She also had anxiety symptoms and excessive worries about handling pain during labor and about the gender of the child.

Clinical Challenges

- Role of antenatal mental health problems on postpartum mental health
- Role of the partner in maternal mental health
- Role of trauma and violence in depression and anxiety during pregnancy and in the postpartum
- Personality factors and postpartum depression

5.3.6 Antenatal Mental Health

Pregnancy and birth are often considered to be stressful life events which may lead to postpartum depression. Several researchers have studied the effects of additional stressful life events—that women experience during pregnancy and the puerperium—on PPD [46]. In one such large, cross-sectional study on the occurrence of antenatal risk factors for PPD in primary care communities, the core risk factors were identified to be antenatal depression, antenatal anxiety, major life events, low social support levels, and a past history of depression [47]. A higher risk was noted where the mother had a history of major/minor depression and antenatal anxiety.

Antenatal Anxiety Several meta-analyses suggest the presence of antenatal anxiety as a significant predictor of postpartum depression [20, 46]. In a cohort survey that was conducted on pregnant women attending a state maternity hospital, women with anxiety disorder (AD) during pregnancy were found to be nearly three times more likely to be affected with postnatal depressive symptoms [48].

Role of Partner in PPD Studies have identified partner support to have a protective effect [47]. A study looking at married women 2 months postpartum identified a lack of help from spouses for childcare and household tasks, as a predictor for the severity of depression [49]. Furthermore, mothers who have received poor spousal support during pregnancy and have delivery complications are prone to severe depression [49]. Studies have consistently shown a negative correlation between PPD and emotional (expressions of caring) and instrumental support (practical help in terms of material aid or assistance with tasks) during pregnancy [20, 50].

5.3.7 Personality and PPD

Maternal personality characteristics such as negative cognitive attributional styles (pessimism, anger, ruminations) are likely to increase the likelihood of postpartum depression [20, 51]. Perfectionism as a trait is linked with high maternal anxiety and has been identified as a risk factor for PPD [47].

There is a high comorbidity of borderline personality disorder (BPD) with depression, dysthymia, and anxiety disorders [52], which in turn increases the risk of developing PPD [53].

Borderline mothers, who have impulse dyscontrol and emotional dysregulation as core features, directly or indirectly impact the infant development and the mother-infant interaction. Studies looking at mother-infant interactions have found that some BPD mothers interact intrusively with their infants and do not adapt to the infant's emotional cues [53].

Intimate Partner Violence and PPD Meta-analyses have also suggested a 1.5–2-fold increased risk of PPD among women exposed to intimate partner violence (IPV), when compared to women who were not exposed to such violence. A significant proportion of women with major depressive disorder, elevated depressive symptoms, and PPD report lifetime exposure to IPV [54]. Abusive experiences, both past and present, can influence women throughout the childbearing cycle. Women with a history of childhood abuse or current partner abuse are at a considerable risk of postpartum mental health problems, and neither pregnancy nor the postpartum period offers protection from abuse [55]. A 3-year follow-up of mothers with postpartum major depressive disorder found that nearly 50% had a history of child sexual abuse. The sexually abused women had significantly higher depression and anxiety scores and greater life stresses compared to the non-abused depressed women. Moreover, the sexually abused women had less improvement in their symptoms over time [56]. Women with a history of childhood abuse or current partner violence are at an increased risk of getting depression and having parenting problems during the postpartum period. Even if their current relationships are not abusive, the partners may not provide mothers with the necessary amount of support. This lack of support has implications on the mothers' physical and mental health and how they care for their babies. Current or past abuse can also affect another important part of the postpartum period which is breastfeeding [57].

A study looking at the prevalence of IPV during pregnancy and its relationship with mental health outcomes such as depression, somatic symptoms, post-traumatic stress disorder (PTSD), and life satisfaction found that women with experiences of physical and psychological violence reported more somatic symptoms, PTSD symptoms, and a lower level of life satisfaction, when compared to those who didn't experience IPV [58].

The Case

Following her admission, Ms. V was started on escitalopram 10 mg which was gradually increased to 20 mg. However, she continued to report suicidal ideas and was quite withdrawn. There was poor infant care and often refusal to breastfeed. She was started on electroconvulsive therapy (ECT) to manage her depression and for suicidality.

The investigation also revealed low hemoglobin concentration (Hb = 9.8 mg/dL). She had elevated TSH (21.09μIU/ml) with anti-TPO antibodies 587 IU/mL. The final clinical impression was one of severe depression with autoimmune thyroiditis and hypothyroidism.

As her depressive symptoms improved, it was noticed that she was not bonding with her baby and would not lift her or soothe her. She reported a lack of maternal feelings and mentioned that she was not "maternal." Her mood swings became more evident and she would quarrel with her mother who was helping her and accuse the nurses of making too many demands of her. She blamed the treating team of focusing more on her infant than on her.

Clinical Challenges

1. Managing suicidal risk
2. Assessing and managing the comorbid medical conditions (anemia and autoimmune thyroiditis) which led to depression, mood swings, tiredness, and fatigue

3. Management of emotionally unstable personality traits which led to poor infant care, impaired mother-infant bonding, and interpersonal problems with her mother and the hospital staff
4. Use of antidepressants during breastfeeding
5. Role of ECT in the management of PPD

A new mother faces various challenges and demands while caring for her newborn: sleep deprivation, providing continued care for the rest of the family; this along with a depressive episode is associated with increased morbidity and, if untreated, can lead to prolonged depression and recurrence of the illness. Studies have suggested that the negative effects of this on a child's development persist even beyond the depressive episode [59].

Most physicians or mother and child healthcare providers recognize the detrimental effects of PPD and agree that screening new mothers helps in the early identification and treatment of mental disorders such as PPD [60, 61]. A woman identified with PPD should be offered treatment choices, which may include pharmacological therapy and psychotherapy discussed below.

Non-pharmacological Treatment Many postpartum women, particularly if breastfeeding, may choose to use non-pharmacological treatments for the management of PPD, in order to avoid the risk of exposure of their breast milk to antidepressants. The various forms of psychotherapies tested for PPD include general counseling or listening visits, interpersonal psychotherapy (IPT), cognitive behavioral therapy (CBT), and brief psychodynamic psychotherapy. Among the psychological interventions, meta-analytical studies have found superiority of IPT over CBT [62]. For women with disruptions in their interpersonal relationships in the perinatal period, a focus on interpersonal problem areas, particularly role transitions and interpersonal disputes, may be well suited [63].

Counseling Related to Infant Feeding Perinatal depression and breastfeeding difficulties are often found to present together; hence, a mother's experience of breastfeeding should be discussed while managing mothers with PPD. Some mothers with depression have reported that breastfeeding has improved their mood symptoms and enhanced mother-infant bonding, whereas others find breastfeeding to be difficult; it is important to simplify feeding plans so as to make mother and infant time enjoyable in the latter group. Arranging a carer to feed the infant at night can help prevent sleep disruptions in the mother [64].

Mothers with Personality Disorders For mothers who have BPD, pregnancy and motherhood are periods of stress, creating a need for intervention. Few approaches include (a) individual psychotherapy focusing on her ability to form and maintain relationships and her current representation of the infant [65]; (b) infant–parent relationship-focused psychotherapy, focusing on understanding attachment themes from the mother's past in the current relationship with the infant and on increasing awareness of the impact of her caregiving on the infant's development [66]; and (c) attachment-focused approach developed by Cohen et al. [67]—also known as watch, wait, and wonder (WWW) therapy—which may be seen as improving parental sensitivity and reflective capacity. This therapy aims to improve mother-infant interaction and promote security of attachment, by promoting maternal capacity to observe and reflect on the meaning of the infant's behavior and emotional communication [68].

5.3.8 Pharmacological Management

Antidepressant treatment of PPD is common among women who breastfeed their infants despite the ambivalence that many women feel about making this choice [69]. A meta-analysis comparing effectiveness of antidepressant drugs with any other treatments (psychological, psychosocial, or pharmacological) found that SSRIs were significantly more effective than placebo for women with PPD, while there was insufficient evidence to conclude whether antidepressants or psychological/psychosocial treatments were more effective [70].

Clinical Factors Affecting Choice of Neuroleptics [64] Clinical factors based on which an antidepressant choice is made include:

- Past treatment response is often the best predictor of future response.
- Family history of psychiatric illness and treatment response.
- Primary symptoms that the medication will be targeting and its potential side effect profile.
- Choosing psychotropic medications with evidence base in lactating women.
- While using any medication in a lactating woman, providers must consider both maternal and infant safety factors.

For moderate-to-severe depression, the benefits of treatment are likely to outweigh the risks of the medication for the mother or the infant. Data from a recent meta-analysis indicated that all antidepressants were detected in milk but that not all were found in infant serum. Nortriptyline, paroxetine, and sertraline were noted to have undetectable serum levels, while citalopram and fluoxetine had infant serum levels which exceeded the recommended 10% maternal level.

Clinical studies of sertraline and paroxetine clearly suggest that transfer of these agents into milk is quite minimal, and virtually no side effects have been reported in numerous breastfed infants. Fluoxetine is considered as a less-preferred SSRI for breastfeeding mothers because there have been three case reports of colic, prolonged crying, vomiting, tremulousness, and other symptoms [71]. There is one case report of seizure activity with bupropion (300 mg PO daily). Doxepin is contraindicated with breastfeeding. Overall, breastfeeding may be safely compatible with antidepressants [72].

If a mother has no history of antidepressant treatment, an antidepressant such as sertraline, which has evidence of presenting lower levels in human milk and infant serum and few side effects, is considered first choice [64].

It is noted that nearly 10–15% of patients diagnosed with unipolar depression will go on to develop bipolar disorder. Making a correct diagnosis in the pregnant or postpartum woman has implications on the treatment of the disorder in pregnancy and the postpartum period. Often, many women, considering pregnancy or in pregnancy, are encouraged to discontinue effective medication out of concern for risks to the fetus, which adds to the challenge in treating them. However, discontinuation of medication places women at an even higher risk of relapse, which has a direct impact on fetal well-being and outcomes [59].

Role of Mood Stabilizers in PPD Research evaluating the use of mood stabilizers in the postpartum period is limited. A few studies support the use of lithium and carbamazepine—but not divalproate—as a prophylactic agent of mood episodes for women with PPD who have a history of bipolar disorder [73]. A prospective cohort study of olanzapine, alone or in combination with an antidepressant or a mood stabilizer for a minimum of 4 weeks following delivery, correlated with a reduced risk of postpartum mood episodes [74]. There is some evidence that quetiapine is effective as a first-line treatment option for management of postpartum bipolar depression. A 14-week open-label study to determine the effectiveness of quetiapine (extended release) as monotherapy for postpartum bipolar II disorder found this drug to significantly improve symptom control and quality of life, with minimal side effects reported [75]. Studies also suggest that quetiapine may be useful as adjunctive therapy to lithium or divalproate providing greater benefit than either lithium or divalproate alone [76]. Olanzapine, risperidone, and quetiapine achieve very low levels in infant plasma, with no evident adverse effects, suggesting that these agents may be safe [77–79].

Pharmacotherapy for BPD, if it is associated with PPD, is used to target cognitive-perceptual symptoms, emotional dysregulation, or impulsive-behavioral dyscontrol. Psychopharmacological treatment may become necessary during episodes of acute decompensation in which suicidal or self-destructive behavior erupts. Some classes of psychotropic drugs have demonstrated efficacy in diminishing symptom severity and optimizing functioning. In many patients, medication helps calm them and allows them to reflect before acting. This treatment might be relevant to psychosocial interventions, once patients have learned to manage themselves, and provides the possibility to discontinue medication.

In a placebo-controlled trial, the atypical antipsychotic olanzapine was superior to placebo in the treatment of borderline psychopathology [80, 81]. Open-label studies have also identified that monotherapeutic treatment with quetiapine was well tolerated and resulted in a marked improvement of impulsive behavior and overall levels of functioning [82].

ECT in PPD A systematic review [83] found that ECT was considered as a treatment choice in severe and refractory depression and for catatonic symptoms in the postpartum period, especially for early treatment response [84]. In a study by Babu et al., among the 34 women with postpartum psychosis who received ECT, 15 were hospitalized with their infants and 10 continued to breastfeed their infants with no clinically observable adverse effects [85].

Assessment of suicidality in the perinatal woman should include specific inquiry about depressed mood, substance abuse, previous suicide attempts, current or previous psychiatric illness, previous trauma, current intimate partner violence, and access to firearms [42].

A good risk assessment (see Table 5.2) and systematic approach (see Fig. 5.2) are key to the management of depression during postpartum period.

Table 5.2 Risk assessment for Mothers with PPD and her infant

Risk to self
Has the mother's oral intake been very poor?
Has the mother been showing severe neglect in self-care?
Has the mother expressed any suicidal ideas/suicidal threats in this episode?
Has the mother attempted suicide or self-harm in this episode?
Has the mother tried to leave the ward or hospital against medical advice?
Risk to the infant
Has the mother been refusing to care or been unable to care for the baby?
Has the mother been refusing or been unable to breastfeed?
Has the mother been expressing any ideas about harming the baby ("I will throw the baby, this baby is a devil, baby is not mine, etc.")?
Has the mother been trying to physically harm the baby (hitting, pinching, handling the baby roughly)?
Has the mother been clinging to the baby excessively (resisting separation)?
Has the mother been neglecting the baby (not responding when the baby cries or is at risk of falling or hurting itself)?
Risk to others and other factors
Has the mother been violent toward other relatives or hospital staff?
Does the mother have any medical illness (hypertension, diabetes, thyroid disorders, anemia)?
Does the mother have an infection (HIV, breast abscess, TB, MRSA, vaginal infection)?
Has the mother faced any form of violence in this episode (assault, evidence of injuries)?
Infant health
Does the baby have any health problems that require care within the first 24 h (diarrhea, respiratory difficulties, high-grade fever)?
Are there any immediate concerns related to infant feeding (does the baby need top feeds)?

5.3.9 Suicide in the Postpartum Period

Suicide has been identified as one of the most common causes of maternal deaths in the first year following delivery, although the incidence remains lower when compared to women during pregnancy. Studies suggest that despite suicidal ideation being common during pregnancy and postpartum, rates of completed suicide are lower, suggesting that this period may actually offer some protective effect.

The UK Confidential Enquiries into Maternal Deaths and Morbidity (2009–2013) has identified suicide to be a leading cause of death in the first 12 months postpartum. It reports a rate of 2.3 deaths (per 100,000 maternities) by suicide, during or up to 1 year after the end of pregnancy. Among 101 women who died by suicide, over

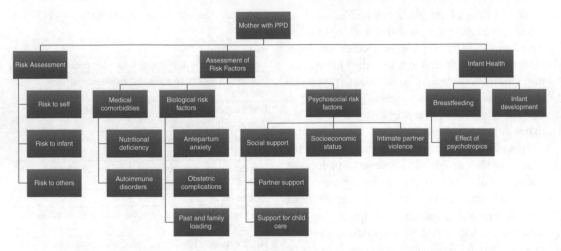

Fig. 5.2 Approach to mothers with postpartum depression

half (57 women) had a diagnosis of recurrent mental health disorder. It was also noted that two women had a prior diagnosis of bipolar disorder and two had schizophrenia. Three out of four of these women had psychiatric care in pregnancy and two had inpatient psychiatric care. However none were referred to specialized perinatal mental health services. The most common prior diagnosis for women who died by suicide was recurrent depressive disorder. All but one of these women had a diagnosis of moderate or severe disorder, and one quarter had psychotic symptoms [86].

A register-based Swedish study on suicide rates in pregnancy and 1-year postpartum reported a suicide ratio of 3.7 per 100,000 live births (1980–2007). Violent suicide methods were common, especially during the first 6 months postpartum [87]. The NSW Australian Department of Health, evaluating a 6-year time period, also found that 73% of suicides by women within a year of birth were conducted by violent means (i.e., jumping from a high place, lying in front of moving objects, gunshots, strangulation, and suffocation) [88]. Having a prior psychiatric illness had a strong correlation with perinatal suicidality. Several studies have identified depression to be associated with postpartum suicidality [89, 90].

A study looking at suicidal ideations (SI) in the postpartum period identified antepartum complications and a past history of depression to be significantly associated with later postpartum SI, among a relatively healthy cohort of postpartum mothers.

This study also noted that heightened self-efficacy and confidence in meeting postpartum demands were associated with lower odds of later SI [91].

Risk factors associated with suicides in the perinatal period were younger maternal age, unpartnered relationship status, unplanned pregnancy, undesired pregnancy or having mixed feelings about pregnancy, shorter illness duration, current or past psychiatric diagnosis, and women who are less likely to be receiving any active treatment at the time of death. Women who have had a postpartum psychiatric admission have a 70 times greater risk of suicide in their first postpartum year. Factors related to delivery include severe vaginal laceration, while planned cesarean delivery was negatively associated. Furthermore, experiencing IPV, including emotional abuse, physical, and/or sexual violence, seems to be more likely associated with suicidal thoughts during pregnancy and after childbirth [92–97].

The role of the multidisciplinary team is crucial in the management of PPD, especially when it is complicated with personality problems and multiple family and partner-related problems.

5.4 A Multidisciplinary Team Approach to Help Ms. V
(See Fig. 5.3)

Following a course of six ECTs, Ms. V gradually improved. Her mood became better, and she appeared more involved in caring for the infant.

Fig. 5.3 Management of postpartum depression

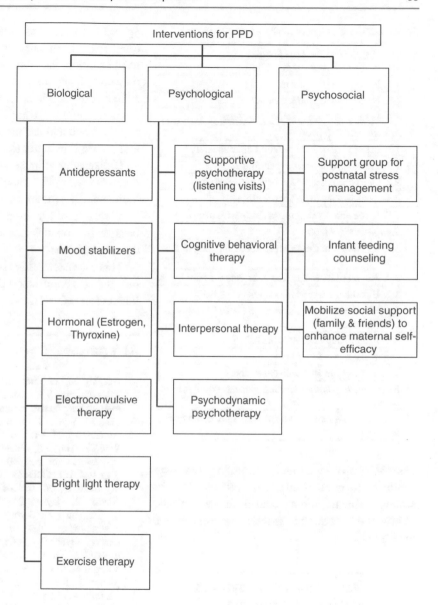

She continued to breastfeed her baby. She had sessions with the psychologists which focused on her earlier traumatic experiences and helped her in regulating her emotions. The psychologist used principles of interpersonal therapy and trauma-focused CBT. In addition, the nursing and social work team helped her in bonding with the infant. A detailed assessment of the problems in bonding using multiple techniques, such as direct observation of play, video recording of brief periods of interaction, and the nurse's observation in the ward, helped in identifying areas that needed intervention (see Table 5.3).

With better control of her own emotions, Ms. V could focus on the infant's needs and bonding exercises, and techniques such as play and infant massage helped her in engaging with the infant. Video feedback and education of appropriate mother-infant interactions were useful tools in helping Ms. V identify areas that she needed to work on.

Assessment of the infant's socio-emotional development indicated adequate progress. The infant had however not gained enough weight, and a pediatric referral was sought for the same.

An important part of her treatment included involving the partner. Educating him about

Table 5.3 Assessment of mother-baby interaction

1. *Care for the baby's basic needs*
1.1. Is she able to *dress* her child?
1.2. Is she able to *bathe* her child?
1.3. Is she able to *feed* her child?
1.4. Is she able to *put her baby to sleep*?
2. *Affectionate behavior*
2.1. Is she able to *hold* her child affectionately?
2.2. Is she able to *comfort* her child?
2.3. Does she engage in affectionate *gazing*?
2.4. Does she try to *talk* to her child?
2.5. Is she able to *cuddle and smile* with baby?
3. *Significant incidents*
3.1. Are there incidents where she is *shouting* at the baby?
3.2. Are there incidents where she *hits* the baby?
3.3. Has the mother tried to *smother* the baby?
3.4. Has the mother tried to *harm the baby* in any other manner?
3.5. Is there any *neglect* of the baby?
4. *Overall assessment of safety*
4.1. Is the infant safe with the mother?
5. *How does the mother handle separation from the baby?*
6. *Was the mother separated from the baby in the last few days?*

Ms. V's problems and addressing his own inability to control anger as well as his substance abuse were useful interventions. Cultural issues such as gender preference were also addressed.

5.5 Management of Thyroiditis and Hypothyroidism

An important part of management was a referral to the endocrinologist and treating the hypothyroidism.

5.6 Conclusion and Take-Home Points

PPD can often be a complex clinical phenomenon with multiple factors contributing to its etiology and treatment nonresponse. A biopsychosocial approach to the understanding of the problem often helps in identifying the various areas that need attention. Personality and medical problems may complicate the presentation and add to possible risk of suicide or chronicity.

Interventions using a multidisciplinary approach and addressing the various contributing factors result in better treatment response.

Unlike other clinical situations in psychiatry, treatment of PPD involves two people—the mother and the infant. In fact perinatal psychiatry is often referred to as mother-infant psychiatry because the infant forms a very important part of the interventions.

This case exemplifies several of the above factors and also emphasizes the need for appropriate liaison and referrals.

References

1. Beeghly M, Weinberg MK, Olson KL, Kernan H, Riley J, Tronick EZ. Stability and change in level of maternal depressive symptomatology during the first postpartum year. J Affect Disord. 2002;71:169–80.
2. Norhayati MN, Hazlina NHN, Asrenee AR, Emilin WMAW, Abbasi S, Chuang CH, et al. Magnitude and risk factors for postpartum symptoms: a literature review. J Affect Disord. 2015;175:34–52. https://doi.org/10.1016/j.jad.2014.12.041.
3. Gavin NI, Gaynes BN, Lohr KN, Meltzer-Brody S, Gartlehner G, Swinson T. Perinatal depression: a systematic review of prevalence and incidence. Obstet Gynecol. 2005;106:1071–83. https://doi.org/10.1097/01.AOG.0000183597.31630.db.
4. Vliegen N, Casalin S, Luyten P. The course of postpartum depression. Harv Rev Psychiatry. 2014;22:1–22. https://doi.org/10.1097/HRP.0000000000000013.
5. Fisher J, Cabral De Mello M, Patel V, Rahman A, Tran T, Holton S, et al. Prevalence and determinants of common perinatal mental disorders in women in low and lower-middle-income countries: a systematic review. Bull World Heal Organ. 2012;90:139–49. https://doi.org/10.2471/BLT.11.091850.
6. Gelaye B, Rondon MB, Araya R, Williams MA. Epidemiology of maternal depression, risk factors, and child outcomes in low-income and middle-income countries. The Lancet Psychiatry. 2016;3:973–82. https://doi.org/10.1016/S2215-0366(16)30284-X.
7. Boyce P, Hickey A. Psychosocial risk factors to major depression after childbirth. Soc Psychiatry Psychiatr Epidemiol. 2005;40:605–12. https://doi.org/10.1007/s00127-005-0931-0.

8. Kozinszky Z, Dudas RB, Csatordai S, Devosa I, Tóth É, Szabó D, et al. Social dynamics of postpartum depression: a population-based screening in south-eastern Hungary. Soc Psychiatry Psychiatr Epidemiol. 2011;46:413–23. https://doi.org/10.1007/s00127-010-0206-2.

9. Quelopana AM, Champion JD, Reyes-Rubilar T. Factors associated with postpartum depression in Chilean women. Health Care Women Int. 2011;32:939–49. https://doi.org/10.1080/07399332.2011.603866.

10. Sword W, Kurtz Landy C, Thabane L, Watt S, Krueger P, Farine D, et al. Is mode of delivery associated with postpartum depression at 6 weeks: a prospective cohort study. BJOG An Int J Obstet Gynaecol. 2011;118:966–77. https://doi.org/10.1111/j.1471-0528.2011.02950.x.

11. Glavin K, Smith L, Sørum R. Prevalence of postpartum depression in two municipalities in Norway. Scand J Caring Sci. 2009;23:705–10. https://doi.org/10.1111/j.1471-6712.2008.00667.x.

12. Goyal D, Gay C, Lee KA. How much does low socioeconomic status increase the risk of prenatal and postpartum depressive symptoms in first-time mothers? Women's Heal Issues. 2010;20:96–104. https://doi.org/10.1016/j.whi.2009.11.003.

13. Patel V, Rodrigues M, DeSouza N. Gender, poverty, and postnatal depression: a study of mothers in Goa, India. Am J Psychiatry. 2002;159:43–7. https://doi.org/10.1176/appi.ajp.159.1.43.

14. Lee DT, Yip AS, Leung TY, Chung TK. Identifying women at risk of postnatal depression: prospective longitudinal study. Hong Kong Med J = Xianggang Yi Xue Za Zhi. 2000;6:349–54.

15. Seguin L, Potvin L, St-Denis M, Loiselle J. Depressive symptoms in the late postpartum among low socioeconomic status women. Birth. 1999;26:157–63. https://doi.org/10.1046/j.1523-536x.1999.00157.x.

16. Gaillard A, Le Strat Y, Mandelbrot L, Kcïta H, Dubertret C, Adouard F, et al. Predictors of postpartum depression: prospective study of 264 women followed during pregnancy and postpartum. Psychiatry Res. 2014;215:341–6. https://doi.org/10.1016/j.psychres.2013.10.003.

17. Dennis C-L, Vigod S. The relationship between postpartum depression, domestic violence, childhood violence, and substance use: epidemiologic study of a large community sample. Violence Against Women. 2013;19:503–17. https://doi.org/10.1177/1077801213487057.

18. Patel V, Araya R, de Lima M, Ludermir A, Todd C. Women, poverty and common mental disorders in four restructuring societies. Soc Sci Med. 1999;49:1461–71.

19. Warner R, Appleby L, Whitton A, Faragher B. Demographic and obstetric risk factors for postnatal psychiatric morbidity. Br J Psychiatry. 1996;168:607–11.

20. O'hara MW, Swain AM. Rates and risk of postpartum depression—a meta-analysis. Int Rev Psychiatry. 1996;8:37–54. https://doi.org/10.3109/09540269609037816.

21. Nielsen Forman D, Videbech P, Hedegaard M, Dalby Salvig J, Secher NJ. Postpartum depression: identification of women at risk. BJOG. 2000;107:1210–7.

22. Boyce PM, Todd AL. Increased risk of postnatal depression after emergency caesarean section. Med J Aust. 1992;157:172–4.

23. Hannah P, Adams D, Lee A, Glover V, Sandler M. Links between early post-partum mood and postnatal depression. Br J Psychiatry. 1992;160:777–80.

24. Johnstone SJ, Boyce PM, Hickey AR, Morris-Yatees AD, Harris MG. Obstetric risk factors for postnatal depression in urban and rural community samples. Aust N Z J Psychiatry. 2001;35:69–74.

25. Räisänen S, Lehto SM, Nielsen HS, Gissler M, Kramer MR, Heinonen S. Fear of childbirth predicts postpartum depression: a population-based analysis of 511 422 singleton births in Finland. BMJ Open. 2013;3:e004047. https://doi.org/10.1136/bmjopen-2013-004047.

26. Nakku JEM, Nakasi G, Mirembe F. Postpartum major depression at six weeks in primary health care: prevalence and associated factors. Afr Health Sci. 2006;6:207–14. https://doi.org/10.5555/afhs.2006.6.4.207.

27. East M. Postpartum anaemia. Are we vigilant enough? Pract Midwife. 2012;15:37–9.

28. Murphy PK, Mueller M, Hulsey TC, Ebeling MD, Wagner CL. An exploratory study of postpartum depression and vitamin D. J Am Psychiatr Nurses Assoc. 2010;16:170–7. https://doi.org/10.1177/1078390310370476.

29. Sontrop J, Campbell MK. Omega-3 polyunsaturated fatty acids and depression: a review of the evidence and a methodological critique. Prev Med (Baltim). 2006;42:4–13. https://doi.org/10.1016/j.ypmed.2005.11.005.

30. Beard JL, Hendricks MK, Perez EM, Murray-Kolb LE, Berg A, Vernon-Feagans L, et al. Maternal iron deficiency anemia affects postpartum emotions and cognition. J Nutr. 2005;135:267–72.

31. Wójcik J, Dudek D, Schlegel-Zawadzka M, Grabowska M, Marcinek A, Florek E, et al. Antepartum/postpartum depressive symptoms and serum zinc and magnesium levels. Pharmacol Rep. 2006;58:571–6.

32. Dahale AB, Chandra PS, Sherine L, Thippeswamy H, Desai G, Reddy D. Postpartum psychosis in a woman with graves' disease: a case report. Gen Hosp Psychiatry. 2014;36:761.e7–8. https://doi.org/10.1016/j.genhosppsych.2014.07.003.

33. Kuijpens JL, Vader HL, Drexhage HA, Wiersinga WM, van Son MJ, Pop VJ. Thyroid peroxidase antibodies during gestation are a marker for subsequent depression postpartum. Eur J Endocrinol. 2001;145:579–84.

34. Salm Ward T, Kanu FA, Robb SW. Prevalence of stressful life events during pregnancy and its association with postpartum depressive symptoms. Arch Womens Ment Health. 2016;20:161–71. https://doi.org/10.1007/s00737-016-0689-2.

35. Kumar R, Robson KM. A prospective study of emotional disorders in childbearing women. Br J Psychiatry. 1984;144:35–47.

36. Manjunath NG, Venkatesh G, Rajanna. Postpartum blue is common in socially and economically insecure mothers. Indian J Community Med. 2011;36:231–3. https://doi.org/10.4103/0970-0218.86527.

37. Miller LJ, LaRusso EM. Preventing postpartum depression. Psychiatr Clin North Am. 2011;34:53–65. https://doi.org/10.1016/j.psc.2010.11.010.

38. Oates M. Suicide: the leading cause of maternal death. Br J Psychiatry. 2003;183:279–81.

39. Meena PS, Soni R, Jain M, Jilowa CS, Omprakash. Cognitive dysfunction and associated behaviour problems in postpartum women: a study from North India. East Asian Arch Psychiatry. 2016;26:104–8.

40. Massoudi P, Hwang CP, Wickberg B. Fathers depressive symptoms in the postnatal period: prevalence and correlates in a population-based Swedish study. Scand J Public Health. 2016. https://doi.org/10.1177/1403494816661652.

41. Behrendt HF, Konrad K, Goecke TW, Fakhrabadi R, Herpertz-Dahlmann B, Firk C. Postnatal mother-to-infant attachment in subclinically depressed mothers: dyads at risk? Psychopathology. 2016;49:269–76. https://doi.org/10.1159/000447597.

42. Lindahl V, Pearson JL, Colpe L. Prevalence of suicidality during pregnancy and the postpartum. Arch Women's Ment Heal. 2005;8:77–87. https://doi.org/10.1007/s00737-005-0080-1.

43. Turkcapar AF, Kadıoğlu N, Aslan E, Tunc S, Zayıfoğlu M, Mollamahmutoğlu L. Sociodemographic and clinical features of postpartum depression among Turkish women: a prospective study. BMC Pregnancy Childbirth. 2015;15:108. https://doi.org/10.1186/s12884-015-0532-1.

44. Supraja TA, Thennarasu K, Satyanarayana VA, Seena TK, Desai G, Jangam KV, et al. Suicidality in early pregnancy among antepartum mothers in urban India. Arch Womens Ment Health. 2016;19:1101–8. https://doi.org/10.1007/s00737-016-0660-2.

45. Orsolini L, Valchera A, Vecchiotti R, Tomasetti C, Iasevoli F, Fornaro M, et al. Suicide during perinatal period: epidemiology, risk factors, and clinical correlates. Front Psych. 2016;7. https://doi.org/10.3389/fpsyt.2016.00138.

46. Robertson E, Grace S, Wallington T, Stewart DE. Antenatal risk factors for postpartum depression: a synthesis of recent literature. Gen Hosp Psychiatry. 2004;26:289–95. https://doi.org/10.1016/j.genhosppsych.2004.02.006.

47. Milgrom J, Gemmill AW, Bilszta JL, Hayes B, Barnett B, Brooks J, et al. Antenatal risk factors for postnatal depression: a large prospective study. J Affect Disord. 2008;108:147–57. https://doi.org/10.1016/j.jad.2007.10.014.

48. Sutter-Dallay AL, Giaconne-Marcesche V, Glatigny-Dallay E, Verdoux H. Women with anxiety disorders during pregnancy are at increased risk of intense postnatal depressive symptoms: a prospective survey of the MATQUID cohort. Eur Psychiatry. 2004;19:459–63. https://doi.org/10.1016/j.eurpsy.2004.09.025.

49. Campbell SB, Cohn JF, Flanagan C, Popper S, Meyers T, Bates JE, et al. Course and correlates of postpartum depression during the transition to parenthood. Dev Psychopathol. 1992;4:29. https://doi.org/10.1017/S095457940000554X.

50. Richman JA, Raskin VD, Gaines C. Gender roles, social support, and postpartum depressive symptomatology. The benefits of caring. J Nerv Ment Dis. 1991;179:139–47.

51. Barnett PA, Gotlib IH. Psychosocial functioning and depression: distinguishing among antecedents, concomitants, and consequences. Psychol Bull. 1988;104:97–126.

52. Pepper CM, Klein DN, Anderson RL, Riso LP, Ouimette PC, Lizardi H. DSM-III-R axis II comorbidity in dysthymia and major depression. Am J Psychiatry. 1995;152:239–47. https://doi.org/10.1176/ajp.152.2.239.

53. Apter-Danon G, Candilis-Huisman D. A challenge for perinatal psychiatry: Therapeutic management of maternal borderline personality disorder and their very young infants. Clin Neuropsychiatry. 2005;2:302–14.

54. Beydoun HA, Beydoun MA, Kaufman JS, Lo B, Zonderman AB. Intimate partner violence against adult women and its association with major depressive disorder, depressive symptoms and postpartum depression: a systematic review and meta-analysis. Soc Sci Med. 2012;75:959–75. https://doi.org/10.1016/j.socscimed.2012.04.025.

55. Kendall-Tackett KA. Depression in new mothers. Binghanton/New York: Haworth Press; 2005.

56. Buist A. Childhood abuse, postpartum depression and parenting difficulties: A literature review of associations. Aust N Z J Psychiatry. 1998;32:370–8. https://doi.org/10.3109/00048679809065529.

57. Kendall-Tackett KA. Violence against women and the perinatal period: the impact of lifetime violence and abuse on pregnancy, postpartum, and breastfeeding. Trauma, Violence, Abus. 2007;8:344–53. https://doi.org/10.1177/1524838007304406.

58. Varma D, Chandra PS, Thomas T, Carey MP. Intimate partner violence and sexual coercion among pregnant women in India: relationship with depression and post-traumatic stress disorder. J Affect Disord. 2007;102:227–35. https://doi.org/10.1016/j.jad.2006.09.026.

59. Pearlstein T. Mood Disorders. In: Rosen-Montella K, editor. Med. Manag. Pregnant Patient. New York: Springer; 2015.

60. Olson AL, Kemper KJ, Kelleher KJ, Hammond CS, Zuckerman BS, Dietrich AJ. Primary care pediatricians' roles and perceived responsibilities in the identification and management of maternal depression. Pediatrics. 2002;110:1169–76.

61. Committee on Psychosocial Aspects of Child and Family Health and Task Force on Mental Health. Policy statement—the future of pediatrics: mental health competencies for pediatric primary care.

Pediatrics. 2009;124:410–21. https://doi.org/10.1542/peds.2009-1061.

62. Bledsoe S, Grote N. Treating depression during pregnancy and the postpartum: a preliminary meta-analysis. Res Soc Work Pract. 2006;16:109–20.

63. Stuart S, O'Hara MW. Treatment of postpartum depression with interpersonal psychotherapy. Arch Gen Psychiatry. 1995;52:75–6.

64. Sriraman NK, Melvin K, Meltzer-Brody S. ABM clinical protocol #18: use of antidepressants in breastfeeding mothers. Breastfeed Med. 2015;10:290–9. https://doi.org/10.1089/bfm.2015.29002.

65. Stevenson J, Meares R. An outcome study of psychotherapy for patients with borderline personality disorder. Am J Psychiatry. 1992;149:358–62. https://doi.org/10.1176/ajp.149.3.358.

66. Lieberman AF, Silverman R, Pawl JH. Infant-parent psychotherapy: Core concepts and current approaches. Handb infant Ment Heal. 2000;83:472–84.

67. Cohen NJ, Muir E, Lojkasek M, Muir R, Parker CJ, Barwick M, et al. Watch, wait, and wonder: testing the effectiveness of a new approach to mother-infant psychotherapy. Infant Ment Health J. 1999;20:429–51. https://doi.org/10.1002/(SICI)1097-0355(199924)20:4<429::AID-IMHJ5>3.0.CO;2-Q.

68. Slade A. Parental reflective functioning: an introduction. Attach Hum Dev. 2005;7:269–81. https://doi.org/10.1080/14616730500245906.

69. Pearlstein TB, Zlotnick C, Battle CL, Stuart S, O'Hara MW, Price AB, et al. Patient choice of treatment for postpartum depression: a pilot study. Arch Womens Ment Health. 2006,9.303–8. https://doi.org/10.1007/s00737-006-0145-9.

70. Molyneaux E, Howard LM, McGeown HR, Karia AM, Trevillion K. Antidepressant treatment for postnatal depression, vol. 20. John Wiley & Sons, Ltd: Chichester, UK; 2014. https://doi.org/10.1002/14651858.CD002018.pub2.

71. Kendall-Tackett K, Hale TW. Review: the use of antidepressants in pregnant and breastfeeding women: a review of recent studies. J Hum Lact. 2010;26:187–95. https://doi.org/10.1177/0890334409342071.

72. Oystein Berle J, Spigset O. Antidepressant use during breastfeeding. Curr Womens Health Rev. 2011;7:28–34. https://doi.org/10.2174/157340411794474784.

73. Viguera AC, Newport DJ, Ritchie J, Stowe Z, Whitfield T, Mogielnicki J, et al. Lithium in breast milk and nursing infants: clinical implications. Am J Psychiatry. 2007;164:342–5. https://doi.org/10.1176/ajp.2007.164.2.342.

74. Sharma V, Smith A, Mazmanian D. Olanzapine in the prevention of postpartum psychosis and mood episodes in bipolar disorder. Bipolar Disord. 2006;8(4):400. https://doi.org/10.1111/j.1399-5618.2006.00335.x.

75. Misri S. Quetiapine treats postpartum bipolar disorder. 11th Can. Psychiatr. Assoc. Annu. Conf., Vancouver, British Columbia, Canada: n.d.

76. Gentile S. Infant safety with antipsychotic therapy in breast-feeding: a systematic review. J Clin Psychiatry. 2008;69:666–73.

77. Yoshida K, Smith B, Craggs M, Kumar R. Neuroleptic drugs in breast-milk: a study of pharmacokinetics and of possible adverse effects in breast-fed infants. Psychol Med. 2016;28:81–91.

78. Lee A, Giesbrecht E, Dunn E, Ito S. Excretion of quetiapine in breast milk. Am J Psychiatry. 2004;161:1715–NaN-1716. https://doi.org/10.1176/appi.ajp.161.9.1715-a.

79. Gilad O, Merlob P, Stahl B, Klinger G. Outcome of infants exposed to olanzapine during breastfeeding. Breastfeed Med. 2011;6:55–8. https://doi.org/10.1089/bfm.2010.0027.

80. Soloff PH. Psychopharmacology of borderline personality disorder. Psychiatr Clin North Am. 2000;23:169–92. ix

81. Zanarini MC, Frankenburg FR. Olanzapine treatment of female borderline personality disorder patients: a double-blind, placebo-controlled pilot study. J Clin Psychiatry. 2001;62:849–54.

82. Perrella C, Carrus D, Costa E, Schifano F. Quetiapine for the treatment of borderline personality disorder; an open-label study. Prog Neuro-Psychopharmacology Biol Psychiatry. 2007;31:158–63. https://doi.org/10.1016/j.pnpbp.2006.08.012.

83. Gressier F, Rotenberg S, Cazas O, Hardy P. Postpartum electroconvulsive therapy: a systematic review and case report. Gen Hosp Psychiatry. 2015;37(4):310. https://doi.org/10.1016/j.genhosppsych.2015.04.009.

84. Focht A, Kellner CH. Electroconvulsive therapy (ECT) in the treatment of postpartum psychosis. J ECT. 2012;28:31–3. https://doi.org/10.1097/YCT.0b013e3182315aa8.

85. Babu GN, Thippeswamy H, Chandra PS. Use of electroconvulsive therapy (ECT) in postpartum psychosis—a naturalistic prospective study. Arch Womens Ment Health. 2013;16:247–51. https://doi.org/10.1007/s00737-013-0342-2.

86. Lives S. Improving mothers' care surveillance of maternal deaths in the UK 2011–13 and lessons learned to inform maternity care from the UK and Ireland confidential enquiries into maternal deaths and morbidity 2009–13. Oxford: University of Oxford; 2015.

87. Esscher A, Essén B, Innala E, Papadopoulos FC, Skalidou A, Sundström Poromaa I, et al. Suicides during pregnancy and 1 year postpartum in Sweden, 1980–2007. Br J Psychiatry. 2016;208(5):462–9.

88. Thornton C, Schmied V, Dennis CL, Barnett B, Dahlen HG. Maternal deaths in NSW (2000–2006) from non-medical causes (suicide and trauma) in the first year following birth. Biomed Res Int. 2013;19:1–6.

89. Johannsen BM, Larsen JT, Laursen TM, Bergink V, Meltzer-Brody S, Munk-Olsen T. All-cause mortality in women with severe postpartum psychiatric disorders. Am J Psychiatr. 2016;173(6):635–42.

90. Pinheiro RT, Da Silva RA, Magalhães PV, Horta BL, Pinheiro KA. Two studies on suicidality in the postpartum. Acta Psychiatr Scand. 2008;118(2):160–3.

91. Bodnar-Deren S, Klipstein K, Fersh M, Shemesh E, Howell EA. Suicidal ideation during the postpartum period. J Women's Health. 2016;25:1219–24.

92. Newport DJ, Levey LC, Pennell PB, Ragan K, Stowe ZN. Suicidal ideation in pregnancy: assessment and clinical implications. Arch Womens Ment Health. 2007;10(5):181–7.

93. Khalifeh H, Hunt IM, Appleby L, Howard LM. Suicide in perinatal and non-perinatal women in contact with psychiatric services: 15 year findings from a UK national inquiry. The Lancet Psychiatry. 2016;3(3):233–42.

94. Celik C, Ozdemir B, Oznur T. Suicide risk among perinatal women who report thoughts of self-harm on depression screens. Obstet Gynecol. 2015;126(1):216–7.

95. Gavin AR, Tabb KM, Melville JL, Guo Y, Katon W. Prevalence and correlates of suicidal ideation during pregnancy. Arch Womens Ment Health. 2011;14(3):239–46.

96. Comtois KA, Schiff MA, Grossman DC. Psychiatric risk factors associated with postpartum suicide attempt in Washington state, 1992-2001. Am J Obstet Gynecol. 2008;199(2):120–e1.

97. Alhusen JL, Frohman N, Purcell G. Intimate partner violence and suicidal ideation in pregnant women. Arch Womens Ment Health. 2015;18(4):573–8.

A Complex Case of Endocrine Disorder: Diabetes Associated with Depression

Nisha Nigil Haroon, Najala Orrell,
Kuppuswami Shivakumar,
and Shabbir Amanullah

6.1 Case Study

A 33-year-old female, single, mother of two, unemployed, a smoker averaging 30 packs per year, currently on social assistance, presented with a 10-year history of poorly controlled diabetes mellitus; her BMI was ≥30 kg/m. She had been seen by a series of specialists and been tried on various medications for diabetes with poor effect. She was more recently started on insulin to better manage her blood sugar levels out of concerns she would develop significant peripheral neuropathy. She was reporting pain in her feet, fatigue, poor concentration, and lack of motivation. The diabetic nurse worked intensely with the patient to address dietary needs and also looked at activation to ensure physical activity. She consistently denied any sadness or hopelessness but would lament on how she had a lot more energy and achieved more when she didn't have diabetes. Her social supports were limited, and she led a fairly isolated lifestyle when compared to her early adulthood years. A referral was made to psychiatry out of concerns that there may be a history of depression. On presentation to psychiatry, she brought both children along with her and insisted they attended the appointment. It became abundantly clear that the children had ADHD from her reports of their school performance and disruptive behavior at home. She went on to talk about a short-lived marriage and its abusive nature. During the interview, she disclosed extensive childhood trauma with neglect and fears that she would never have enough to eat, and hence, she would eat as much as she could when she had food. This explains the poor response to the dietary intervention, and she always lived in a state of fear of being deprived. The children seemed well fed, but there was very little control that she was able to control on the children who were aged 13 and 9. On further probing, it emerged that she ran away from home and worked in fast-food joints but was fired when they found she was stealing food. Following the birth of her first child, she had anhedonia, poor sleep, poor appetite, and irritability. This unfortunately seemed to tie in with marital discord, and, as such, depression was

N.N. Haroon, MD, MSc, Dip NB, CCD, DM (✉)
Department of Internal Medicine, Northern Ontario
School of Medicine (NOSM), Sudbury, ON, Canada
e-mail: nigilharoon@nosm.ca

N. Orrell, MD
Medical student, Schoool of Medicine, Royal College
of Surgeons in Ireland, Dublin, Ireland

K. Shivakumar, MD, MPH, MRCPsych(UK), FRCPC
Department of Psychiatry, Northern Ontario School
of Medicine Psychiatry Department,
Sudbury, ON, Canada

S. Amanullah, MD, DPM, FRCPsych(UK),
CCT,FRCPC
University of Western Ontario, Woodstock General
Hospital University of Western Ontario,
Woodstock, ON, Canada

never diagnosed. Following this, she was diagnosed with diabetes a year later. She endorsed issues with mood, poor self-esteem, irritability, poor concentration, sadness, loneliness, and, over the last 2 years, hopelessness. She denied at any point in time suicidal thoughts or behavior and tearfully said "I would like to be able to take care of my children and be a good mom." An impression of postpartum onset of major depressive disorder was made, and patient was started on antidepressants. Bupropion was chosen, and the patient was followed up both in psychiatry and a specialized, eating disorders clinic while having therapy for grief and abuse. The case above highlights the sometimes very complicated nature of depression in individuals with endocrine disorders and the critical need for a high index of suspicion. Over a period of time, the patient showed better engagement in diabetes management, better blood sugar control, and improved mood, and she was able to find a job albeit part time. Her blood sugar was controlled with oral hypoglycemics, and insulin was discontinued. After 1 year, she reported good self-esteem; the children were less disruptive and showed better performance in school.

6.2   Epidemiology

6.2.1   What Is the Epidemiology of the Depression in Diabetic Patients?

The comorbidity of diabetes and depression has long been recognized to exist. The chance of people with diabetes to have depression is double than that of the normal population. Most studies suggest that one in five people with type 2 diabetes mellitus (T2DM) have depression. A recent study based on US National Health and Nutrition Examination Survey (NHANES) 2005–2012 data reported a prevalence of 11% (95% CI 8.9–12.2%) for clinically relevant depression and 4% (95% CI 3.4–5.1%) for clinically significant depression [1].

6.2.2   What Are the Relationships Between Diabetes and Depressive Disorders?

Patients with type 2 diabetes experience several adverse outcomes if they have concomitant depression. Depression in people with diabetes can result in increased risk for early mortality, chronic kidney disease as well as microvascular and macrovascular complications [2–4]. A prospective longitudinal study done by Lin and colleagues suggested that patients with type 2 diabetes had a 36% higher risk of developing microvascular events such as blindness, end-stage renal disease, amputations, and renal failure deaths (hazard ratio 1.36 [95% CI 1.05–1.75]) [5]. The risk of macrovascular events such as myocardial infarction, stroke, cardiovascular procedures, and deaths were 24% higher when compared to diabetic patients without depression (hazard ratio 1.24 [95% CI: 1.0–1.54]) [5]. Cummings et al. recently reported a significantly higher incidence of stroke (HR 1.57 [95% CI 1.05, 2.33] vs. 1.01 [0.79, 1.30]) and death due to cardiovascular disorder (1.53 [1.08, 2.17] vs. 1.12 [0.90, 1.38]) in people with diabetes than those without diabetes [2]. According to the results of ACCORD-MIND trial, diabetes patients with depression showed a greater cognitive decline [6]. The effect of depression on the risk of cognitive decline was not affected by the presence of vascular disease, baseline cognition, age, or control of vascular risk factors such as hyperglycemia, hypertension, and dyslipidemia [6] indicating a direct link between diabetes and depression. Depression in diabetes has been consistently linked to mortality [7]. A recent meta-analysis confirmed that the mortality risk was estimated to be 76% higher in patients with diabetes and depression in comparison with diabetic patients without depression (HR = 1.76, 95% CI 1.45–2.14). The risk was independent of the presence of diabetes complications and vascular factors [7]. Coexistence of diabetes and depression can affect glycemic outcomes, dietary patterns, self-care, and quality of life in people with diabetes. In addition, the presence of depression contributes to higher utilization of health-care resources, loss of productivity (at an individual level), inferior quality of life, and even disability in people with diabetes. These unfavorable health outcomes are mediated through factors such as inability to adhere to a healthy diet, poor eating habits, missing meals, altered sleep patterns, lack of exercise, weight gain, smoking, inadequate glucose monitoring, poor compliance with antidiabetic medications, and poor glycemic status. Most often, treatment of depression receives less attention as more focus is given on optimizing glycemic control and preventing vascular complications. Furthermore, depression is frequently missed or diagnosed very late in patients with diabetes, as there is an overlap of symptoms. Patients with diabetes often complain of fatigue, insomnia, and low mood, and these symptoms are dismissed as occurring secondary to diabetes.

6.2.3   Is there a Causative Link Between Depression and Type 2 Diabetes?

The causative link between depression and type 2 diabetes is complex and potentially bidirectional. Evolving data suggest that both diseases might be originating from common biological mecha-

nisms [8] (Fig. 6.1). Genetic factors, immune dysregulation, endocrine consequences of stress, and disturbances of circadian rhythm have been proposed as causative factors for diabetes and depression. A genetic correlation is postulated as some of the single-nucleotide polymorphisms related to diabetes have been linked to depression as well [8]. Epigenetic mechanisms such as DNA methylation known to alter the metabolic adaptations in the intrauterine environment of the fetus are also considered to influence the pathogenesis of both the conditions. Immune-related causes for diabetes and depression include dysregulation of innate immunity and acute-phase inflammatory response. Inflammatory cytokines such as CRP and interleukin-6 potentiate the apoptosis of pancreatic β cells and mediate insulin resistance, triggering the onset of diabetes. Similar immune dysregulation activates the hypothalamic-pituitary axis, increases oxidative stress in the brain, and lowers the production of serotonin causing depression [8]. Chronic stress, HPA-axis dysregulation, and resultant hypercortisolemia play a significant role in the onset of diabetes and depression. Excess cortisol can not only increase the release of free fatty acids but also impair the ability of insulin to transport glucose to the cell surface. This results in insulin resistance. In addition, hypercortisolemia can impair hippocampal

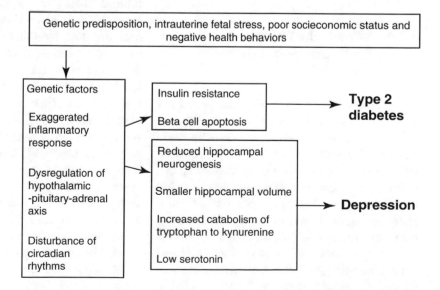

Fig. 6.1 Shared pathogenetic pathways of diabetes and depression Arrow included to indicate bidirectional relationship

neurogenesis and cause reduction in hippocampal volume [8].

Several factors have been shown to predict the coexistence of diabetes and depression. Age < 65 years, female gender, low income, lower educational level, marital status, sedentary lifestyle, smoking, body mass index (≥30 kg/m), altered sleep behavior, recent hospitalization, dyslipidemia, and vascular comorbidities have been shown to trigger the onset of depression in people with type 2 diabetes [1].

Depression is often unrecognized in patients with type 2 diabetes despite the availability of validated screening tools such as Patient Health Questionnaire-9 (PHQ-9) [9].

Diagnostic cutoff scores between 8 and 11 are suggested to diagnose major depression in the general population [9]. PHQ-9 is now recognized as screening tool for depressive symptoms in individuals with type 2 diabetes [10]. PHQ-9 was found to have adequate diagnostic properties for detecting major depressive disorders. Most studies suggest cutoff scores between 8 and 11 for the diagnosis of depression in patients with type 2 diabetes. A recent study by Janssen and colleagues reported a cutoff value of 5 as this provided a sensitivity of 92.3% and specificity of 70.4% [10]. However this needs further validation.

6.2.4 What Is the Treatment for Depression in Diabetic Patients?

Treatment of depression is often delayed or not prioritized in patients with type 2 diabetes. Significant advances have been made in the pharmacotherapy of diabetes in the past two decades. However data on the safety of antidepressant use in diabetes is conflicting. More research is needed to analyze the long-term efficacy of non-pharmacological interventions such as cognitive behavioral therapy. It is important that physicians be aware of careful selection of antidepressants in patients with type 2 diabetes. Many of the side effects of antidepressants can be exaggerated in diabetic patients. Use of first-line antidepressants are associated with side effects such as weight gain, postural dizziness, urinary retention, arrhythmias, and sexual dysfunction. This is not desirable in patients with type 2 diabetes as they are already on polypharmacy and may experience postural hypotension and cardiac arrhythmias due to autonomic neuropathy, sexual dysfunction due to diabetic neuropathy, and weight gain due to insulin treatment with insulin and sulfonylureas. The potential interaction between newer antidiabetic agents and antidepressants should be addressed as well. Also, there are concerns that certain antidepressants might worsen beta-cell dysfunction, insulin resistance, and hyperglycemia [11, 12]. This is likely mediated by weight gain. The degree of weight gain differs significantly between various antidepressive agents. For instance, a large-scale population-based study by Blumenthal and colleagues recently showed antidepressants such as bupropion, amitriptyline, and nortriptyline are associated with less weight gain compared to citalopram [13].

A Cochrane review published in 2012 concluded that psychological and pharmacological interventions show moderate benefits on the management of depression in patients with type 2 diabetes [14]. The conclusions of this meta-analysis were based on interventions that lasted from 3 weeks to 12 months and outcomes observed for up to 6 months after treatment. Both cognitive behavioral therapy and antidepressants have a statistical significant effect on decreasing depressive symptoms in patients with diabetes (Table 6.1). Eleven studies evaluated antidepressant therapy and the related outcomes. In terms of glycemic control, five pharmacological studies were pooled into a meta-analysis, which showed a statistical beneficial. Short-term benefits (up to 6 months) on glycemic outcomes (HBA1c) were observed with the use of antidepressants but not with psychological interventions. Among the antidepressants used, serotonin selective inhibitors showed the most benefit. Neither intervention showed benefit on a long-term glycemic control (Table 6.1). One may debate that improving patients' mood should correlate to an improve-

Table 6.1 Psychological vs. pharmacological treatment in patients with type 2 diabetes mellitus and depression

	Psychological interventions	Antidepressants
Short-term depression remission	Or 2.88; 95% CI 1.58–5.25 N = 647; 4 trials	Or 2.50; 95% CI 1.21–5.15; N = 136; 3 trials
Medium-term depression remission	Or 2.49; 95% CI 1.44–4.32 N = 296; 2 trials	Not studied
Short-term and long-term depression severity	Showed benefits but data showed significant heterogeneity	Moderate benefit on short-term Depression severity SMD −0.61; 95% CI −0.94 to −0.27; N = 306; 7 trials SSRI: SMD −0.39; 95% CI −0.64 to −0.13; P = 0.003; n = 241; 5 trials
Glycemic control	Results are hetcrogcneous and inconclusive.	Short-term glycemic control improved (mean difference for HbA1c −0.4%; 95% CI −0.6 to −0.1; N = 238; 5 trials
Health-related quality of life (HRQoL)	Did not improve significantly (3 trials)	No significant benefit (single trial)
Adherence	Not enough data	No significant benefit (single trial)

HRQoL health-related quality of life, *SMD* standardized mean difference
Outcomes were analyzed 1–6 months after completion of treatment regimen

ment in their overall quality of life. However, there is lack of conclusive data on the effect of psychological therapy and antidepressants on quality of life. The beneficial effects of psychological and pharmacological interventions on factors such as adherence to antidepressive and antihyperglycemic medications, long-term depression, and long-term glycemic outcomes need to be studied [14].

Conclusion

Type 2 diabetes and depression often coexist and seem to share the same biological pathways of origin. More effort is needed to diagnose depression in people with diabetes. Validated questionnaires such as PHQ-9 can be used even in outpatient settings to screen diabetic people for depression. More research is needed to know the long-term metabolic effects of cognitive behavioral treatment and antidepressant drugs.

Disclosure Statement None related to this presentation.

References

1. Wang Y, Lopez JM, Bolge SC, Zhu VJ, Stang PE. Depression among people with type 2 diabetes mellitus, US National Health and Nutrition Examination Survey (NHANES), 2005–2012. BMC Psychiatry. 2016;16:88.
2. Cummings DM, Kirian K, Howard G, Howard V, Yuan Y, Muntner P, Kissela B, Redmond N, Judd SE, Safford MM. Consequences of comorbidity of elevated stress and/or depressive symptoms and incident cardiovascular outcomes in diabetes: results from the reasons for geographic and racial differences in stroke (REGARDS) study. Diabetes Care. 2016;39(1):101–9.
3. Novak M, Mucsi I, Rhee CM, Streja E, Lu JL, Kalantar-Zadeh K, Molnar MZ, Kovesdy CP. Increased risk of incident chronic kidney disease, cardiovascular disease, and mortality in diabetic patients with comorbid depression. Diabetes Care. 2016;39(11):1940–7.
4. Aguilar A. Diabetes: depression is associated with renal complications. Nat Rev Nephrol. 2016;12(8):444.
5. Lin EH, Rutter CM, Katon W, Heckbert SR, Ciechanowski P, Oliver MM, Ludman EJ, Young BA, Williams LH, McCulloch DK, Von Korff M. Depression and advanced complications of diabetes: a prospective cohort study. Diabetes Care. 2010;33(2):264–9.
6. Sullivan MD, Katon WJ, Lovato LC, Miller ME, Murray AM, Horowitz KR, Bryan RN, Gerstein HC, Marcovina S, Akpunonu BE, Johnson J, Yale JF, Williamson J, Launer LJ. Association of depression with accelerated cognitive decline among patients with type 2 diabetes in the ACCORD-MIND trial. JAMA Psychiat. 2013;70(10):1041–7.
7. Hofmann M, Köhler B, Leichsenring F, Kruse J. Depression as a risk factor for mortality in individu-

als with diabetes: a meta-analysis of prospective studies. PLoS One. 2013;8(11):e79809.

8. Moulton CD, Pickup JC, Ismail K. The link between depression and diabetes: the search for shared mechanisms. Lancet Diabetes Endocrinol. 2015;3(6):461.

9. Manea L, Gilbody S, McMillan D. Optimal cut-off score for diagnosing depression with the patient health questionnaire (PHQ-9): a meta-analysis. CMAJ. 2012;184(3):E191–6.

10. Janssen EP, Köhler S, Stehouwer CD, Schaper NC, Dagnelie PC, Sep SJ, Henry RM, van der Kallen CJ, Verhey FR, Schram MT. The patient health questionnaire-9 as a screening tool for depression in individuals with type 2 diabetes mellitus: the Maastricht study. J Am Geriatr Soc. 2016;64(11):e201–6. doi: 10.1111/jgs.14388. Epub 2016 Oct 26.

11. Barnard K, Peveler RC, Holt RI. Antidepressant medication as a risk factor for type 2 diabetes and impaired glucose regulation: systematic review. Diabetes Care. 2013;36(10):3337–45.

12. Noordam R, Aarts N, Peeters RP, Hofman A, Stricker BH, Visser LE. Selective serotonin reuptake inhibitors decrease pancreatic insulin secretion in older adults and increase the risk of insulin dependence in type 2 diabetes patients. J Clin Psychiatry. 2016;77(9):e1124–9.

13. Blumenthal SR, Castro VM, Clements CC, Rosenfield HR, Murphy SN, Fava M, Weilburg JB, Erb JL, Churchill SE, Kohane IS, Smoller JW, Perlis RH. An electronic health records study of long-term weight gain following antidepressant use. JAMA Psychiat. 2014;71(8):889–96.

14. Baumeister H, Hutter N, Bengel J. Psychological and pharmacological interventions for depression in patients with diabetes mellitus and depression. Cochrane Database Syst Rev. 2012;12:CD008381.

A Complex Case of Opiates and Related Pathologies

Jennifer L. Pikard, Sarah Penfold,
and M. Nadeem Mazhar

7.1 Chapter Objectives

- Provide an overview of epidemiology and risk factors for opioid use disorder
- Assess neurobiology and effects of opioids
- Review specific pharmacological and psychosocial interventions tailored to individual needs
- Focus on issues related to management of opioid use disorder with comorbid PTSD

7.2 Case Presentation

A 28-year-old female, Jane, is referred by her family physician to your outpatient addiction psychiatry practice for assessment of anxiety and opioid misuse. On history, Jane reports that she was sexually assaulted in a public restroom 3 years ago. Since then, she avoids public restrooms and does not leave her apartment at night. She avoids watching television because any news stories or depictions of assault trigger vivid images of her trauma. She also endorses frequent nightmares and insomnia. Jane states that she is always "on edge" and easily startled. She was diagnosed with posttraumatic stress disorder (PTSD) and prescribed sertraline for her symptoms 1 year ago but discontinued the medication after a month, as she didn't find that it helped.

Jane first tried hydromorphone, offered by a friend, a year ago and found that it calmed her, so she started using 2–3 tablets of 8 mg per day. Over the last 6 months, her use has increased to 8–10 tablets (64–80 mg) per day. She denies intravenous or intranasal use. Jane finds it difficult to control her opioid use, even after losing her job as a sales associate because she was stealing from her workplace to pay for her hydromorphone. She has taken out loans and borrowed money from family members to sustain her use. She signed into a detoxification center 6 weeks ago and experienced significant withdrawal symptoms such as muscle aches, feeling hot and cold, diarrhea, nausea, sweating, insomnia, increased anxiety, and restlessness. She found the symptoms to be intolerable and left the detoxification center after 3 days to resume opioid use.

You diagnose Jane with opioid use disorder and posttraumatic stress disorder. She has heard about methadone and would like to explore medication options to help her discontinue hydromorphone.

7.2.1 What Are Opioids/Opiates?

The term "opiates" and "opioids" have been used interchangeably throughout the literature. The term opioids encompass a class of a wide variety

J.L. Pikard, MD, MSc • S. Penfold, MD
M. Nadeem Mazhar, MD, FRCPC (✉)
Department of Psychiatry, Queen's University,
Kingston, ON, Canada

© Springer International Publishing AG, part of Springer Nature 2018
K. Shivakumar, S. Amanullah (eds.), *Complex Clinical Conundrums in Psychiatry*,
https://doi.org/10.1007/978-3-319-70311-4_7

Table 7.1 Pharmacokinetics of common opioids [2, 3]

Substance	Pharmacokinetics	Onset (mins)	Peak (mins)	Duration (h)	Half-life (h)
Codeine (PO)	Mu agonist	30–60	60–90	3–4	2–4
Hydrocodone (PO)	Mu agonist	30–60	60–90	4–6	4
Oxycodone (PO)	Mu agonist	30–60	60–90	3–4	2–3
Meperidine (PO)	Mu agonist	30–60	60–90	2–4	2–3
Morphine (PO)	Mu agonist	30–60	60–90	3–6	2–4
Fentanyl (TD)	Mu agonist	12–16 h	24 h	48–72	>24
Methadone (PO)	Mu agonist	30–60	2–6 h	24–48	8–60
Buprenorphine (SL)	Agonist-antagonist	30–60	1–4 h	8–12	24–37
Pentazocine (PO)	Agonist-antagonist	15–30	60–180	3–4	2–3

of drugs, both natural and alkaloid compounds derived directly from the resin of the opium poppy (termed opiates, including morphine and heroin) as well as synthetic compounds (including oxycodone and hydromorphone). All members of the opioid drug class have agonistic effects on the mu receptor in the brain [1]. Although opioids are prescribed to control pain and can be used to diminish cough or relieve diarrhea, they also generate feelings of euphoria, peacefulness, and sedation that may lead to someone to continue taking these medications or drugs despite the development of serious consequences. Opioids have been known to cause such adverse effects as respiratory depression, which can lead to death [1]. For the purpose of this chapter, the term "opioid" will be used to describe any drug/medication that is an agonist of the mu opioid receptor in the brain Table 7.1.

7.2.2 How Do You Assess and Diagnose Opioid Use Disorder?

Opioid use disorder is described in the DSM-5 as "a problematic pattern of opioid use leading to clinically significant impairment or distress, as manifested by at least two criteria, occurring within a 12-month period." These criteria include such patterns as opioids being taken in larger amounts or over a longer period than was intended or a persistent desire or unsuccessful efforts to cut down or control opioid use. A great deal of time must be spent in activities necessary to obtain the opioid, use the opioid, or recover

from its effects or cravings or a strong desire or urge to use opioids. Recurrent opioid use resulting in a failure to fulfill major role obligations at work, school, or home and continued opioid use despite having persistent or recurrent social or interpersonal problems caused or exacerbated by the effects of opioids are also part of the DSM-5 criteria. Diagnosing opioid use disorder becomes apparent when important social, occupational, or recreational activities are given up or reduced because of opioid use and when recurrent opioid use occurs in situations in which it is physically hazardous. Those who continue to use opioids despite knowledge of having a persistent or recurrent physical or psychological problem that is likely to have been caused or exacerbated by the substance can be thought to be one part of the criteria for the disorder [4].

Both tolerance and withdrawal are important components of the criteria for opioid use disorder. Tolerance, is defined by either a need for markedly increased amounts of opioids to achieve intoxication/desired effect or a when a markedly diminished effect is achieved with continued use of the same amount of an opioid. It is important to note here that this criterion is not considered to be met for those taking opioids solely under appropriate medical supervision. Withdrawal is manifested by a characteristic opioid withdrawal syndrome, which consists of the presence of either cessation or reduction in opioid use that has been heavy and prolonged or administration of an opioid antagonist after a period of opioid use. Withdrawal syndrome also includes three or more symptoms such as dysphoric mood, nausea or vomiting, muscle aches, lacrimation or rhinorrhea, pupillary dilation, piloerection, or sweating. Withdrawal of opioids or closely related substances may be taken to relieve or avoid withdrawal symptoms, and it is important to note that this criterion is not considered to be met for those individuals taking opioids solely under appropriate medical supervision as well [4].

While not part of the formal DSM-5 criteria, assessment for opioid use disorder should also include completion of a patient's medical history including screening for concomitant medical conditions such as pregnancy and trauma and infectious diseases such as hepatitis, HIV, and tuberculosis. A physical examination should be part of the comprehensive assessment process along with laboratory tests including complete blood count, liver function tests, hepatitis C, HIV, and other sexually transmitted infections. Testing for pregnancy should be done in women of childbearing age [4].

7.2.3 What Is the Epidemiology of Opioid Use Disorder?

Opioid use disorder can commence at any age, but problems with the disorder are most commonly observed in adolescence and early 20s [1]. Age of onset is an important predictor of risk and clinical severity, and age of first use is correlated with a higher prevalence of dependence and worsening consequences. Those who are using opioids as their primary substance of abuse tend to have an earlier age of onset of any substance abuse compared with those who may abuse alcohol or marijuana first. Age of onset for opioid use disorder as their primary drug of abuse has also been found to be much earlier than those who switch from other substances. Those adolescents with earlier onset of prescription opioid or heroin use also have a more rapid progression to injection heroin use [1].

The 12-month prevalence of opioid use disorder is estimated to be around 0.37% among adults age 18 years and older in community populations. There are increased prevalence rates in males compared to females (0.49% versus 0.26%), with the male-to-female ratio typically being 1.5:1 for opioids other than heroin (e.g., those opioids available by prescription) and 3:1 for heroin itself. The number of people using prescription opioids has more than doubled between 1975 and 2008, while marijuana use and alcohol abuse have decreased or plateaued [1]. The prevalence decreases with age, with the prevalence highest (0.82%) among adults age 29 years or younger and decreasing to 0.09% among adults age 65 years and older [4].

While the socioeconomic status of youth instigating opioid use has increased over time, the prevalence of opioid addiction is highest in white males [1]. Among adults, the prevalence among Native Americans is 1.25%, Asian or Pacific Islanders is 0.35%, and Hispanics is 0.39%. The 12-month prevalence in European countries in community populations between the ages of 15 and 64 years is between 0.1% and 0.8%, and the average prevalence of opioid use in the European Union and Norway is between 0.36% and 0.44% [4].

Morbidity and mortality in relation to opioid use have increased since 2001 with a 2.5-fold increase in mortality from prescription opioids and a fivefold increase in mortality from heroin overdose. In the United States, drug overdoses have surpassed motor vehicle incidents as the country's leading accidental cause of death with prescription opioids accounting for 75% of the prescription overdoses. Opioids have been one of the most common drugs used in suicide attempts, and the prevalence of hepatitis C virus has become particularly worrisome in those aged 16–21 years [1].

7.2.4 What Is the Main Mechanism of Action for Opioids?

Opioid peptides and their receptors are expressed throughout the pain-related circuits in the central nervous system and in the brain structures related to reward and emotion [5]. Neurons originate in a part of the brain called the arcuate nucleus and project to two parts of the brain called the ventral tegmental area (VTA), the site of dopamine cell bodies, and the nucleus accumbens. Opioid neurons release endogenous opioids in the brain, which mediate natural rewards and are involved (particularly in the VTA and nucleus accumbens) in the motivational aspects of dependence and aversive states [6].

Four different opioid receptors, mu (μ), delta (δ), kappa (κ), and opioid receptor like-1 (ORL-1), have been identified so far. Mu receptors in the VTA are critically involved in reinforcement and are also involved in drug dependence. Actions on mu receptor systems also activate central dopamine reward pathways with mood-enhancing and euphoric effects. Kappa receptors induce dysphoria, counteract mu receptors, and are involved in stress-related drug intake. Delta receptors are involved in emotional control [6].

Exogenous opioids are also thought to act at mu, delta, and kappa receptors, most particularly at mu receptors. Specifically, mu and possibly delta receptors in the VTA and nucleus accumbens mediate the positive reinforcement properties of exogenous opioids [6]. Even so, some studies have implicated all four receptors in multiple behavioral effects including analgesia, reward, depression, anxiety, and addiction [5].

7.2.5 What Are the Common Comorbid Medical and Psychiatric Comorbidities with Opioid Use Disorder?

Opioid use disorder is associated with multiple medical and psychiatric comorbidities. Medically, opioid use has shown slowing of the gastrointestinal tract and decreased gut motility, which has shown to be the cause of constipation. Opioids have also been shown to be associated with a lack of mucous membrane secretions causing dry mouth. Pupillary constriction may cause visual disturbances [4].

For those who inject opioids, puncture marks, called "track marks," which are sclerosed veins, may develop into peripheral edema. Some may start injecting subcutaneously when veins become severely sclerosed which could lead to complications such as cellulitis or other infec-

tions such as abscesses. Serious, however rare, infections such as tetanus and *Clostridium botulinum* can be acquired through contaminated needles. Other infections from contaminated needles may occur throughout the body and include conditions such as bacterial endocarditis, hepatitis, and HIV. Tuberculosis is also common [4].

Mortality rates from infections maybe as high as 1.5–2% per year. Those who sniff opioids may irritate the nasal mucosa and even perforate the nasal septum. Difficulties in sexual functioning including erectile dysfunction for males or disturbances in reproductive function and irregular menses in women are common [4].

Psychiatrically, opioid use disorder is often associated with other substance use disorders, which may be taken to reduce the symptoms of opioid withdrawal or cravings for opioids. These include tobacco, alcohol, cannabis, stimulants, and benzodiazepines. Those with opioid use disorder are also at risk for developing mild to moderate depression that meets the criteria for dysthymia or major depressive disorder. The symptoms may even exacerbate a preexisting primary depressive disorder. Periods of low mood are common during chronic use and even more so with psychosocial stressors. Insomnia is common during withdrawal. Those with antisocial personality disorder more commonly develop opioid use disorder than those in the general population. Those with posttraumatic stress disorder also show increased rates of opioid use disorder. One significant risk factor for a substance-related disorder is a history of conduct disorder in childhood or adolescence, especially the development of opioid use disorder [4].

7.2.6 What Are the Pharmacological Treatment Options Available for Opioid Withdrawal and Relapse Prevention in Opioid Use Disorder?

Treatment with opioid agonist/antagonist therapy for opioid withdrawal and relapse prevention has been found to be more effective than non-pharmacological interventions or detoxification approaches. There are both individual and societal benefits in the treatment of opioid use disorder for withdrawal and relapse prevention, and medications are gaining more widespread adaptation [1, 7]. Methadone, buprenorphine-naloxone, and naltrexone continue to show reduction in opioid withdrawal, relapse, improve treatment adherence, and decreased overdose in opioid users [1].

7.2.6.1 Methadone

Methadone is a synthetic long-acting opioid full agonist, which has high affinity for the mu receptor. It is known to reach peak levels in 2–6 h after oral ingestion and remains bound to its receptors for 24–48 h after administration [8]. It inhibits ascending pain pathways preventing withdrawal symptoms and decreases opioid cravings. It also reduces the euphoric effects of opioid use by maintaining high levels of opioid tolerance and stabilizes psychosocial functioning. In this way, methadone, in once-daily dosing, stabilizes the cycles of euphoria seeking compounded by opioid withdrawal, which could lead to a loss of control. This is the concept of "narcotic blockade" [8].

The general dosage range is between 40 and 100 mg/day, but between 40 and 60 mg/day is often sufficient to block opioid withdrawal symptoms, and higher doses are generally reserved for craving prevention [6]. Once a stable dose has been determined, in most cases, the patient is maintained on this dose without further need for dose titration. Methadone has proven its effectiveness in the treatment of opioid use disorder both in terms of treatment retention and opioid use [7, 8]. In this way, methadone can be used to treat opioid withdrawal as well as a maintenance treatment for relapse prevention. Maintenance treatment is typically 1–2 years but can be longer.

Notable side effects of methadone include constipation, excess sweating, drowsiness, and decreased libido. QT prolongation is also an adverse effect to be monitored. Interactions with several medications also metabolized by hepatic cytochrome P450 (CYP) 3A4 must also be considered [8].

7.2.6.2 Buprenorphine-Naloxone

Buprenorphine-naloxone (Suboxone) is a sublingual high-affinity partial mu agonist and an antagonist at the kappa receptor. Due to its partial agonist properties, there is a ceiling to its agonist effect including analgesia and respiratory depression, and so buprenorphine-naloxone appears to be safer in overdose compared to methadone. However, if given in the presence of opioids, withdrawal will occur. The usual dose of buprenorphine-naloxone is between 8 and 24 mg daily; however it has been found to be less effective than methadone at doses above 60 or 80 mg, and thus, methadone may be more appropriate for patients who are dependent on large doses of opioids [8]. Like methadone, buprenorphine-naloxone can be used for withdrawal as well as relapse prevention [6]. Patients who have failed at buprenorphine-naloxone treatment may be switched to methadone maintenance treatment; however switching from methadone to buprenorphine is clinically more difficult [9]. Side effects of buprenorphine-naloxone include headache and the more common opioid-related side effects such as constipation, sweating, and decreased libido.

Some of the indications for buprenorphine-naloxone treatment as opposed to methadone include patients with prolonged QTc interval or those at higher risk for methadone toxicity. Those who might be at a higher risk for toxicity might be elderly patients or those taking benzodiazepines or other sedating drugs, those with heavy alcohol consumption, COPD or other respiratory illness, and patients with lower tolerance to opioids (e.g., on codeine or less than daily opioid use). Also, patients with good prognoses who may be able to successfully taper off opioid agonist treatment after 6–12 months may benefit from this treatment. Literature indicates that buprenorphine-naloxone has a milder withdrawal syndrome and may be easier to discontinue than methadone treatment.

7.2.6.3 Naltrexone

Naltrexone is another pharmacological option available in the treatment of opioid use disorder. It is a high-affinity opioid receptor antagonist that causes a potent blockade of opioid effects. It is a derivative of naloxone and has an affinity for the mu receptor that is 20 times that of morphine [8]. It blocks the euphoric effects of opioids, which diminishes its reinforcing aspects. It is prescribed as oral formulation in which peak plasma concentration is achieved within 1 h, and antagonistic effects can last for up to 72 h. In the United States, it is also available as an extended-release intramuscular formulation administered on a monthly basis. Opioid antagonists have no addictive potential or tolerance. It is used in highly motivated individuals or those bound to adhere to treatment to help with relapse prevention [8].

When deciding on a treatment regimen with their patients, clinicians need to take into consideration factors such as patient preference, previous history of treatment, and treatment setting when deciding between the use of methadone, buprenorphine-naloxone, and naltrexone while making a shared decision with each patient about treatment of addiction involving opioid use [10].

7.2.7 What Other Options Could Have Been Used to Treat Opioid Withdrawal When Jane Was in the Inpatient Detoxification Facility?

Opioid withdrawal management with medications is recommended over abrupt cessation of opioids. A thorough medical history and physical examination focusing on signs and symptoms associated with opioid withdrawal should be part of clinical management. Validated clinical scales that measure withdrawal symptoms such as the Clinical Opiate Withdrawal Scale (COWS) or Subjective Opioid Withdrawal Scale (SOWS) may be used to assist in the evaluation of opioid withdrawal [11].

The COWS is an 11-item scale that can be used to reproducibly rate common signs and symptoms of opioid withdrawal and assess the level of physical dependence on opioids. It includes signs/symptoms such as resting pulse rate, gastrointestinal upset, sweating, tremor, restlessness, yawning, pupil size, anxiety/irritability, bone/joint aches, piloerection, and rhinorrhea/epiphora. The SOWS is a 16-item scale answered by the patient seen in Table 7.2. Mild withdrawal would be considered a score of 0–10, moderate withdrawal 11–20, and severe withdrawal 21–30 [11].

7.2.8 Clonidine

There is some evidence to support off-label use of the medication clonidine for the treatment of opioid withdrawal, although it is not approved by the Food and Drug Administration (FDA) in the United States. Clonidine may be used orally or transdermally at doses of 0.1–0.3 mg every 6–8 h up to a maximum dose of 1.2 mg daily as part of treatment for opioid withdrawal symptoms. It acts centrally

Table 7.2 The subjective opioid withdrawal scale [11]

	Not at all	A little	Moderately	Quite a bit	Extremely
I feel like anxious	0	1	2	3	4
I feel like yawning	0	1	2	3	4
I'm perspiring	0	1	2	3	4
My eyes are tearing	0	1	2	3	4
My nose is running	0	1	2	3	4
I have goose flesh	0	1	2	3	4
I am shaking	0	1	2	3	4
My bones and muscles ache	0	1	2	3	4
I feel restless	0	1	2	3	4
I feel nauseous	0	1	2	3	4
My muscles twitch	0	1	2	3	4
I have cramps in my stomach	0	1	2	3	4
I feel like shooting up now	0	1	2	3	4

Maximum score = 64

via alpha-2 adrenergic receptors as an antihypertensive agent to suppress withdrawal symptoms such as vomiting, diarrhea, cramps, and sweating when an opioid is stopped abruptly [6]. The maximum amount of clonidine is often limited by its hypotensive effects. However, it does not reduce other symptoms of opioid withdrawal such as insomnia, distress, and drug cravings and therefore can be combined with symptomatic treatment for withdrawal such as nonsteroidal anti-inflammatory medications (NSAIDs) for pain, loperamide for diarrhea, benzodiazepines for anxiety, and ondansetron or other agents for nausea.

Other treatment options for opioid withdrawal in an inpatient setting include using methadone where a tapering schedule could be used beginning at doses between 20 and 30 mg per day, decreasing daily with discontinuation of the drug in 6–10 days. The use of buprenorphine and low dose oral naltrexone has shown promise to manage withdrawal in and inpatient setting, but more research is required before they can be accepted into standard practice [10].

7.2.9   Is There a Role for Psychosocial Treatment in Conjunction with Medications for the Treatment of Opioid Use Disorder?

Psychosocial treatment is recommended in combination with any of the above medication options to treat opioid use disorder. Psychosocial interventions can vary from psychosocial needs assessment, supportive counselling, and referrals to community services [10]. Standardized approaches used in adjunctive counselling can include (1) motivational interviewing which is a directive, patient-centered approach that focuses on changing unhealthy behavior by enhancing intrinsic motivation to change by exploring and resolving ambivalence; (2) cognitive behavioral therapy (CBT), a structured, goal-directed, problem-focused therapy centering on identification and modification of thoughts contributing to drug use; and/or (3) intensive outpatient treatment programs constituting a higher level of care

with participation in group therapy and individual counselling on a more frequent basis [8].

7.2.10   What Pharmacological Interventions Are Used to Treat PTSD?

The Canadian Clinical Practice Guidelines for the Pharmacological Management of Anxiety, Posttraumatic Stress, and Obsessive-Compulsive Disorders were developed to assist clinicians and other health-care workers with diagnosis and treatment of anxiety and related disorders and to provide evidence-based recommendations. Table 7.3 outlines the recommended first-line, second-line, third-line, adjunct, and not recommended treatments as provided by the Canadian Clinical Practice Guidelines for PTSD [12].

Table 7.3 Recommendations for the pharmacological treatment of PTSD from the Canadian clinical practice guidelines for anxiety, PTSD, and OCD [12]

First line	Fluoxetine	Sertraline
	Paroxetine	Venlafaxine XR
Second line	Fluvoxamine	Phenelzine
	Mirtazapine	–
Third line	Amitriptyline	Aripiprazole
	Bupropion SR	Carbamazepine
	Buspirone	Desipramine
	Duloxetine	Escitalopram
	Imipramine	Lamotrigine
	Memantine	Moclobemide
	Quetiapine	Reboxetine
	Risperidone	Tianeptine
	Topiramate	Trazodone
Adjuncts (second line)	Eszopiclone	Risperidone
	Olanzapine	–
Adjuncts (third line)	Aripiprazole	Gabapentin
	Clonidine	Levetiracetam
	Pregabalin	Quetiapine
	Reboxetine	Tiagabine
Adjuncts (not recommended)	Bupropion SR	Topiramate
	Guanfacine	Zolpidem
Not recommended	Alprazolam	Citalopram
	Clonazepam	Desipramine
	Divalproex	Olanzapine
	Tiagabine	–

7.3   Case Presentation

After an informed discussion, Jane consents to a trial of buprenorphine-naloxone. You arrange to see her in 3 days. Urine drug testing comes back positive for hydromorphone. She reports 48 hours of abstinence, endorses symptoms of opioid withdrawal, and scores high on the Clinical Opiate Withdrawal Scale (COWS). Her starting dose was 4 mg of buprenorphine-naloxone. Over the next 2 weeks, the dose is gradually increased to 12 mg, and she remains on this dose for 3 months. She is eventually able to discontinue hydromorphone use.

During one of her follow-up visits, Jane informs you that she is pregnant and would like to discuss the safety of buprenorphine-naloxone treatment during pregnancy.

7.3.1   What Particular Issues Need to Be Considered in the Management of a Pregnant Woman with Opioid Use Disorder?

Treatment of women who are pregnant with opioid use disorder improves both maternal and fetal outcomes [13]. Pregnant women physically dependent on opioids should receive treatment using methadone or buprenorphine monoproduct (Subutex) versus withdrawal management or abstinence as detoxification gives potential risks to both mother and fetus [14]. Methadone, however, remains the standard of care. Where there is some evidence of safety, there is insufficient evidence to recommend the combination buprenorphine-naloxone formulation at this time.

The pharmacokinetics of methadone is affected by pregnancy with the need for increased or split dosing required as the pregnancy progresses due to larger plasma volume and decreased plasma protein binding as well as increased methadone metabolism during pregnancy. As a result of this, the dose may need to be increased during pregnancy, and women may experience mild withdrawal symptoms unless dose adjustment is accounted for. Methadone crosses the placenta with approximately 31%

reaching the fetus at term. Adverse effects of methadone during pregnancy include nausea, constipation, and reduction in fetal heart rate variability with the less common effects of QT prolongation, somnolence, and respiratory depression but usually at doses higher than 100 mg/day [13].

Buprenorphine monoproduct (sublingual preparation) a partial mu agonist and k antagonist does not require the same dose adjustment during pregnancy and therefore can be a more convenient substitute to methadone although is considered to be an alternative to methadone by the American College of Obstetricians and Gynecologists [14]. Mothers being treated with methadone or buprenorphine monoproduct for opioid use disorder should be encouraged to breastfeed, and pregnant women with opioid use disorder should be cared for by both an obstetrician and addiction specialist [10].

The prevalence of opioid use disorder among women who are pregnant has increased more than fourfold since 2002. The use of opioids during pregnancy can lead to such complications as increased rates of placental abruption, intrauterine fetal demise, preterm delivery, and a higher likelihood of having a low-birth weight baby [13]. The incidence of neonatal opioid withdrawal syndrome (NOWS) has risen since the year 2000, and an estimate of 5.9% of women use illicit drugs during pregnancy. With marijuana being the most common substance of abuse, prescription opioids, stimulants, heroin, and psychotropic drugs follow. It is proposed that women who use opioids during pregnancy may not obtain prenatal care, and therefore many neonates who are exposed to opioids in utero are at risk for NOWS. Previous studies have shown that between 21% and 94% of neonates exposed to opioids in utero will develop withdrawal signs and symptoms that are severe enough to warrant pharmacological treatment once born [14].

Neonatal opioid withdrawal syndrome may develop based on the timing and quantity of the opioids transferred into the developing brain of the fetus. Several scales have been developed to assess the neonate's withdrawal signs and symptoms. Withdrawal scales such as the Lipsitz Withdrawal Scale consists of assigning a score of 0–3 for each of the following 11 symptoms: tremors, irritability, reflexes, stool, muscle tone, skin abrasions, tachypnea, sneezing, yawning, vomiting, and fever. A score of greater than 4 is required to administer medication to the neonate and is scored every 3 h.

The Modified Finnegan Neonatal Assessment Tool (see Table 7.4) includes scores for central nervous system disturbances such as sleeping after feeding, hyperactive Moro reflex, continued or excessing high-pitched crying, or increased muscle tone/excoriation/myoclonic jerks/generalized convulsions; metabolic/vasomotor or respiratory disturbances such as mottling, sweating, sneezing, nasal flaring/stuffing; and gastrointestinal disturbances such as excessive sucking or poor feeding, regurgitation versus projectile vomiting, and loose stools versus watery stools [15, 16]. It is scored within 2 h of life and continues to be scored every 4 h to determine if pharmacotherapy should be used for neonatal withdrawal. Pharmacotherapy should be initiated when a score of 8 or greater is achieved or when the sum of 3 consecutive Finnegan scores is 24 or greater. Non-pharmacotherapy could include swaddling, rocking, minimal sensory or environmental stimulation, temperature stability, or feeding.

The treatment for neonatal opioid withdrawal has historically been a combination of opium with alcohol. Formulations of morphine, methadone, and, most recently, buprenorphine are currently used. Morphine appears to be the most commonly used and is administered every 3–4 h due to its short half-life, and while there is no evidence of current optimal oral morphine regimen, the safe average dose is between 0.06 and 0.24 mg/kg/day [17] based on the Finnegan score. Methadone's longer half-life may allow for outpatient therapy; however further studies are warranted to determine treatment regimens and comparisons with other treatments currently. Buprenorphine also has limited data but has shown a shorter hospital length of stay; however in the literature, infants required adjunct therapy with phenobarbital, and more studies are also

Table 7.4 Modified finnegan score [15]

Central nervous system dysfunction	
High-pitched cry	2
High-pitched cry >2 h	3
Sleeps less than 3 h after feeding	1
Sleeps less than 2 h after feeding	2
Sleeps less than 1 h after feeding	3
Mild tremors when disturbed	1
Marked tremors when disturbed	2
Mild tremors when undisturbed	3
Marked tremors when undisturbed	4
Increased muscle tone	2
Excoriation of the skin	1
Myoclonic jerks in sleep	3
Generalized convulsion	5
Autonomic dysfunction	
Sweating	1
Temperature 37.5–38.0 degrees C	1
Temperature > 38 degrees C	2
Frequent yawning	1
Mottling	1
Nasal stuffiness	2
Sneezing	1
Gastrointestinal dysfunction	
Frantic sucking	1
Poor feeding	2
Regurgitation	2
Projectile vomiting	3
Loose stools	2
Watery stools	3
Respiratory dysfunction	
Tachypnea >60/min	1
Tachypnea >60/min with retractions	2
Total score (minimum 0, maximum 37)	

Table 7.5 Methadone versus buprenorphine in neonatal opioid withdrawal syndrome [17]

Methadone	Buprenorphine
Full mu receptor agonist	Partial mu receptor antagonist
Possible faster time to withdrawal	Possible slower time to withdrawal
Increased severity with benzodiazepines	Lower peak Finnegan scores
	Shorter hospital stays
	Shorter duration of treatment

required before it is to become the mainstay of treatment Table 7.5.

7.3.2 How Would You Assess and Manage Comorbid Psychiatric Disorders in Individuals with Opioid Use Disorder?

Firstly, a comprehensive assessment focusing on mental health status should evaluate whether the patient is stable. A clinician should consider hospitalization and immediate referral for treatment as an inpatient if one presents with suicidal or homicidal ideation for safety. Careful monitoring of medications will be required in patients with a history of suicidal ideation or attempts. Reassessment of psychiatric disorders using a detailed mental status examination should occur after stabilization with methadone, buprenorphine-naloxone, or naltrexone. Pharmacotherapy can be used in conjunction with psychosocial interventions in patients with opioid use disorder and a comorbid psychiatric disorder, with particular attention to potential interactions between medications being used to treat comorbid conditions.

7.3.3 What Is the Etiological Relationship Between PTSD and SUD and Related Neurobiological Factors in Comorbid PTSD and SUD?

Posttraumatic stress disorder (PTSD) and substance use disorder (SUD) are common and well-recognized psychiatric disorders with common comorbidities. Among individuals with SUD, the lifetime prevalence of PTSD ranges from 25–52% with the prevalence of PTSD being between 15% and 42% [18]. Those with both disorders tend to have a more severe clinical profile than those with either disorder alone and tend to have a lower general functioning, poorer well-being, and worse outcome across a variety of measures. Comorbidity with PTSD and SUD is associated with poorer treatment adherence and shorter periods of abstinence from substances than having SUD alone.

Several theories have been offered to explain the nature and high comorbidity of PTSD and SUD. One theory postulates that with the increased use of substances, one might be more vulnerable to the exposure of a trauma. A second theory describes that those with PTSD tend to self-medicate with substances eventually leading to a substance use disorder, known as the "self-medication hypothesis." A third relates the two disorders as stemming from two separate but shared etiologies with common risks including personality traits such as impulsivity, genetic factors, and environmental factors such as trauma [18]. Coping styles and emotional (dys)regulation are also factors that could contribute to an individual developing either PTSD or SUD.

7.3.4 What Is "Seeking Safety" and Discuss Its Role as a Psychosocial Intervention in Women with PTSD and Comorbid Substance Use Disorder (SUD)?

Seeking Safety is one of the first empirically studied, integrative treatment approaches developed specifically for those with a dual diagnosis of posttraumatic stress disorder and substance use disorder. It is a manual-based 25-topic cognitive behavioral group therapy protocol treatment with evidence to support significant improvements in substance use, trauma-related symptoms, suicide risk, suicidal thoughts, social adjustment, family functioning, problem solving, depression, cognitions about substance use, and didactic knowledge related to the treatment in patients with PTSD and comorbid substance use disorder [19].

The model was specifically designed for complex trauma clients with comorbid conditions with a list of over 80 safe coping skills applied to the disorders. These sessions can be conducted in any order and in a wide range of settings, which allow for its flexibility. Each topic has multiple handouts, and the patient can be invited to choose commitments (homework) that are meaningful for them, instilling a sense of success and accomplishment [20]. It has been shown in a wide range of the literature to be an effective treatment modality for those with a dual diagnosis of PTSD and substance use disorder.

7.4 Summary

Opioid use disorder is a problematic pattern of opioid use leading to clinically significant impairment or distress resulting in social and/or occupational impairment. The 12-month prevalence of opioid use disorder is estimated to be around 0.37% among adults age 18 years and older in community populations. The most commonly used opioids for pain management act on mu opioid receptors for analgesic effects. Actions on mu receptor systems also activate central dopamine reward pathways with mood-enhancing and euphoric effects.

Treatment with opioid agonist therapy or antagonist therapy is more effective than non-pharmacological interventions or detoxification approaches in opioid use disorder. Medication options include (1) methadone, a long-acting mu opioid full agonist; (2) buprenorphine-naloxone, a sublingual partial mu agonist; and (3) naltrexone, a high-affinity opioid receptor antagonist that causes a potent blockade of opioid effects. There is evidence to support off-label use of clonidine for the treatment of opioid withdrawal symptoms. Psychosocial treatment is recommended in combination with any of the medication options to treat opioid use disorder.

Pregnant women physically dependent on opioids should receive treatment using methadone (standard of care) or buprenorphine monoproduct versus withdrawal management or abstinence. Care for women who are pregnant with opioid use disorder should be provided by both an obstetrician and addiction specialist. Neonatal opioid withdrawal syndrome can be clinically scored using several scales, and infants suffering from withdrawal are best treated with morphine until their symptoms dissipate.

Pharmacotherapy can be used in conjunction with psychosocial interventions in patients with opioid use disorder and a co-occurring psychiatric disorder, with attention to potential interactions between medications being used to treat the co-occurring conditions. First-line medications for treatment of PTSD include fluoxetine, paroxetine, sertraline, and venlafaxine XR. Posttraumatic stress disorder (PTSD) and substance use disorder (SUD) are common and well-recognized psychiatric disorders with common comorbidities. *Seeking Safety* is a manual-based 25-topic cognitive behavioral group therapy protocol treatment with evidence to support significant improvements in substance use and trauma-related symptoms in individuals with PTSD and comorbid substance use disorder.

Disclosure Statement "The authors have nothing to disclose."

References

1. Sharma B, Bruner A, Barnett G, Fishman M. Opioid use disorders. Child Adolesc Psychiatr Clin N Am. 2016;25:473–87.
2. Bateman N. Opioids Med. 2012;40(3):141–3.
3. Comerford D. Techniques of opioid administration. Anesth Intensive Care Med. 2011;12(1):16–20.
4. American Psychiatric Association. Diagnostic and statistical manual of mental disorders. 5th ed. Arlington, VA: Am Psychiatr Assoc; 2013.
5. Al-Hasani R, Michael R. Bruchas. Molecular mechanisms of opioid receptor-dependent signaling and behavior. Anesthesiology. 2011;115(6):1363–81.
6. Stahl SM. Essential psychopharmacology online. 2008. Retrieved September 3, 2016 from "http://stahlonline.cambridge.org/violence.jsf" http://stahlonline.cambridge.org/violence.jsf.
7. Terault JM, Butner JL. Non-medical prescription opioid use and prescription opioid use disorder: a review. Yale J Biol Med. 2015;88:227–33.
8. Tetrault JM, Fiellin DA. Current and potential pharmacological treatment options for maintenance therapy in opioid dependent individuals. Drugs. 2012;72(2):217–28.
9. College of Physicians and Surgeons of Ontario (CPSO) methadone maintenance treatment program standards and clinical guidelines 4th edition February 2011 accessed on August 26, 2016 at: "http://www.cpso.on.ca/policies-publications/cpgs-other-guidelines/methadone-program/mmt-program-standards-and-clinical-guidelines" http://www.cpso.on.ca/policies-publications/cpgs-other-guidelines/methadone-program/mmt-program-standards-and-clinical-guidelines.
10. Kampman K, Jarvis M. American Society of Addiction Medicine (ASAM) national practice guidelines for the use of medications in the treatment of addiction involving opioid use. J Addict Med. 2015;9(5):1–10.
11. Handelsman L, Cochrane K, Aronson M, et al. Two new rating scales for opiate withdrawal. Am J Alcohol Abuse. 1987;13:293–308.
12. Katzman M, Bleau P, Blier P, Chokka P, Kjernisted K, Van Ameringen M. Canadian clinical practice guidelines for the management of anxiety, posttraumatic stress and obsessive-compulsive disorders. BMC Psychiatry. 2014;14(1):S1.

13. Goodman D, Milliken C, Theiler R, Nordstrom B, Akerman S. A multidisciplinary approach to the treatment of co-occurring opioid use disorder and posttraumatic stress disorder in pregnancy: a case report. J Dual Diagn. 2015;11(3–4):248–57.

14. ACOG Committee on Health Care for Underserved Women and American Society of Addiction Medicine. ACOG committee opinion no. 524: opioid abuse, dependence, and addiction in pregnancy. Obstet Gynecol. 2012;119(5):1070–6.

15. Finnegan L, Connaughton J, Kron R, Emich J. Neonatal abstinence syndrome: assessment and management. J Addict Dis. 1975;2(1–2):141–58.

16. D'Apolito K. Neonatal opiate withdrawal: pharmacologic management. Newborn Infant Nurs Rev. 2009;9(1):62–9.

17. Sutter M, Leeman L, His A. Neonatal opioid withdrawal syndrome. Subst Abuse During Pregnancy. 2014;41(2):317–34.

18. Roberts N, Roberts P, Jones N, Bisson J. Psychological interventions for post-traumatic stress disorder and comorbid substance use disorder: a systematic review and meta-analysis. Clin Psychol Rev. 2015;38:25–38.

19. Najavits L, Roger D, Weiss S, Shaw S, Muenz L. "seeking safety": outcome of a new cognitive-behavioral psychotherapy for women with posttraumatic stress disorder and substance dependence. J Trauma Stress. 1998;11(3):437–56.

20. Schmitz M. The case: treating Jared through seeking safety. J Clin Psychol In Session. 2013;69(5):490–3.

A Complex Case of Stimulants and Related Pathologies

8

Sarah Penfold, Jennifer L. Pikard, and M. Nadeem Mazhar

8.1 Case Presentation

A 26-year-old patient, John, is referred to your outpatient psychiatric clinic by his family physician for diagnostic clarification and treatment recommendations. John is currently on probation, having been released from jail 2 months ago, following a 6-month incarceration for assault.

John has a history of attention deficit hyperactivity disorder (ADHD), diagnosed by a child psychiatrist when John was 7 years old. John was treated with methylphenidate throughout elementary school, but he stopped taking the medication in grade 9 when he felt it was no longer effective.

In grade 12, John was expelled from school because of frequent truancy and aggressive behaviors. He went on to work in construction but rarely lasted a few months on a job before being fired or laid off. Former co-workers and bosses have told John that he has "anger problems" and "problems with authority."

John first started using cocaine when he was 18 years old. He would initially snort cocaine powder and later went on to smoking "crack cocaine." John spent $300,000 of an inheritance on cocaine use in less than a year. He has struggled financially since then and has resorted to

selling drugs, theft, and recently prostitution to fund his addiction.

For the last 2 years, John has been smoking and injecting methamphetamine. He describes a pattern of "binging" for several days, "crashing" for 2–3 days, and then repeating the cycle of use. He has not had any prolonged periods of abstinence from stimulant use, aside from his time in prison.

John reports feelings of "depression" and low motivation during brief periods of abstinence and/or withdrawal. Six months ago, John was brought to the hospital by police and admitted for 5 days because he believed that the government was using helicopters and drones to spy on him.

While John recognizes that he has a problem, previous attempts to control or decrease his methamphetamine use have been unsuccessful. You diagnose John with stimulant use disorder, amphetamine-type, and ADHD.

8.2 Discussion

Stimulants, also called psychostimulants, are defined as a class of substances that stimulate the central nervous system (CNS), leading to effects such as excitation, elevated mood, and increased alertness [1].

In the *Diagnostic and Statistical Manual of Mental Disorders*, 5th Edition (DSM-5), stimulants include cocaine, amphetamines, and amphetamine-type substances, such as dextroamphetamine,

S. Penfold, MD • J.L. Pikard, MD, MSc
M. Nadeem Mazhar, MD, FRCPC (✉)
Department of Psychiatry, Queen's University,
Kingston, ON, Canada
e-mail: mir_mazhar@yahoo.com

© Springer International Publishing AG, part of Springer Nature 2018
K. Shivakumar, S. Amanullah (eds.), *Complex Clinical Conundrums in Psychiatry*,
https://doi.org/10.1007/978-3-319-70311-4_8

methamphetamine, ephedrine, and methylpheni-date, as well as plant-derived stimulants, such as khat. Bath salts are a synthetically prepared sub-stance, which is an amphetamine stimulant similar to khat. These stimulants may be taken either orally nasally or intravenously, and many prescription substances are sold on the black market. The effects of amphetamines and other stimulants are similar to that of cocaine. Cocaine may be taken in many preparations (e.g., coca leaves, freebase, and crack), and each varies in levels of potency, speed of onset, and purity. Alterations with levamisole which has significant lethality have been reported recently [2].

While substances such as caffeine and nico-tine stimulate the CNS and are, therefore, classi-fied as psychostimulants, the DSM-5 separates them into their own diagnoses in the substance use disorder classification [2]. This is likely due to the fact that the clinical features of intoxica-tion, withdrawal, and disordered use of caffeine and nicotine differ significantly from the clinical picture associated with cocaine and amphetamine-type substance use disorders.

8.2.1 Diagnosis of Stimulant Use Disorder According to DSM-5

Stimulant use disorder is defined, according to the DSM-5, as "a maladaptive pattern of stimu-lant use causing clinically significant impair-ment or distress." As with other substance use disorders in the DSM-5, the diagnosis is applied if a patient has two or more of the following symptoms, occurring within a 12-month period: recurrent stimulant use resulting in a failure to fulfill major role obligations, recurrent stimulant use in situations where it is hazardous, or contin-ued use despite persistent or recurrent social/interpersonal problems associated with stimu-lant use.

Two particular criteria that are important to the diagnosis of substance use disorder include tolerance and withdrawal. Tolerance is defined either by a need for increased amounts of the stimulant in order to achieve intoxication or desired effect or a diminished effect with contin-ued use of the same amount of the stimulant.

Withdrawal is manifested by a characteristic withdrawal syndrome, which includes symp-toms such as dysphoric mood, fatigue, vivid or unpleasant dreams, insomnia or hypersomnia, increased appetite, or psychomotor retardation or agitation. It is important to know that the cri-teria for tolerance and withdrawal are not con-sidered to be met for those taking stimulant medications under appropriate medical supervision.

Other criteria for stimulant use disorder include using increasing quantities of the sub-stance over a longer period of time than intended; persistent desire or unsuccessful attempts to decrease or control use; spending significant time acquiring, using, or recovering from the effects of stimulants; giving up on or limiting important activities in favor of using stimulants; continued use despite knowledge of ongoing physical or psychological harm caused by or worsened by stimulants; and craving or strong desire or urge to use stimulant(s) [2].

8.2.2 Prevalence of Stimulant Use and Stimulant Use Disorder

Results from the 2008 National Survey on Drug Use and Health (NSDUH) reported a lifetime prev-alence of cocaine use in the United States of 14.7%; 0.7% of survey respondents reported cocaine use in the past month [3]. With regard to nonmedical amphetamine-type substance use, NSDUH reported a lifetime prevalence of 8.5%; 0.4% of respondents were current (past month) users [3].

With regard to stimulant use disorder, the 12-month US prevalence is estimated to be 0.3% and 0.2%, for cocaine and amphetamine-type substances, respectively [2]. Rates of stimulant use disorder are higher in men (0.4%) as com-pared to women (0.1%) [1]. Male to female ratio of intravenous stimulant use is 3:1 or 4:1, but rates become more balanced among non-injection users. Those aged 18–29 years have a 12-month prevalence of 0.4% compared to 45–64-year-olds (0.1%). High school children using illegal prescription stimulants occurred in 5–9% with 5–35% of college-age people reporting use over the past year [2].

8.2.3 Main Risk and Prognostic Factors for Stimulant Use Disorder

According the DSM-5, comorbid psychiatric conditions such as ADHD, bipolar disorder, schizophrenia, antisocial personality disorder, and other substance use disorders increase the risk for developing a stimulant use disorder. Growing up in an unstable home environment, exposures to community violence during childhood, and social association with dealers and stimulant users have been identified as environmental risk factors. Stimulant use disorder affects all ethnic, socio-economic, gender, and age groups [2].

8.2.4 The Neurophysiologic Mechanism of Stimulants

Cocaine and amphetamine-like substances increase monoamine (dopamine, serotonin, and norepinephrine) neurotransmitter activity, though their mechanisms of action differ [4]. The properties of cocaine and amphetamine-type substances quickly penetrate the blood-brain barrier. Through competitive inhibition, cocaine functions as a monoamine reuptake inhibitor, increasing synaptic availability of neurotransmitters by preventing their reuptake across the presynaptic membrane [5].

The mechanism of amphetamine-type substances involves reversal, rather than blockade, of monoamine transport across the presynaptic membrane; neurotransmitters are released into the synapse, in exchange for amphetamine, which is taken up by the transporter [4]. Once inside the cell, amphetamines potentiate redistribution of neurotransmitters, from intracellular vesicles into the cytosol; proposed mechanisms for this effect include amphetamine acting as a substrate at the vesicular monoamine transporters or disrupting vesicular pH gradient by acting as a weak base [5]. In addition, amphetamines enhance monoaminergic transmission via inhibition of monoamine oxidase (MAO) and by increasing the activity of tyrosine hydroxylase, the rate-limiting dopamine synthetic enzyme [5].

As with other potential substances of abuse, the pleasurable and rewarding, and therefore reinforcing, effects of stimulants involve the dopaminergic pathways of the CNS reward circuit, comprised of the ventral tegmental area, the nucleus accumbens, and the prefrontal cortex [4]. Stimulants exert their effects, then, via transient increases in dopamine availability throughout this pathway, which is called the "brain reward pathway" [5].

Norepinephrine and serotonin levels in the nucleus accumbens are also increased following administration of stimulants, though the role of these neurotransmitters in behavioral reinforcement of stimulant use is poorly understood and thought to be far less central than dopamine [5].

8.2.5 Clinical Features of Stimulant Intoxication, Withdrawal, and Overdose and the Features of Chronic Stimulant Use

In the acute phase of stimulant intoxication, rapid release of neurotransmitters leads to euphoria, increased energy and libido, elated mood, and increased self-confidence [4]. The acute adrenergic effects of stimulants lead to increased heart rate and blood pressure, in a dose-responsive manner; escalating doses can intensify euphoria but increase the likelihood of unpleasant effects such as insomnia, irritability, confusion, panic attacks, paranoia and hallucinations, impulsivity, and grandiosity [4]. Adverse adrenergic effects, such as hyperpyrexia, hyperreflexia, tremor, diaphoresis, tachycardia, hypertension, and tachypnea, can also occur [6].

Stimulant withdrawal manifestations include hypersomnolence, increased appetite, depression, lethargy, fatigue, anxiety, irritability, and intense stimulant cravings [7].

Manifestations of stimulant overdose include respiratory failure, cardiac ischemia or arrhythmias, seizures, cerebral infarct or hemorrhage, and rhabdomyolysis [6].

It is estimated that 10–15% of stimulant users will eventually become dependent [8]. Chronic stimulant use is often characterized by binge-abstinence cycles. Up to half of chronic stimulant users report psychotic symptoms, which can persist for years following abstinence [9]. Common psychotic symptoms include persecutory delusions and tactile hallucinations (called "formication"). Some users will repetitively pick at their skin in response to tactile hallucinations, and some engage in "punding," a behavior characterized by compulsive involvement in mechanical tasks such as collecting, sorting, and assembling and disassembling objects [10].

8.2.6 Potential Medical Complications Associated with Stimulant Use Disorder

Stimulant abuse has potential adverse effects on all organ systems. These widespread effects are mediated by one, or more, of the following mechanisms: excess nervous system stimulation (primarily through increased dopaminergic, glutaminergic, and adrenergic activity), ischemia (through vasoconstriction, vasospasm, endothelial damage, and clotting effects), direct toxicity, and other mechanisms [4].

Neurological complications of stimulant abuse include seizures, hemorrhagic and non-hemorrhagic strokes, and movement disorders such as acute dystonia and akathisia. Within the cardiovascular system, infarctions, arrhythmias, myocarditis, and cardiomyopathy can occur. Respiratory hazards include pulmonary edema and respiratory failure. Renal failure can occur secondary to rhabdomyolysis and/or direct toxicity. Reproductive complications, such as placental abruption and low birth weights, have been associated with stimulant abuse [11].

Lifestyle factors related to stimulant use disorder can also affect physical health. The combination of neglect, bruxism, high sugar intake, and malnutrition can lead to a condition known as "meth mouth," characterized by gingival recession, periodontal decay, and dental caries [12].

Stimulant abuse is associated with sexual risk-taking behaviors, such as unprotected sex and exchanging drugs for sex, thus placing users at higher risk of sexually transmitted infections [13]. Impulsivity and involvement in illegal activities may also increase the risk of suffering injuries related to physical violence.

A number of medical complications of stimulant abuse relate to routes of administration. Intravenous (IV) use increases the risk of infectious diseases such as HIV, HCV, and HBV, and snorting can lead to sinus infections and nasal septum perforations.

8.3 Case Presentation Continuation

John occasionally borrows or buys methylphenidate from friends with prescriptions. John reports that methylphenidate improves his energy levels, focus, and overall well-being. He insists that he would not use street drugs if he was prescribed with methylphenidate or some other stimulant medications.

8.3.1 The Role of Prescribed Psychostimulant Medications for the Treatment of Stimulant Use Disorder

A 2013 Cochrane review studied the efficacy of psychostimulants, including dexamphetamine, methylphenidate, and modafinil, in the treatment of amphetamine abuse or dependence. Psychostimulants did not reduce amphetamine use or amphetamine craving, nor did they increase the likelihood of sustained abstinence. There is currently no evidence to support psychostimulants as replacement therapy for amphetamine abuse or dependence [14].

8.3.2 Is it Possible that John's Risk of Stimulant Use Disorder was Increased by the Fact That He was Prescribed with Stimulants for ADHD in Childhood?

A large-scale longitudinal study, the Massachusetts General Hospital (MGH) Longitudinal Studies of ADHD, found that children diagnosed with ADHD treated with stimulants were significantly less likely to develop addictive disorders [15]. Based on current evidence, it does not appear that stimulants, when taken as prescribed, lead to abuse; in fact, some studies suggest that treating children diagnosed with ADHD with stimulants may help reduce the risk of subsequent substance use disorder later in life [16].

8.3.3 What Is the Relationship Between ADHD and Substance Use Disorders?

ADHD is an independent risk factor for substance use disorders [16]. Longitudinal studies have estimated that children diagnosed with ADHD are twice as likely to go on to develop a substance use disorder, as compared to children without ADHD [15] with those diagnosed with ADHD having been found to be 6.2 times more likely to have a substance use disorder as compared to controls [17]. Adults with ADHD have estimated substance use disorder rates of 47%, as compared to 38% among controls [18].

The rates of ADHD among treatment-seeking adolescents and adults with substance use disorder have been found to be 34% and 35%, respectively, rates which are significantly higher than those reported in the general US population [16, 19].

8.3.4 How Would You Approach Management for a Patient Diagnosed with Stimulant Use Disorder and Comorbid ADHD?

Management of patients with both stimulant use disorder and ADHD involves prioritizing treatment—and, ideally, stabilization—of the stimulant use disorder. In cases where ADHD symptoms appear to be as, or more, functionally impairing than the stimulant use disorder symptoms, concomitant treatment may be warranted.

Currently, no pharmacological agents are approved for the treatment of stimulant use disor-

der. There is evidence, however, in support of psychosocial interventions for the treatment of stimulant use disorders. Cognitive behavioral therapy (CBT), contingency management (CM), and motivational interviewing (MI) can be effective both in reducing stimulant use and decreasing the harms associated with stimulant use disorder [20].

Cognitive behavioral therapy is a structured form of psychotherapy, which applies principals of learning and conditioning to educate, support, and motivate individuals. With regard to the treatment of stimulant use disorder, the treatment goals for CBT would be to teach skills for achieving abstinence and preventing relapse [21]. CBT interventions have been associated with reductions in self-reported stimulant use, and this effect can be sustained for a year, or more, post treatment [21].

Contingency management applies operant conditioning, in that positive reinforcements, such as vouchers or cash, reward desirable behaviors such as abstinence, attending treatment, or providing drug-negative urine samples [21]. There is strong evidence for CM interventions across substance use disorders including stimulant use disorder, though the degree to which the effects of treatment persist after the reinforcements are no longer available [21] is unclear.

Motivational interviewing is a directive, patient-centered approach to counseling that aims to assist patients to explore and address ambivalence related to behavior change. While evidence for effectiveness of motivational interviewing (MI) in addiction research literature has been strongest for the treatment of alcohol-related problems, there is evidence to support MI interventions for individuals with methamphetamine dependence [22].

For patients who achieve sustained remission of stimulant use disorder, reevaluation of ADHD is warranted, as ADHD symptoms can be exacerbated, or even induced, in the context of acute intoxication and/or chronic abuse [23]. If ADHD symptoms persist and continue to be functionally impairing, it is reasonable to consider pharmacotherapy.

8.3.5 How Do You Determine the Optimal Addiction Treatment Setting for a Patient with Stimulant Use Disorder?

The American Society of Addiction Medicine (ASAM) criteria are a set of guidelines to aid practitioners in the assessment, placement, and disposition of patients with substance use and co-occurring disorders [24]. ASAM's criteria apply six dimensions to address in the biopsychosocial assessment of an individual. These dimensions include intoxication and withdrawal potential, biomedical conditions and complications, emotional and cognitive conditions, readiness to change, relapse potential and recovery environment.

Through this strength-based multidimensional assessment, the ASAM criteria address patient needs, obstacles, and liabilities, as well as the patient's strengths, assets, resources, and support structure. The guidelines also outline five broad levels of care along a continuum; patients can move up and down in terms of intensity of services, which could vary from Outpatient services to residential treatment [24].

8.4 Case Presentation Continuation

John agreed to attend residential treatment for 90 days. After completing the program, he has continued to attend Narcotics Anonymous meetings and follows up with an addiction counselor on a weekly basis.

One year later, John is re-referred to your clinic after asking his family physician to prescribe methylphenidate for ADHD. He reports abstinence from stimulants for 1 year. His abstinence has been confirmed by regular urine drug testing. John has enrolled in adult education to complete his remaining high school credits and reports struggling in class and with homework due to inattention and inability to organize his thoughts. He complains of a subjective feeling of restlessness in class and notes that he makes many careless mistakes on assignments. He also has difficulty arriving to class on time because he often forgets something at home.

8.4.1 What Concerns Would You Have with Regard to Prescribing Psychostimulant Medications to John?

It is important to be aware of the potential for misuse, diversion, and abuse of prescribed stimulant medications. Misuse and diversion practices are relatively common, particularly among adolescents and young adults [25]. Short-acting stimulants are most likely to be misused and/or diverted, as compared to longer-acting stimulants. All professionals who prescribe stimulants for ADHD should be vigilant about signs of diversion and misuse [26].

8.4.2 After a Discussion of Potential Risks and Benefits, You Decide to Initiate ADHD Medication. Which Treatment Approach Would You Consider, Given John's Past History of Substance Use Disorder?

In adults with ADHD and a history of substance use disorder (SUD), non-stimulant agents (e.g., atomoxetine), antidepressants (e.g., bupropion), and extended-release or longer-acting stimulants (e.g., lisdexamfetamine (Vyvanse)) are preferred treatments, given their lower abuse liability and diversion potential. Individuals with ADHD and current, or past, history of SUD should be monitored frequently. Safe and effective treatment incorporates the following: treatment adherence assessments, questionnaires, random toxicology screens as indicated, and coordination of care with other caregivers [27].

8.4.3 Which Precautions Can Be Taken to Reduce the Potential for Diversion and Misuse of Prescribed Psychostimulant Medications?

Stimulant preparation has an impact on the potential for misuse and diversion, and there is growing evidence to support the use of extended-release stimulant preparations, especially in populations at higher risk to misuse or divert their stimulants. For example, less misuse of extended- compared to immediate-release methylphenidate has been reported [23]. There is evidence to suggest that lisdexamfetamine, a prodrug stimulant that is metabolized in vivo to d-amphetamine, has less potential for intravenous or intranasal abuse compared to equipotent d-amphetamine [26]. Physicians who prescribe stimulants for the treatment of ADHD should directly caution all patients against diversion and inform them of the legal and health risks of diversion and, when appropriate, work with other caregivers to reinforce this message.

8.4.4 What "Red Flags" Might Alert You to Potential Medication Misuse and/or Diversion of Prescription Medications and How Could You Address the Issue?

The following behaviors, organized into three broad categories, should alert physicians to the potential for misuse, abuse, and/or diversion:

1. Escalating the dose (e.g., requesting higher doses, running out early)
2. Altering the route of delivery (e.g., biting, crushing controlled-release tablets, snorting, or injecting oral tablets)
3. Engaging in illegal activities (e.g., double-doctoring, prescription fraud, and buying, selling, and stealing drugs)

When prescribing controlled substances, it is recommended that physicians clarify the conditions necessary for continued prescribing. This can include preconditions such as monitoring practices to detect possible aberrant drug-related behaviors (e.g., urine drug screening) and requiring a treatment agreement.

Treatment agreements are formal and explicit written agreements between physicians and patients that delineate key aspects regarding therapy adherence. An agreement often includes the following tenets:

- The physician will only prescribe if the patient agrees to stop all other controlled substances.
- The patient will use the drug only as directed.
- The patient acknowledges that all risks of taking the drug have been fully explained to him or her.
- The patient will use a single pharmacy of their choice to obtain the drug.

A treatment agreement can be an effective tool for ensuring proper utilization of controlled substances. These agreements may be particularly helpful for patients at higher risk for prescription drug misuse or abuse. By entering into a treatment agreement, a patient is fully aware of what is expected of them and knows the consequences of nonadherence to the agreement; the physician may discontinue prescribing controlled substances [28].

8.5 Summary

Stimulant use disorder is a pattern of amphetamine-type substance, cocaine, or other stimulant use leading to clinically significant impairment or distress and social and/or occupational dysfunction. The US prevalence of stimulant use disorder is 0.2–0.3%. The pleasurable and rewarding effects of stimulants are mediated by dopamine activity in the reward pathways of the CNS. There are considerable physical, psychological, and social hazards associated with stimulant use disorder.

Current evidence does not support psychostimulant medications as replacement therapy for stimulant use disorders. When treating patients with both ADHD and stimulant use disorder, both disorders must be taken into consideration, but treatment of the stimulant disorder should be prioritized. There is evidence for cognitive behavioral therapy, contingency management, community reinforcement, and motivational interviewing for the treatment of stimulant use disorder. The ASAM criteria can be applied to tailor addiction treatment settings to individual patient needs.

It is important to consider the potential for misuse, abuse, and diversion of prescribed stimulants. With regard to the treatment of ADHD in patients with previous substance use disorders, non-stimulant medications or long-acting and/or prodrug stimulant preparations are preferable, due to lower abuse, misuse, and diversion potential. Assessment of treatment adherence, random toxicology screens as indicated, and collaboration contribute to safe and effective stimulant-prescribing practices. A number of "red flags" (frequent dose escalations, altering the route of delivery, involvement in illegal activities) can alert a prescriber to the potential for aberrant use of prescribed stimulants. A treatment agreement can be an effective tool for ensuring proper use of prescribed stimulants for patients at risk for prescription drug misuse or abuse.

References

1. Favrod-Coune T, Broers B. The health effect of psychostimulants: a literature review. Pharmaceuticals. 2010;3(7):2333–61.
2. American Psychiatric Association. Diagnostic and statistical manual of mental disorders. Washington, DC: American Psychiatric Association; 2000.
3. Substance Abuse and Mental Health Services Administration. Results from the 2008 National Survey on Drug Use and Health: National Findings (Office of Applied Studies, NSDUH Series H-36, HHS Publication No. SMA 09-4434). Rockville: 2009.
4. Ciccarone D. Stimulant abuse: pharmacology, cocaine, methamphetamine, treatment, attempts at pharmacotherapy. Prim Care. 2011;38(1):41–58.
5. Taylor SB, Lewis CR, Olive MF. The neurocircuitry of illicit psychostimulant addiction: acute and chronic effects in humans. Subst Abuse Rehabil. 2013;4:29–43.
6. Gay GR. Clinical management of acute and chronic cocaine poisoning. Ann Emerg Med. 1982;11(10):562–72.
7. McGregor C, Srisurapanont M, Jittiwutikarn J, Laobhripatr S, Wongtan T, White JM. The nature, time course and severity of methamphetamine withdrawal. Addiction. 2005;100(9):1320–9.
8. Anthony JC, Warner LA, Kessler RC. Comparative epidemiology of dependence on tobacco, alcohol, controlled substances, and inhalants: basic findings from the National Comorbidity Survey. Exp Clin Psychopharmacol. 1994;2(3):244.
9. Flaum M, Schultz SK. When does amphetamine-induced psychosis become schizophrenia? Focus. 2003;1(2):205–10.
10. Fasano A, Barra A, Nicosia P, Rinaldi F, Bria P, Bentivoglio AR, Tonioni F. Cocaine addiction: from habits to stereotypical-repetitive behaviors and punding. Drug Alcohol Depend. 2008;96(1):178–82.
11. Phupong V, Darojn D. Amphetamine abuse in pregnancy: the impact on obstetric outcome. Arch Gynecol Obstet. 2007;276(2):167–70.
12. Curtis EK. Meth mouth: a review of methamphetamine abuse and its oral manifestations. Gen Dent. 2005;54(2):125–9.
13. Molitor F, Truax SR, Ruiz JD, Sun RK. Association of methamphetamine use during sex with risky sexual behaviors and HIV infection among non-injection drug users. West J Med. 1998;168(2):93.
14. Pérez-Mañá C, Castells X, Torrens M, Capellà D, Farre M. Efficacy of psychostimulant drugs for amphetamine abuse or dependence. Cochrane Database Syst Rev. 2013;2(9):CD009695.
15. Biederman J, Monuteaux MC, Spencer T, Wilens TE, MacPherson HA, Faraone SV. Stimulant therapy and risk for subsequent substance use disorders in male adults with ADHD: a naturalistic controlled 10-year follow-up study. Am J Psychiatr. 2008;165(5):597–603.
16. Kollins SH. ADHD, substance use disorders, and psychostimulant treatment current literature and treatment guidelines. J Atten Disord. 2008;12(2):115–25.
17. Katusic SK, Barbaresi WJ, Colligan RC, Weaver AL, Leibson CL, Jacobsen SJ. Psychostimulant treatment and risk for substance abuse among young adults with a history of attention-deficit/hyperactivity disorder: a population-based, birth cohort study. J Child Adolesc Psychopharmacol. 2005;15(5):764–76.
18. McGough JJ, Smalley SL, McCracken JT, Yang M, Del'Homme M, Lynn DE, Loo S. Psychiatric comorbidity in adult attention deficit hyperactivity disorder: findings from multiplex families. Am J Psychiatr. 2005;162(9):1621–7.
19. Kessler RC, Adler L, Barkley R, Biederman J, Conners CK, Demler O, Faraone SV, Greenhill LL, Howes MJ, Secnik K, Spencer T. The prevalence and correlates of adult ADHD in the United States: results from the national comorbidity survey replication. Am J Psychiatr. 2006;163(4):716–23.

20. Park TM, Haning WF. Stimulant use disorders. Child Adolesc Psychiatr Clin N Am. 2016;25(3):461–71.
21. Lee NK, Lee NK, Rawson RA, Lee NK, Rawson RA. A systematic review of cognitive and behavioural therapies for methamphetamine dependence. Drug Alcohol Rev. 2008;27(3):309–17.
22. Polcin DL, Bond J, Korcha R, Nayak MB, Galloway GP, Evans K. Randomized trial of intensive motivational interviewing for methamphetamine dependence. J Addict Dis. 2014;33(3):253–65.
23. Harstad E, Levy S. Attention-deficit/hyperactivity disorder and substance abuse. Pediatrics. 2014;134(1):e293–301.
24. American Society of Addiction Medicine [Internet]. What is the ASAM Criteria. [cited 2016 Aug 15]. Available from: http://www.asam.org/quality-practice/guidelines-and-consensus-documents/the-asam-criteria/about

25. Wilens TE, Adler LA, Adams J, Sgambati S, Rotrosen J, Sawtelle R, Utzinger L, Fusillo S. Misuse and diversion of stimulants prescribed for ADHD: a systematic review of the literature. J Am Acad Child Adolesc Psychiatry. 2008;47(1):21–31.
26. Download Guidelines – CADDRA – Canadian ADHD Resource Alliance [Internet]. Caddra.ca. 2016 [cited 18 September 2016]. Available from: http://www.caddra.ca/practice-guidelines/download.
27. Wilens TE, Morrison NR. The intersection of attention-deficit/hyperactivity disorder and substance abuse. Curr Opin Psychiatry. 2011;24(4):280–5.
28. Prescribing Drugs|Policy|Policies & Publications| College of Physicians and Surgeons of Ontario [Internet]. Cpso.on.ca. 2016 [cited 1 September 2016]. Available from: http://www.cpso.on.ca/Policies-Publications/Policy/Prescribing-Drugs#2.Specific.

A Complex Case of Psychiatric Issues Associated with HIV Disorder

9

Alana Rawana and Kuppuswami Shivakumar

Case History

A 39-year-old Italian-Canadian male, father of two young children, with a history major depressive disorder and IV drug use (opioids) presented to the family clinic after being notified that he has HIV. He was notified of the HIV infection 2 weeks ago after completing anonymous HIV testing. He acquired the infection via unprotected intercourse with a female partner whom also contracted HIV months previous. The patient is worried about how his diagnosis will affect his future relationships and about who will take care of his young children in the future if the infection progresses given he is their sole care provider. Currently, the patient's sister is a source of support for the patient's family and she is aware of the diagnosis. The patient has not used IV drugs for 2 years. The patient reports he has had a sore throat for the past 2 weeks and has experienced increased fatigue over the past month. Patient also reports starting an SSRI for low mood 2 months ago. He is taking sertraline 100 mg per day for depressed mood. On physical examination, patient has nontender lymphadenopathy primarily involving the posterior cervical lymph nodes. The patients CD4 count is currently 320 cells/ microL.

9.1 Epidemiology of Mental Disorders among HIV Patients Focusing on the Most Common Psychiatric Disorders

Commonly seen mental disorders in patients with HIV include:
Delirium
Major depression
Bipolar disorders including mania
PTSD
Anxiety disorders
Neurocognitive disorders
Substance abuse or dependence
HIV-associated dementia

Mental health disorders among individuals with HIV are common. Overall, in the United States, nearly half of individuals with HIV have a psychiatric disorder [9]. The most common psychiatric disorders among those with HIV are major depressive disorder and substance use disorder [9, 17, 71]. HIV has also been linked to an increased likelihood of having comorbid anxiety and/or psychosis [35, 71].

A. Rawana, HBSc, MA (Clinical Psychology) (✉)
Northern Ontario School of Medicine, Thunder Bay, ON, Canada
e-mail: arawana@nosm.ca

K. Shivakumar, MD, MPH, MRCPsych(UK), FRCPC
Department of Psychiatry, Northern Ontario School of Medicine (NOSM), Sudbury, ON, Canada
e-mail: kshivakumar@hsnsudbury.ca

© Springer International Publishing AG, part of Springer Nature 2018
K. Shivakumar, S. Amanullah (eds.), *Complex Clinical Conundrums in Psychiatry*,
https://doi.org/10.1007/978-3-319-70311-4_9

9.1.1 Delirium

Delirium is highly prevalent in HIV-infected patients with an estimated prevalence of 40–65% and a major cause of mortality. Delirium symptoms can be characterized by changes in alertness or global impairment of cognition with disorientation; impairment of recent memory and abstract thinking; sleep-wake cycle disturbances; psychomotor disturbances including hypo or hyperactivity; and emotional changes such as anxiety, irritability, fear, depression, euphoria and apathy. Numerous factors can contribute to delirium in HIV patients including metabolic abnormalities, infection, sepsis, hypoxemia, anaemia and various CNS manifestations seen in HIV patients. A patient who is diagnosed with delirium should be considered as a medical emergency and given a full diagnostic work to exclude various general medical complications associated with HIV infection. In this group of patients, delirium treatment can be associated with major treatment challenge and high mortality (Fig. 9.1).

9.1.2 Depression

With regard to depression, studies have shown that a patient with HIV is 2X–7X more likely to experience depression than those who do not have HIV [18, 76]. In fact, between 5% and 45% of HIV-positive people experience depression at some point in their life [3, 15]. It is noteworthy, however, that many individuals with HIV are diagnosed with major depressive disorder before they contract HIV [3], implying that depression could be a risk factor to contracting the disease. The etiology of depression among HIV patients is multifactorial, and various HIV-related conditions have been associated with the development of depression including HIV-related infection, malignancy and the medications used in HIV patients. Medications including efavirenz, interferon, metocloproamide, anabolic steroids and propranolol may produce major depression or depressive syndromes.

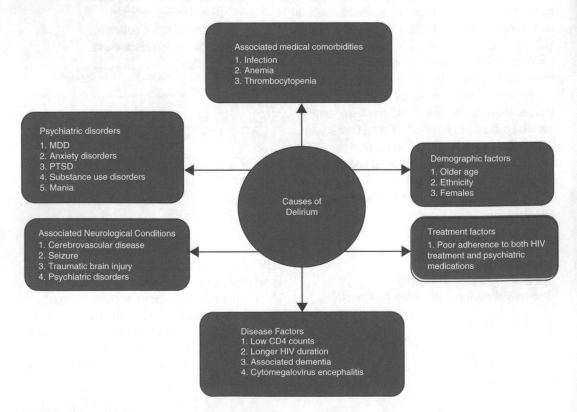

Fig. 9.1 Causes of delirium

9.1.3 Mania

Mania can occur in two distinct patterns among those with HIV. It can occur in those with HIV who have comorbid Bipolar I or as a separate manifestation called "aids mania". Among those with both bipolar and HIV, manic episodes involving, for example, grandiosity, flight of ideas and involvement in risky activities can range from producing devastating effects on one's life to mildly affecting one's functioning outside of their manic episodes [70]. Aids mania, in contrast, appears as a late manifestation of aids where mania, typically in the form of increased irritability, generally arises in those whom have never had bipolar nor experienced mania before [70] (Table 9.1).

9.1.4 Schizophrenia

Research indicates that the prevalence of comorbid HIV with schizophrenia ranges from 4% to 19% [12, 19]. It has also been suggested that those with schizophrenia may be more likely to contract HIV than those without schizophrenia given their higher likelihood towards engaging in high risk behaviours such as unprotected intercourse with multiple partners and injection drug use [16, 56]. It is unclear whether HIV can increase one's risk of developing schizophrenia, but it appears plausible when considering the neural diathesis-stress model of the development of schizophrenia [88]. This model posits that those predisposed to developing schizophrenia may have an abnormality in dopamine (DA) neurotransmission that may be exacerbated by the cortisol release associated with an environmental stressor [88]. In line with this hypothesis, it is plausible that the stress associated with receiving the diagnosis of HIV or managing the illness could trigger symptoms of schizophrenia in those who are predisposed to schizophrenia. Research has yet to support this hypothesis. The diagnosis of schizophrenia may affect the course of HIV. For instance, those with both HIV and schizophrenia may be less equipped to cope with the stresses of the diagnosis and may be less able to afford care associated with the illness, there-

Table 9.1 Common symptoms of depression and bipolar disorder in HIV-infected patients

Commonly seen symptoms of depression and bipolar disorder in HIV-infected patients		
	Differential diagnosis	Assessment tools
Depressive symptoms		
Low or depressed mood Loss of interest Sleep difficulties Loss of appetite Poor concentration Memory Non-specific somatic symptoms Excessive tiredness	Rule out bipolar disorder Dysphoria from PTSD Substance use disorder HIV-associated neurocognitive disorder	Center for epidemiological studies Depression scale Hospital anxiety and depression scale Phq-9 Hamilton scale for depression
Bipolar symptoms		
Mania Grandiose feelings Sleep difficulties Pressure of speech Flight of ideas Distractibility Excessive involvement in pleasurable activities	Manic or hypomanic symptoms induced by metabolic disturbances Endocrine disorders Neurological disorders Mania or hypomania associated with systemic infection Mania or hypomania associated with illicit or prescribed medication including ART (antiretroviral treatment)	Mood disorders questionnaire (MDQ) Jung mania rating scale

Adapted from Cozza et al. [23]

fore they may not fare as well as compared to those with HIV alone [80]. Furthermore, those with schizophrenia and HIV have a higher rate of morbidity and mortality than compared to those with HIV alone [85].

9.1.5 Substance Abuse or Dependence

In terms of the epidemiology of substance use issues among those with HIV, approximately 40% of those with HIV have a substance use problem involving a substance other than marijuana [9]. Common substances reported to be used among individuals with HIV include alcohol, heroin, and cocaine. Amphetamine use appears to be increasingly used by this population [1]. The lifetime prevalence for alcohol use disorders and other drug use disorders among HIV patients compared with the lifetime prevalence of general population is much higher. It is also common to see an increased HIV-related mortality, morbidity and lower treatment adherence at antiretroviral therapy among the patients with substance abuse disorders and HIV.

9.1.6 Anxiety Disorders

Individuals with HIV are also more likely to have anxiety and psychotic disorders compared to the general population. Approximately 15.8% of those receiving care for HIV also have a generalized anxiety disorder while 10.5% meet criteria for panic disorder [9]. Adjustment disorder is one of the most common psychiatric disorders seen in HIV patients, especially during the early course of the illness [69].

9.1.7 Psychosis

The prevalence rate of new-onset psychosis among HIV-positive individuals ranges between 0.5% and 15% [19, 55]. New-onset of psychotic disorders among HIV patients are commonly seen in the late stages of the disease, and this may be associated with neurocognitive disorders. Common symptoms of psychosis include delusions of grandeur, somatic and persecution typically presenting during the late stages of HIV [38]. The etiology of psychosis in HIV infection is complex and multifactorial, and this may be part of the comorbid psychiatric conditions associated with HIV such as major depressive disorders, bipolar disorder, delirium, neurocognitive disorders or medication side effects.

9.1.8 Post-traumatic Stress Disorder

The lifetime prevalence rate of post-traumatic stress disorder (PTSD) has been found to be as high as 40% among those with HIV [53]. It has been posited that PTSD may develop after the diagnosis of a life-threatening illness such as HIV [53]. This may be the case particularly in those with HIV who lack adequate coping skills, social support or access to appropriate mental health services to help them manage with their illness. Furthermore, many individuals with HIV have been found to have had experienced traumatic events that triggered PTSD before the HIV diagnosis [65]. Given that research studies have produced mixed results as to whether HIV causes PTSD, more research is needed to better elucidate the relationship between the two conditions [44]. A better understanding of the relationship between HIV and PTSD is important so that healthcare providers may develop trauma prevention programmes targeting high-risk groups such as those with HIV and thus help potentially decrease rates of morbidity and mortality associated with the disease.

9.2 Pathogenesis of Mental Disorders in HIV

The pathogenesis of mental disorders in HIV is complex and varies widely depending on the type of mental disorder. For example, study findings have shown that factors such as stress, immune cell functioning, inflammation and medication interactions contribute to the development of various mental illnesses [18, 25, 40, 50, 86]. With regard to stress, individuals diagnosed with HIV are often faced many stressors in addition to the health complications that may arise throughout their illness. For instance, those diagnosed with HIV often deal with the stigma associated with the disease; make major lifestyle decisions; adjust to treatment regimens; determine when and who to disclose their illness to; and deal with changes in family, partner or friendship dynamics following diagnosis [78, 89]. Those with HIV are more likely to develop a comorbid psychiatric disorder such as depression and anxiety than compared to those who are HIV negative because they must endure many additional stressors [18].

Immune cell dysfunction can also contribute to the development of mental illness among those diagnosed with HIV. For example, the biological mechanism of HIV, monocytes and lymphocytes entering the brain along with the production and release of inflammatory cytokines has been found to contribute to the pathogenesis of HIV-associated dementia (HAD) [57]. More specifically, macrophages, microglia and astrocytes interact with each other to release cytokines such as IL-1β, TNF-α and arachidonic acid, which are neurotoxic to the brain and said to contribute to the development of HAD [31].

Mania is another symptom of mental illness that can occur in those with HIV. Mania may be related to a comorbid bipolar disorder, caused by substance use or secondary to HIV infection, HIV medication, or HIV-related infection [14, 42, 61]. The exact mechanism of how HIV infection is related to the development of manic symptoms is unclear; however, it has been posited that HIV is neurotoxic and disrupts brain structure and function which leads to manic symptoms [51, 66]. Another study highlighted the potential role of CD4 cells in the pathogenesis of mania secondary to HIV. The study findings found that those with HIV had lower CD4 counts than compared to those without manic symptoms [51]. Therefore, perhaps CD4 cells may influence whether a patient with HIV experiences symptoms of mania or not.

Certain antiretroviral medications have been found to cause mental illness. For example, mania has developed secondary to the use of antiretroviral medications such as zidovudine and didanosine [14, 54]. In contrast, one study found that if antiretroviral medication was able to reach the CNS it was protective effect against the development of manic symptoms among those with HIV [58]. More studies with larger sample sizes would be helpful to better elucidate the relationship between mania and antiretroviral medication.

9.3   Psychosocial and Behavioural Risk Factors for Depression and Anxiety

There are a number of factors that may predispose individuals with HIV to developing depression and anxiety. Nakimuli-Mpungu et al. [60] examined risk factors for depression among those with HIV living in Southern Uganda. Their research findings showed that HIV-positive patients with depressive disorders were more likely to have difficulty adhering to their antiretroviral medication regimens, have less social support and were less likely to have feelings of self-efficacy compared to those with HIV whom did not have depression [60]. According to their study, those with HIV and comorbid depression were also more likely to have tuberculosis and experience manic episodes than those with HIV and no depression [60]. In another study involving HIV-positive individuals in Uganda, research findings showed that factors such as being female, a family history of psychiatric illness, the use of poor coping strategies, alcohol use, stress and food insecurity were predictive of major depressive disorder [45]. In terms of factors that correlated with anxiety, Pappin et al. [67] found HIV-positive patients who experienced adverse effects from their antiretroviral medications, engaged in avoidant coping styles or were subjected to stigma related to their diagnosis were more likely to develop symptoms of anxiety.

9.4   Assessing Depression and Other Comorbid Psychiatric Conditions: The Role of Screening Instruments

According to the research literature, depression affects approximately 4–40% of those living with HIV [17, 59, 69]. Currently, there is no gold standard for examining depression among HIV-positive individuals. Typically the diagnosis of depression among people living with HIV in clinical settings is made with information obtained from a clinical interview based on either the International Classification of Diseases (ICD;

[92]) or Diagnostic and Statistical Manual of Mental Disorders criteria (DSM 5; [5]). A structured clinical interview such as the Structured Clinical Interview for the DSM-5 (SCID, [28]) or the Composite International Diagnostic Interview [91] is the most commonly used assessment when examining depression in research settings [82]. Symptom severity scales are often utilized to monitor change in symptomology over a course of time. The Center for Epidemiologic Studies Depression Scale (CES-D-20; [72]) and the Beck Depression Inventory [8] are symptom severity scales that have been used extensively with HIV populations.

The CES-D-20 is a well-validated tool used to examine depression in the general population [72]. Zhang et al. [94] tested both the shorter version of the CES-D-20 and the CES-D-10, with HIV-positive people in British Columbia, Canada, and found the internal consistency reliability coefficient to be adequate with a coefficient alpha of 0.88. Furthermore, the researchers found high levels of sensitivity (with 95% CI) at 91% and specificity (with 95% CI) at 92% [94]. Therefore, the study determined that the shortened 10-item CES-D scale was adequate and comparable to the CES-D-20 in its utility when examining depression symptoms among those with HIV.

Kalichman et al. [43] used the Beck Depression Inventory II (BDI II; [7]) to examine depression among those with the HIV infection. The items on the BDI II can be split into two subscales: affective symptoms and somatic symptoms of depression. It is important to note that while the BDI is a very common tool to use to examine depression, research findings suggest that the BDI places more emphasis on somatic symptoms compared to other measures of depression [82]. To illustrate, Kalichman et al. [43] found, via factor analysis, that there was a positive relationship between somatic symptoms of depression, the number of acquired immunodeficiency syndrome diagnoses and the number of HIV-related symptoms. There was also an inverse relationship between somatic symptoms of depression rating and the number of T-helper cells [43]. These findings indicate that one's level of depression may

be strongly linked to the disease status and symptomology. Thus, when using the BDI to assess depression symptoms in those with HIV, it is important to consider the patient's symptomology, diagnostic information and life stressors and how these factors may be influencing their depression score. The Hamilton Rating Scale for Depression (HAM-D; [36, 37]) also emphasises somatic depression symptoms as compared to other measures of depression such as the CES-D-20 [82].

Another study examined the use of two other measures of depression symptom severity called the Patient Health Questionnaire-9 (PHQ-9) [46] and its short version Patient Health Questionnaire-2 (PHQ-2) [47] with those with HIV living in Western Kenya. The PHQ-9 and PHQ-2 are a nine-item and a two-item measure, respectively, both based on the Diagnostic and Statistical Manual of Mental Disorders, 4th edition's (DSM-IV; [4]) criteria for depressive disorders. The researchers found that both measures have adequate psychometric properties when used with this population. The coefficient alpha for the PHQ-9 was reported to be 0.78 and when using a cut-off point ≥ 3, the PHQ-2 was shown to have high sensitivity (91.1%) and moderate specificity (76.8%) for diagnosing PHQ-9 major depressive disorder. It is important to note that more studies must be conducted to confirm the measure's utility with other HIV populations beyond those residing in Western Kenya.

Despite the lack of a gold standard for examining depression among those with HIV in the clinical setting, it appears that a clinical interview based on the DSM-5 or ICD-10 criteria is the best method for diagnosing depression. Additionally, the BDI II, CES-D-20, CES-D-10, PHQ-9 and PHQ-2 may be helpful tools when monitoring depression symptoms over time. Patient demographics, culture, stage of HIV disease, life stressors and symptomology should all be considered when choosing an interpreting the measurement tool of depression in those with HIV.

In order to assess for other comorbid psychiatric conditions among HIV-positive individuals, the research literature suggests to first begin by taking a thorough history, which includes information obtained from both the patient, and collateral sources regarding the patient's health status, and history of medications, illnesses, substance abuse, and sexual behaviours [27]. The clinician should also perform a mental status examination, the Folstein-McHugh Mini-Mental Status Examination [29], and determine the patient's level of executive function [27]. Screening questionnaires that assess a broad range of psychiatric illnesses may be helpful among those with HIV. The General Health Questionnaire [32] can be useful when used to examine mental illness among HIV-positive individuals. It is a common clinical practice to use a combination of assessment tools such as General Health Questionnaire and Becks Depression Inventory to increase the case detection. Any mental health concerns that arise during the clinician's initial assessment should be further assessed using more specific measurement tools.

Case History Continued

- Eight years later the patient relapses with IV drugs (opioids) and reports that he has been injecting opioids for the past month.
- Patient reports having difficulty adhering to the treatment regimen and that he has been taking his antiretroviral medication intermittently.
- HIV associated dementia develops with deficits in fine motor speed, information-processing speed, executive functioning and apraxia.
- The patient's CD4 counts are <200 cells/microL.
- Magnetic resonance imaging (MRI) and T2-weighted images show cerebral atrophy of the caudate in the basal ganglia.

9.5   HIV-Associated Neurocognitive Dysfunction (Hand)

HIV associated neurocognitive dysfunction refers to neurocognitive impairment that is either symptomatic or asymptomatic [10]. There are three main subtypes of HAND: Asymptomatic neurocognitive impairment (ANI), mild neurocognitive disorder (MND) and HIV associated dementia (HAD) [21]. Asymptomatic neurocognitive impairment is diagnosed when neurocognitive decline is evident in at least two domains (i.e., work, activities of daily living) but there is no functional impairment [2]. In contrast, MND and HAD are described as the presence of minor and major neurocognitive impairment, respectively, with the presence of functional decline [10]. HIV associated dementia also typically involves motor abnormalities such as tremors, gait ataxia and loss of fine motor skills, and behavioural problems such as mania and emotional lability [10, 57].

In order to determine whether the patient has HAND, a clinician should first characterize the degree of functional impairment, take a thorough history of the symptoms, determine whether the patient is on antiretroviral treatment and, if possible, obtain collateral information from family members or from those close to the patient. The clinician should also develop a differential diagnosis for HAND including disorders such as substance use disorder, major depressive disorder and schizophrenia. A patient's level of cognitive impairment can be characterized by using bedside cognitive testing and, if necessary, neuropsychological testing [2]. Some options for bedside cognitive testing include using the MiniMental Status Exam (MMSE) [2], the Montreal Cognitive Assessment (MoCA) [62] and the International HIV Dementia Screen [21].

These measures are not specific for HAND; however, the tools can be quite helpful when assessing cognitive decline in those with HIV [74]. There is no standard battery to use to assess neurocognitive impairment in those with HAND; however, literature suggests repeating assessments at least biannually in order to better understand changes patient's cognitive functioning [21]. The next step in the investigation for HAND depends on the stage of HIV and whether the patient is on antiretroviral medication. Those with more severe cognitive decline and who are not on medication for their HIV are more likely to benefit from neuroimaging, an examination of biomarkers of inflammation, and a lumbar puncture to determine the extent of central nervous system (CNS) involvement. Staging and assessment of HIV can be completed by performing a complete blood count, electrolytes, urea, fasting blood glucose, creatinine, liver function tests, amylase and lipid panel, and screening for syphilis, hepatitis A, B, C, and sexually transmitted diseases [27].

Researchers have yet to find sufficient evidence for using these above-mentioned modalities and laboratory diagnostics with those receiving antiretroviral therapy to help understand the degree of CNS involvement [2]. Instead, these tests are useful to help rule out other diseases that may be the contributing to the observed neurocognitive decline. In the past, indicators such as viral load were strongly linked to HAND, particularly HAD; however since the advent of combination antiretroviral therapies, the viral load is less indicative of cognitive decline because of antiretroviral medication's influence on viral load [90]. Furthermore, among those that are not receiving antiretroviral therapy, CD4 levels also appears to have some utility, particularly in determining whether a patient with HAND has or will develop HAD [90]. Neuroimaging (MRI), cerebral spinal fluid analysis and certain laboratory investigations such as B12 levels are typically reserved to help rule out other diseases that may be the contributing to the observed neurocognitive decline.

9.6 Treatment of Major Psychiatric Disorders in HIV Infected People

The following is a guideline on treatment major psychiatric disorders in HIV-infected individuals. This section highlights key tools to aid in clinicians' decision-making when they are developing treatment plans for those with HIV and comorbid mental illness.

9.6.1 Antidepressants

The use of psychopharmacological management techniques for patients with HIV and depressive symptoms is a common method of treatment often used in combination with psychotherapeutic

intervention (McDaniel et al. 2000). There are some considerations that must be taken into account before starting psychopharmacological treatment such as antidepressants. For instance, clinicians should determine whether the depressive symptoms can be ameliorated using other means besides the use of antidepressants. For instance, the patient's depressive mood may be due to recent changes in the patient's medical condition, new life stressors or side effects of other medications which need to be addressed by the clinician.

In addition, before starting an antidepressant in those with HIV, the patient's medication profile including over-the-counter products, recreational medications and natural remedies should be reviewed in order to predict any drug-drug interactions, particularly if the patient is on a complex cocktail of HIV medications [26]. Serotonin reuptake inhibitors, tricyclic antidepressants and psychostimulants have all been shown to be beneficial in treating depressive symptoms among those with HIV [64]. It has been suggested that patients with HIV should be prescribed these medications in a similar fashion as when prescribing to another medically ill population with careful attention paid to the dose of medication prescribed and route of administration selected (McDaniel et al. 2000). Low doses of antidepressants should be given initially and slowly titrated up with careful monitoring along the way [26].

Significant interactions between certain antidepressants and antiretroviral medication have been documented. Typically, either the antidepressant or the antiretroviral medication increases the presence of the other medication in the patient's system by affecting drug metabolism pathways [84]. Patients should be routinely monitored for side effects of antidepressant medication such as insomnia and loss of appetite or weight, and side effects should be treated aggressively. One reason to treat side effects aggressively is because untreated depression among those with HIV leads to lower levels of adherence to HIV medication thus worsening the patient's symptoms, which is often more debilitating than the side effects of the antidepressant [64] (Table 9.2).

Table 9.2 Commonly used antidepressant medications in the HIV patients

Antidepressant	Comments
Selective Serotonin Reuptake Inhibitors(SSRI's)	
Citalopram	Potential for arrhythmia in doses over 60 mg Prolongation of QTc intervals
Fluoxetine	Prolongation of QTc intervals with certain ART drugs Very long-acting metabolite
Fluvoxamine	High discontinuation rate due to insomnia, gastrointestinal disturbance, anorexia behavioural changes, and sedation [33]
Selective Norepinephrine Reuptake Inhibitors(SNRI's)	
Desvenlafaxine	Low likelihood of interactions with HIV antiretrovirals Potential for hypertension, weight gain, and sexual dysfunction
Venlafaxine (extended release)	Prolongation of QTc intervals Ritonavir may increase serum levels of venlafaxine Potential for hypertension and weight gain
*Levomilnacipran**	Weight neutral Potential for: hypertension and sexual dysfunction Serum levels of levmilnacipran may be increased by protease inhibitors
Duloxetine	Potential for: hypertension Sexual dysfunction
Novel Antidepressants	
Mirtazapine	Potential for weight gain Anti-nausea Sedation Least potential for clinical interactions with ART
Trazodone	Sedating effect Often used a sleep aid Protease inhibitors may increase serum levels
Tricyclic Antidepressants(TCA's)	
Amitriptyline	Known for multiple side-effects such as constipation, dry mouth, weight gain Toxicities include arrhythmia, Potential for anticholinergic delirium All protease inhibitors may increase TCA serum levels to toxicity Use therapeutic drug monitoring
Doxepin	Features in common with TCA

*preferentially inhibiting reuptake of NE over 5-HT
Adapted from Cozza et al. [23]

Table 9.3 Commonly used anxiolytics

Anxiolytic	Comments
Benzodiazepines such as clonazepam	Can be prescribed for relatively mild-to-moderate cases of anxiety Used as a sleep aid Treating delirium Can be used as a first-line agent for the treatment of anxiety in patients with HIV
Non-benzodiazepine anxiolytics such as buspirone	Potent CYP3A4 inhibitors may increase buspirone serum levels

Adapted from Cozza et al. [23]

9.6.2   Anxiolytics

Anxiolytics, particularly benzodiazepines, are commonly prescribed to treat anxiety among those with HIV [87]. Research studies have shown the possibility of a significant interaction arising when a patient takes benzodiazepines along with antiretroviral medication [34]. For example, ritonavir, an antiretroviral medication, can inhibit the effects of the CYP3A enzyme; which breaks down the short-acting benzodiazepine alprazolam leading to a disruption in the clearance of alprazolam [34]. At this time, more research is needed to further examine the use of psychotropic medication such as anxiolytics among those with HIV to determine the best practice guidelines (Table 9.3).

9.6.3   Mood Stabilizers

Preliminary research findings have shown the benefits of mood stabilizers among those who are HIV positive. One study by Parenti et al. [68] treated ten HIV-positive homosexual men with lithium carbonate, and eight of the patients withdrew from the study because they developed drug toxicity. In contrast, pilot studies have found that mood stabilizers such as lithium and valproic acid are well tolerated and may even improve cognitive functioning when used in conjunction with antiretroviral therapy ([48, 77]. Researchers also studied the use of anticonvulsants in treating acute manic episodes in those who are HIV positive. Romanelli et al. [73] found that anticonvulsants may interact with anti-

Table 9.4 Common side effects of mood stabilizers

Mood stabilizer	Comments
Lithium	Lithium is exclusively dependent on renal excretion
	If renal function is compromised or if there is hyponatremia, lithium levels can be affected
	Common side effects include fatigue, slower cognition, weight gain and skin changes
	Symptoms of lithium toxicity (serum levels >1.5 mEq/L) include tremor, nausea, vomiting, diarrhoea, vertigo and confusion which may mimic HIV symptoms
	Plasma levels >2.5 mEq/L require haemodialysis and may lead to seizure, coma, cardiac arrhythmia and permanent neurological damage [20]
Valproic acid	Prone to complicated drug interactions such as hepatotoxicity, thrombocytopenia, hyperammonemia, weight gain and metabolic syndrome
	Lowering VPA serum levels may be seen due to metabolic induction by ritonavir and lopinavir/ritonavir combination [24]
Carbamazepine	Potent pan-inducer with the potential to reduce the levels of protease inhibitors and NNRTIs [63, 93]
Lamotrigine	Used for bipolar and unipolar depression but it has not been extensively studied in persons with HIV

Adapted from Cozza et al. [23]

Table 9.5 Common side effects of antipsychotics

Antipsychotic	Comments
Aripiprazole	Less risk of EPS, metabolic syndrome and QT interval prolongation
	Potential of increasing aripiprazole's serum levels when used with inhibitors such as protease inhibitors
Asenapine (Saphris)	QTC prolongation
	Not recommended in patients with severe hepatic impairment
Brexpiprazole	Increased risk of akathisia
Clozapine	Risk of agranulocytosis
	Cardiac risks: Bradycardia, syncope QTc prolongation, myocarditis/cardiomyopathy, orthostatic hypotension
	Risk of seizures
Olanzaepine	Co-administration of fosamprenavir/ritonavir may reduce olanzapine levels
Paliperidone	Risk of QTc prolongation
	Gastrointestinal narrowing and dysphagia
Quetiapine	Associated with QTc prolongation

Adapted from Cozza et al. [23]

retroviral medication by competing for protein binding, affecting drug metabolism and increasing viral load [73]. More research is needed to better understand the safety and efficacy of using mood stabilizers among those with HIV (Table 9.4).

9.6.4 Antipsychotics

According to a study by Hill and Lee [39], typical antipsychotics such as haloperidol and chlorpromazine appear to be initially helpful in treating delirium and improving cognitive functioning among those with HIV; however, this change appears to be short lived and dissipates within 24–48 h. Caution should be taken when prescrib-

ing antipsychotics to those with HIV because studies have indicated that HIV-positive individuals are particularly susceptible to developing extrapyramidal side effects following the initiation of antipsychotics [41]. Studies have also indicated the potential benefit of using atypical antipsychotics such as clozapine and risperidone to treat HIV related psychosis [49, 79]. Similar to the field of research examining mood stabilizers and anxiolytics among those with HIV, research aimed at understanding the use of antipsychotics with those receiving care for HIV is quite limited at the moment (Table 9.5).

9.6.5 Non-Pharmacological Approaches in HIV Associated Psychiatric Disorders

Psychotherapy for those with HIV and psychiatric manifestations is often prescribed alone or in conjunction with psychopharmacological treatments. Cognitive behavioural therapy (CBT), a type of psychotherapy, has shown promising results among those with HIV and mental illness such as depression, substance use issues and anxiety. In fact, Clucas et al. [22] conducted a systematic review of interventions for anxiety in people with HIV and found that, in general, CBT and cognitive behavioural stress management interventions were more effective in treating anxiety than pharmacological interventions.

Cognitive behavioural therapy involves teaching patients skills so that they are able to change their maladaptive thoughts and behaviours to be more adaptive [30]. A study by Safren et al. [75] found CBT given to those with HIV and depression over the course of 10–12 sessions was helpful in both increasing adherence to medication and decreasing depressive symptoms. It was also reported that improvements were maintained at the 1 year follow-up. Interestingly, telephone-based CBT also appears to show merit when used with individuals with HIV suffering from major depressive disorder [11]. A randomized control study found telephone CBT to be just as effective as face-to-face CBT. The results of the study also indicated that telephone CBT increased patient adherence to HIV medication to a greater extent than compared to face-to-face CBT [11]. Another study examined the effectiveness of CBT, contingency management and CBT with contingency management among homosexual and bisexual men with HIV who abused methamphetamines [81]. Contingency management involves the use of positive reinforcement to reshape the behaviour of an individual and in the case of the study, to decrease the use of methamphetamines. The study found the combination of CBT and contingency management and contingency management alone both significantly reduced drug use among participants as compared to CBT alone.

Another psychotherapy called interpersonal psychotherapy (IPT) also appears to be effective in treating mental illness among those with HIV [52]. Interpersonal psychotherapy involves examining how the patient's mental illness affects their interpersonal context. Often the patient's past and current relationships are examined to identify how their mental illness has influenced their relationships and what interpersonal changes can be made in the future. Studies have tested interpersonal psychotherapy with groups of HIV-positive individuals, and researchers have generally found

that this type of psychotherapy was helpful in reducing depression symptoms [6, 13, 83].

Disclosure Statement The authors do not have any disclosures.

References

1. Altice F, Kamarulzaman A, Soriano VV, Schechter M, Friedland GH. Treatment of medical, psychiatric, and substance-use comorbidities in people infected with HIV who use drugs. Lancet. 2010;376(9738):367–87. Retrieved from: https://doi.org/10.1016/S0140-6736(10)60829-X
2. Antinori A, Arendt G, Becker JT, Brew BJ, Byrd DA, Cherner M, Clifford DB, Cinque P, Epstein LG, Goodkin K, Gisslen M. Updated research nosology for HIV-associated neurocognitive disorders. Neurology. 2007;69(18):1789–99. Retrieved from: http://dx.doi.org/10.1212/01.WNL.0000287431.88658.8b
3. Atkinson JH, Heaton RK, Patterson TL, Wolfson T, Deutsch R, Brown SJ, Summers J, Sciolla A, Gutierrez R, Ellis RJ, Abramson I. Two-year prospective study of major depressive disorder in HIV-infected men. J Affect Disord. 2008;108(3):225–34. Retrieved from: https://doi.org/10.1016/j.jad.2006.04.013
4. American Psychiatric Association. (2000). Diagnostic and statistical manual of mental disorders, 4th ed. Washington, DC: American Psychiatric Association; text rev. https://doi.org/10.1176/appi.books.9780890423349.
5. American Psychiatric Association. Diagnostic and statistical manual of mental disorders. 5th ed. Washington, DC: American Psychiatric Association; 2013.
6. Bass J, Neugebauer R, Clougherty KF, Verdeli H, Wickramaratne P, Ndogoni L, Speelman L, Weissman M, Bolton P. Group interpersonal psychotherapy for depression in rural Uganda: 6-month outcomes. Br J Psychiatry. 2006;188(6):567–73.
7. Beck AT, Steer RA, Brown GK. Beck depression inventory-II. San Antonio: Psychological Corporation; 1996. p. 490–8.
8. Beck AT, Ward CH, Mendelson M, Mock J, Erbaugh J. An inventory for measuring depression. Arch Gen Psychiatry. 1961;4:561–71.
9. Bing EG, Burnam MA, Longshore D, Fleishman JA, Sherbourne CD, London AS, et al. Psychiatric disorders and drug use among human immunodeficiency virus–infected adults in the United States. Arch Gen Psychiatry. 2001;58(8):721–8. https://doi.org/10.1001/archpsyc.58.8.721.
10. Blackstone K, Moore DJ, Franklin DR, Clifford DB, Collier AC, Marra CM, Gelman BB, McArthur JC, Morgello S, Simpson DM, Ellis RJ. Defining neurocognitive impairment in HIV: deficit scores versus clinical ratings. Clin Neuropsychol. 2012;26(6):894–908. Retrieved from: https://doi.org/10.1080/13854046.2012.694479

11. Blank MB, Himelhoch SS, Balaji AB, Metzger DS, Dixon LB, Rose CE, Oraka E, Davis-Vogel A, Thompson WW, Heffelfinger JD. A multisite study of the prevalence of HIV with rapid testing in mental health settings. Am J Public Health. 2014;104(12):2377–84. https://doi.org/10.2105/AJPH.2013.301633.

12. Blank MB, Mandell DS, Aiken L, Hadley TR. Co-occurrence of HIV and serious mental illness among Medicaid recipients. Psychiatr Serv. 2002;53(7):868–73.

13. Bolton P, Bass J, Neugebauer R, Verdeli H, Clougherty KF, Wickramaratne P, Speelman L, Ndogoni L, Weissman M. Group interpersonal psychotherapy for depression in rural Uganda: a randomized controlled trial. JAMA. 2003;289(23):3117–24.

14. Brouillette MJ, Chouinard G, Lalonde R. Didanosine-induced mania in HIV infection. Am J Psychiatry. 1994;151:1839–40.

15. Brown GR, Rundell JR, McManis SE, Kendall SN, Zachary R, Temoshok L. Prevalence of psychiatric disorders in early stages of HIV infection. Psychosom Med. 1992;54(5):588–601.

16. Bühler B, Hambrecht M, Löffler W, an der Heiden W, Häfner H. Precipitation and determination of the onset and course of schizophrenia by substance abuse—a retrospective and prospective study of 232 population-based first illness episodes. Schizophr Res. 2002;54(3):243–51. Retrieved from: https://doi.org/10.1016/S0920-9964(01)00249-3

17. Ciesla JA, Roberts JE. Meta-analysis of the relationship between HIV infection and risk for depressive disorders. Am J Psychiatr. 2001;158(5):725–30. Retrieved from: https://doi.org/10.1176/appi.ajp.158.5.725

18. Chandra PS, Desai G, Ranjan S. HIV & psychiatric disorders. Indian J Med Res. 2005;121(4):451.

19. Chandra PS, Krishna VA, Ravi V, Desai A, Puttaram S. HIV related admissions in a psychiatric hospital a five year profile. Indian J Psychiatry. 1999;41(4):320.

20. Chen G, Shen W, Lu M. Implication of serum concentration monitoring in patients with lithium intoxication. Psychiatry Clin Neurosci. 2004;58(1):25–9.

21. Clifford DB, Ances BM. HIV-associated neurocognitive disorder. Lancet Infect Dis. 2013;13(11):976–86. Retrieved from: https://doi.org/10.1016/S1473-3099(13)70269-X

22. Clucas C, Sibley E, Harding R, Liu L, Catalan J, Sherr L A systematic review of interventions for anxiety in people with HIV. Psychol Health Med. 2011;16(5):528–47. Retrieved from: https://doi.org/10.1080/13548506.2011.579989

23. Cozza et al, Psychopharmacological treatment issues in HIV/AIDS Psychiatry , Chapter 42, Comprehensive Textbook of AIDS Psychiatry: A Paradigm for Integrated Care. (By Cohen et al). Oxford University Press, New York, NY .2017.

24. Cozza K, Swanton E, Humphreys C. Hepatotoxicity in combination with valproic acid, ritonavir, and nevirapine: a case report. Psychosomatics. 2000;41(5):452–3.

25. Cruess DG, Evans DL, Repetto MJ, Gettes D, Douglas SD, Petitto JM. Prevalence, diagnosis, and pharmaco-logical treatment of mood disorders in HIV disease. Biol Psychiatry. 2003;54(3):307–16.

26. Farber EW, McDaniel JS. Clinical management of psychiatric disorders in patients with HIV disease. Psychiatry Q. 2002;73(1):5–16. Retrieved from: https://doi.org/10.1023/A:1012836516826

27. Fernandez F, Ruiz P, editors. Psychiatric aspects of HIV/AIDS. Philadelphia: Lippincott Williams & Wilkins; 2006. p. 355–64.

28. First MB, Williams JBW, Karg RS, Spitzer RL. Structured clinical interview for DSM-5 disorders, clinician version (SCID-5-CV). Arlington: American Psychiatric Association; 2015.

29. Folstein MF, Folstein SE, McHugh PR. Mini-mental state: a practical method for grading the cognitive state of patients for the clinician. J Psychiatr Res. 1975;12(3):189–98.

30. Fulk LJ, Kane BE, Phillips KD, Bopp CM, Hand GA. Depression in HIV-infected patients: allopathic, complementary, and alternative treatments. J Psychosom Res. 2004;57(4):339–51. Retrieved from: https://doi.org/10.1016/j.jpsychores.2004.02.019

31. Genis P, Jett M, Bernton EW, Boyle T, Gelbard HA, Dzenko K, Keane RW, Resnick L, Mizrachi Y, Volsky DJ. Cytokines and arachidonic metabolites produced during human immunodeficiency virus (HIV)-infected macrophage-astroglia interactions: implications for the neuropathogenesis of HIV disease. J Exp Med. 1992;176(6):1703–18.

32. Goldberg DP, Hillier VF. A scaled version of the general health questionnaire. Psychol Med. 1979;9(01):139–45. https://doi.org/10.1017/s0033291700021644. Cambridge Univ Press

33. Grassi B, Gambini O, Scarone S. Notes on the use of fluvoxamine as a treatment of depression in HIV-1-infected subjects. Phamacopsychiatric. 1995;28(3):93–4.

34. Greenblatt DJ, Harmatz JS, von Moltke LL, Wright CE, Durol AL, Harrel-Joseph LM, Shader RI. Comparative kinetics and response to the benzodiazepine agonists triazolam and zolpidem: evaluation of sex-dependent differences. J Pharmacol Exp Ther. 2000;293(2):435–43.

35. Halstead S, Riccio M, Harlow P, Oretti R, Thompson C. Psychosis associated with HIV infection. Br J Psychiatry. 1988;153(5):618–23. https://doi.org/10.1192/bjp.153.5.618.

36. Hamilton M. A rating scale for depression. J Neurol Neurosurg Psychiatry. 1960;23(1):56.

37. Hamilton MA. Development of a rating scale for primary depressive illness. Br J Clin Psychol. 1967;6(4):278–96.

38. Harris MJ, Jeste DV, Gleghorn A, Sewell DD. New-onset psychosis in HIV-infected patients. J Clin Psychiatry. 1991;52(9):369–76.

39. Hill L, Lee KC. Pharmacotherapy considerations in patients with HIV and psychiatric disorders: focus on antidepressants and antipsychotics. Ann Pharmacother. 2013;47(1):75–89.

40. Holland JC, Tross S. The psychosocial and neuropsychiatric sequelae of the acquired immunodeficiency syndrome

and related disorders. Ann Intern Med. 1985;103(5):760–4. https://doi.org/10.7326/0003-4819-103-5-760.

41. Hriso E, Kuhn T, Masdeu JC, Grundman M. Extrapyramidal symptoms due to dopamine-blocking agents in patients with AIDS encephalopathy. Am J Psychiatr. 1991;148:1558–61.

42. Johannessen DJ, Wilson LG. Mania with cryptococcal meningitis in two AIDS patients. J Clin Psychiatry. 1988;49(5):200–1.

43. Kalichman SC, Sikkema KJ, Somlai A. Assessing persons with human immunodeficiency virus (HIV) infection using the Beck depression inventory: disease processes and other potential confounds. J Pers Assess. 1995;64(1):86–100.

44. Kelly B, Raphael B, Judd F, Perdices M, Kernutt G, Burnett P, Dunne M, Burrows G. Posttraumatic stress disorder in response to HIV infection. Gen Hosp Psychiatry. 1998;20(6):345–52. Retrieved from: https://doi.org/10.1016/S0163-8343(98)00042-5

45. Kinyanda E, Hoskins S, Nakku J, Nawaz S, Patel V. Prevalence and risk factors of major depressive disorder in HIV/AIDS as seen in semi-urban Entebbe district, Uganda. BMC Psychiatry. 2011;11(1):205. https://doi.org/10.1186/1471-244X-11-205.

46. Kroenke K, Spitzer RL, Williams JB. The phq-9. J Gen Intern Med. 2001;16(9):606–13. https://doi.org/10.1046/j.1525-1497.2001.016009606.x.

47. Kroenke K, Spitzer RL, Williams JB. The patient health Questionnaire-2: validity of a two-item depression screener. Med Care. 2003;41:1284–92.

48. Letendre SL, Woods SP, Ellis RJ, Atkinson JH, Masliah E, van den Brande G, Durelle J, Grant I, Everall I. HNRC group. Lithium improves HIV-associated neurocognitive impairment. AIDS. 2006;20(14):1885–8.

49. Lera G, Zirulnik J. Pilot study with clozapine in patients with HIV-associated psychosis and drug-induced parkinsonism. Mov Disord. 1999;14(1):128–31. https://doi.org/10.1002/1531-8257(199901)14:1<128::AID-MDS1021>3.0.CO;2-J.

50. Licinio J, Wong ML. The role of inflammatory mediators in the biology of major depression: central nervous system cytokines modulate the biological substrate of depressive symptoms, regulate stress-responsive systems, and contribute to neurotoxicity and neuroprotection. Mol Psychiatry. 1999;4(4):317–27.

51. Lyketsos CG, Schwartz J, Fishman M, Treisman G. AIDS mania. J Neuropsychiatry Clin Nseurosci. 1997;9(2):277–9.

52. Markowitz JC, Klerman GL, Perry SW. Interpersonal psychotherapy of depressed HIV-positive outpatients. Psychiatr Serv. 1992;43(9):885–90.

53. Martin L, Kagee A. Lifetime and HIV-related PTSD among persons recently diagnosed with HIV. AIDS Behav. 2011;15(1):125–31.

54. Maxwell S, Scheftner WA, Kessler HA, Busch K. Manic syndrome associated with zidovudine treatment. JAMA. 1988;259(23):3406–7. https://doi.org/10.1001/jama.1988.03720230018014.

55. McDaniel JS, Blalock AC. Mood and anxiety disorders. New Dir Stud Leadersh. 2000;2000(87):51–6.

56. Meyer-Bahlburg H, Nat R, Sugden R, Horwath E. Sexual activity and risk of HIV infection among patients with schizophrenia. Am J Psychiatry. 1994;1(51):229. Retrieved from: https://doi.org/10.1176/ajp.151.2.228

57. Minagar A, Shapshak P, Fujimura R, Ownby R, Heyes M, Eisdorfer C. The role of macrophage/microglia and astrocytes in the pathogenesis of three neurologic disorders: HIV-associated dementia, Alzheimer disease, and multiple sclerosis. J Neurol Sci. 2002;202(1):13–23. Retrieved from: https://doi.org/10.1016/S0022-510X(02)00207-1

58. Mijch AM, Judd FK, Lyketsos CG, Ellen S, Cockram A. Secondary mania in patients with HIV infection: are antiretrovirals protective? J Neuropsychiatry Clin Neurosci. 1999;11(4):475–80. Retrieved from: https://doi.org/10.1176/jnp.11.4.475

59. Morrison MF, Petitto JM, Have TT, Gettes DR, Chiappini MS, Weber AL, Brinker-Spence P, Bauer RM, Douglas SD, Evans DL. Depressive and anxiety disorders in women with HIV infection. Am J Psychiatr. 2002;159(5):789–96.

60. Nakimuli-Mpungu E, Musisi S, Katabira E, Nachega J, Bass J. Prevalence and factors associated with depressive disorders in an HIV+ rural patient population in southern Uganda. J Affect Disord. 2011;135(1):160–7. Retrieved from: https://doi.org/10.1016/j.jad.2011.07.009

61. Nakimuli-Mpungu E, Musisi S, Mpungu SK, Katabira E. Primary mania versus HIV-related secondary mania in Uganda. Am J Psychiatr. 2006;163(8):1349–54.

62. Nasreddine ZS, Chertkow H, Phillips N, Whitehead V, Collin I, Cummings JL. The Montreal cognitive assessment (moca). Neurology. 2004;62(7):A132.

63. Okulicz J, Grandits GA, French JA, et al. The impact of enzyme-inducing antiepileptic drugs on antiretroviral drug levels: a case-control study. Epilepsy Res. 2013;103(2–3):245–53.

64. Olatunji BO, Mimiaga MJ, O'Cleirigh C, Safren SA. A review of treatment studies of depression in HIV. Top HIV Med. 2006;14(3):112.

65. Olley BO, Zeier MD, Seedat S, Stein DJ. Posttraumatic stress disorder among recently diagnosed patients with HIV/AIDS in South Africa. AIDS Care. 2005;17(5):550–7. Retrieved from: https://doi.org/10.1080/09540120412331319741

66. Owe-Larsson B, Sall L, Salamon E, Allgulander C. HIV infection and psychiatric illness. Afr J Psychiatry. 2009;12(2):115–28.

67. Pappin M, Wouters E, Booysen FL. Anxiety and depression amongst patients enrolled in a public sector antiretroviral treatment programme in South Africa: a cross-sectional study. BMC Public Health. 2012;12(1):244. https://doi.org/10.1186/1471-2458-12-244.

68. Parenti DM, Simon GL, Scheib RG, Meyer WA, Sztein MB, Paxton H, DiGioia RA, Schulof RS. Effect of lithium carbonate in HIV-infected patients with immune dysfunction. JAIDS J Acquir Immune Defic Syndr. 1988;1(2):119–24.

69. Perkins DO, Stern RA, Golden RN, Murphy C, Naftolowitz D, Evans DL. Mood disorders in HIV infection: prevalence and risk factors in a nonepicenter of the AIDS epidemic. Am J Psychiatry. 1994;151(2):233.

70. Pieper AA, Treisman GJ. Depression, mania, and schizophrenia in HIV-infected patients. In: UpToDate. 2017. https://www.uptodate.com/contents/depression-mania-and-schizophrenia-in-hiv-infected-patients?source=search_result&search=schizophrenia%20hiv%20mania&selectedTitle=1~150. 7 May 2017.

71. Rabkin JG, Ferrando SJ, Jacobsberg LB, Fishman B. Prevalence of axis I disorders in an AIDS cohort: a cross-sectional, controlled study. Compr Psychiatry. 1997;38(3):146–54. Available at: https://doi.org/10.1016/S0010-440X(97)90067-5. https://doi.org/10.1016/S0010-440X(97)90067-5

72. Radloff LS. The CES-D scale: a self report depression scale for research in the general population. Appl Psychol Meas. 1977;1:385–401.

73. Romanelli F, Jennings HR, Nath A, Ryan M, Berger J. Therapeutic dilemma: the use of anticonvulsants in HIV-positive individuals. Neurology. 2000;54(7):1404–7. http://dx.doi.org/10.1212/WNL.54.7.1404

74. Sacktor NC, Wong M, Nakasujja N, Skolasky RL, Selnes OA, Musisi S, Robertson K, McArthur JC, Ronald A, Katabira E. The international HIV dementia scale: a new rapid screening test for HIV dementia. AIDS. 2005;19(13):1367–74.

75. Safren SA, O'cleirigh C, Tan JY, Raminani SR, Reilly LC, Otto MW, Mayer KH. A randomized controlled trial of cognitive behavioral therapy for adherence and depression (CBT-AD) in HIV-infected individuals. Health Psychol. 2009;28(1):1.

76. Satz P, Myers HF, Maj M, Fawzy F, Forney DL, Bing EG, Richardson MA, Janssen R. Depression, substance use, and sexual orientation as cofactors in HIV-1 infected men: cross-cultural comparisons. Treat Drug Dependent Individuals Comorbid Mental Disord. 1997;1:130.

77. Schifitto G, Peterson DR, Zhong J, Ni H, Cruttenden K, Gaugh M, Gendelman HE, Boska M, Gelbard H. Valproic acid adjunctive therapy for HIV-associated cognitive impairment: a first report. Neurology. 2006;66(6):919–21. Retrieved from: http://dx.doi.org/10.1212/01.wnl.0000204294.28189.03

78. Siegel K, Schrimshaw EW. Perceiving benefits in adversity: stress-related growth in women living with HIV/AIDS. Soc Sci Med. 2000;51(10):1543–1554. Retrieved from: https://doi.org/10.1016/S0277-9536(00)00144-1

79. Singh AN, Golledge H, Catalan J. Treatment of HIV-related psychotic disorders with risperidone: a series of 21 cases. J Psychosom Res. 1997;42(5):489–93. Retrieved from: https://doi.org/10.1016/S0022-3999(96)00373-X

80. Sewell DD. Schizophrenia and HIV. Schizophr Bull. 1996;22(3):465–73. Retrieved from: https://doi.org/10.1093/schbul/22.3.465

81. Shoptaw S, Reback CJ, Peck JA, Yang X, Rotheram-Fuller E, Larkins S, Veniegas RC, Freese TE, Hucks-Ortiz C. Behavioral treatment approaches for methamphetamine dependence and HIV-related sexual risk behaviors among urban gay and bisexual men. Drug Alcohol Depend. 2005;78(2):125–34. Retrieved from: https://doi.org/10.1016/j.drugalcdep.2004.10.004

82. Simoni JM, Safren SA, Manhart LE, Lyda K, Grossman CI, Rao D, Mimiaga MJ, Wong FY, Catz SL, Blank MB, DiClemente R. Challenges in addressing depression in HIV research: assessment, cultural context, and methods. AIDS Behav. 2011;15(2):376–88.

83. Swartz HA, Markowitz JC. Interpersonal psychotherapy for the treatment of depression in HIV-positive men and women. In J. C. Markowitz (Ed.), Review of psychiatry series. Interpersonal psychotherapy (pp. 129-155). Arlington, VA, US: American Psychiatric Association.

84. Thompson A, Silverman B, Dzeng L, Treisman G. Psychotropic medications and HIV. Clin Infect Dis. 2006;42(9):1305–10. Retrieved from: https://doi.org/10.1086/501454

85. Torrey EF. Surviving schizophrenia: a family manual. rev. ed. New York: Perennial Library; 1988.

86. Uddin M, Aiello AE, Wildman DE, Koenen KC, Pawelec G, de Los SR, Goldmann E, Galea S. Epigenetic and immune function profiles associated with posttraumatic stress disorder. Proc Natl Acad Sci. 2010;107(20):9470–5.

87. Vitiello B, Burnam MA, Bing EG, Beckman R, Shapiro MF. Use of psychotropic medications among HIV-infected patients in the United States. Am J Psychiatr. 2003;160(3):547–54. Retrieved from: https://doi.org/10.1176/appi.ajp.160.3.547

88. Walker EF, Diforio D. Schizophrenia: a neural diathesis-stress model. Psychol Rev. 1997;104(4):667.

89. Whetten K, Reif S, Whetten R, Murphy-McMillan LK. Trauma, mental health, distrust, and stigma among HIV-positive persons: implications for effective care. Psychosom Med. 2008;70(5):531–8. https://doi.org/10.1097/PSY.0b013e31817749dc.

90. Woods SP, Moore DJ, Weber E, Grant I. Cognitive neuropsychology of HIV-associated neurocognitive disorders. Neuropsychol Rev. 2009;19(2):152–68. Retrieved from: https://doi.org/10.1007/s11065-009-9102-5

91. World Health Organisation. Composite International Diagnostic Interview (CIDI): a) CIDI-interview (version l.O), b) CIDI-user manual, c) CIDI-training manual d) CIDI-computer programs. Geneva: World Health Organisation; 1990.

92. World Health Organization. International statistical classification of diseases and related health problems. Geneva: World Health Organization; 2004.

93. Wynn GW, Armstrong S. Neurology: antiepileptic drugs. In: Wynn GW, Oesterheld J, Cozza KL, Armstrong S, editors. Clinical manual of drug interaction principles for medical practice. Arlington: American Psychiatric Publishing; 2009. p. 325–52.

94. Zhang W, O'Brien N, Forrest JI, Salters KA, Patterson TL, Montaner JSG, et al. Validating a shortened depression scale (10 item CES-D) among HIV-positive people in British Columbia, Canada. PLoS One. 2012;7(7):e40793. https://doi.org/10.1371/journal.pone.0040793.

Conundrums in Managing Early Stages of Schizophrenia

10

Lena Palaniyappan, Priyadharshini Sabesan, Ross Norman, and Alkomiet Hasan

10.1 Introduction

Schizophrenia is conceptualized as a neurodevelopmental disorder with varying trajectories of clinical course. While a substantial number of patients demonstrate meaningful recovery with current interventions, a large number continue to experience recurrent relapses and/or unrelenting functional deficits [38]. The onset of first episode appears to be a critical period of intervention that can positively alter the outcomes, the trajectory of which, once established, remains relatively stable over long follow-up periods [29]. Several clinical challenges can appear during this critical period. In this chapter, we raise some of these issues and present relevant current evidence to navigate through these challenges.

L. Palaniyappan, MBBS, FRCPC, PhD (✉)
R. Norman, PhD
PEPP Program, London Health Sciences Centre, Robarts Research Institute and Department of Psychiatry, University of Western Ontario, London, ON, Canada
e-mail: lpalaniy@uwo.ca; rnorman@uwo.ca

P. Sabesan, MBBS, MRCPsych
Urgent Care and Ambulatory Mental Health, London Health Sciences Centre and University of Western Ontario, London, ON, Canada
e-mail: priyadharshini.sabesan@lhsc.on.ca

A. Hasan, MD
Department of Psychiatry and Psychotherapy, Klinikum der Universität München, Ludwig-Maximilians Universität München, Munich, Germany
e-mail: alkomiet.hasan@med.uni-muenchen.de

10.2 Case Example: Early Psychosis

Rick is a 19-year-old single, white man who left home only a year ago to pursue a sought-after computer science course at a well-regarded university. When returning home for summer break, he consulted his parent's GP with notable anxiety, slight insomnia, concentration problems, and vaguely formed concerns about artificial intelligence and deep web assassins. The GP noted that his parents were concerned about his lack of enthusiasm to engage with his friends and a preference to stay at home, using his iPad and game consoles. He admitted that he missed several assignment deadlines at his course and will be retaking these classes in the next year. The GP started him on escitalopram with a view of treating depressed mood and anxiety. No further diagnostics or psychotherapy was initiated.

Rick continued to be subdued, with a pattern of isolation from parents and social contacts for nearly 3 months. One week prior to his anticipated return to the university, Rick divulged to his parents that their home is going to be attacked by "DDoS" (distributed denial of service), a web-based attack organized by a group involved in systematic hacking. Rick felt that he was being targeted due to their suspicion that Rick could build an X-breed quantum computer that solves the challenges of virtual storage security. He insisted his parents to switch off their Wi-Fi transmitter to avoid being scrutinized further by the hackers. He erased his Facebook and Instagram profiles in the next few days. He also repeatedly insisted his father buy a lead case for the Wi-Fi transmitter. Furthermore, he refused to leave his parents' home as he was aware that he is in big danger. He was convinced that he was observed at the supermarket some days before. His parents drove him to the emergency department, where he was seen by an ER physician. After initial physical screening and risk profiling, the physician prescribed lorazepam 1 mg BD and discharged him back to his GP's care, with an urgent referral to the early intervention in psychosis (EIP) team.

The next day, he was evaluated by an EIP psychiatrist. Upon PANSS-8 [6] administration, it was noted that Rick had high scores on delusions, unusual thought content, social withdrawal, and blunted affect. He also had lack of spontaneity and conceptual disorganization. On the Calgary Depression Scale (CDS; [1]), he had notable self-depreciation and early awakening. The depressive symptoms did not qualify for a diagnosis of major depressive episode. On the Young Mania Rating Scale [53], he scored on delusions/hallucinations, low insight, and insomnia. On Clinical Global Impression (CGI; [24]), the EIP psychiatrist noted that Rick scored 6 (severely Ill) in overall severity of schizophrenia. At this stage his weight was 66 Kg, height was 178 cm, and his fasting glucose, lipid profile, liver, thyroid, and renal function were within normal limits. Urine toxicology was positive for cannabis and benzodiazepines.

The psychiatrist also evaluated his premorbid adjustment, focusing on academic and social domains. Rick had a fairly uneventful childhood apart from a caution issued at high school for 2 weeks of unexplained absence, with subsequent disclosure of cannabis use near the school campus. Rick admitted being exposed to it on a fairly regular basis (at least once a week) since the age of 15. He described feeling intensely paranoid on some occasions when he consumed more than usual amounts. He denied using any other psychoactive substances.

Several prognostic factors were evaluated during the initial assessment. Rick was the only child in a stable family. His father ran a successful car dealership. His mother worked as a medical secretary. When Rick was born, his father was 28 years old. His mother, who was 29 at that time, developed an episode of postpartum mania requiring hospitalization after his birth; she later had five other episodes with mixed depression and anxiety, none requiring hospitalization, but was treated with lithium prophylaxis. Rick achieved motor and language milestones without notable delay and performed well at school without any notable conduct issues or academic failures. His physical health profile was unremarkable, except for a history of childhood asthma treated using salbutamol inhalers and occasional nebulization.

Rick's parents were keen to obtain a brain scan to confirm the suspected diagnosis of schizophrenia. The psychiatrist explained that there is no need for routinely prescribing diagnostic imaging for first-episode psychosis, in the absence of signs and symptoms suggestive of intracranial pathology. Following a discussion regarding various antipsychotic medications, Rick was started on aripiprazole at a dose of 5 mg initially, titrated to 20 mg on the basis of weekly reviews of response and tolerance. Rick showed a rapid response in the first 2 weeks at a dose of 12.5 mg/day; his CGI dropped to 4, and he expressed a reduction in his preoccupation with DDoS. Unfortunately, he started exhibiting significant restlessness and wanted to stop this treatment by the third week. His psychiatrist reduced his dose from 20 mg to 12.5 mg and prescribed propranolol 90 mg/day to counteract the akathisia.

Rick had to postpone his return to university by 2 months. A nurse case manager attached to the EIP team coordinated the arrangements with his university and regularly monitored his weight and symptom profile over the next 6 months. She also arranged for the family to attend psychoeducational sessions on FEP, negative symptoms, cannabis use, and the effects of antipsychotics.

Rick continued to have some features of reduced motivation but successfully reestablished *his routines upon return to the university. But after 4 months of continued treatment, he decided to stop his antipsychotic drug and "experiment" again with the "occasional" weed. At present, Rick and his parents continue to engage with EIP and have a written crisis plan in place should a relapse occur.*

10.3 Discussion

Rick's case raises several conundrums faced by a clinician when treating first episode of psychosis. These include (1) identifying the prodrome at the primary care clinic, (2) deciding the treatment setting at an early stage, (3) the issue of choosing an appropriate antipsychotic drug, and (4) ensuring continuation of treatment after symptom resolution. We invoke relevant evidence to address these issues in the following sections.

10.3.1 Identifying and Managing the At-Risk State

The majority of individuals who develop schizophrenia or related psychotic illnesses have shown identifiable early signs or prodrome such as mood changes and social withdrawal [37]. Such phenomena also occur in individuals, particularly young people, who do not develop psychosis and are not, therefore, specific risk indicators. With the increasing interest in intervening to prevent the onset of schizophrenia spectrum disorders, there has been much effort to identify profiles associated with high likelihood of their later development. Such high-risk indices have typically focused on three presentations: the presence of peculiarities of thinking or perception such as heightened suspiciousness or thought disorganization which resembles positive symptoms of psychosis but at an attenuated level; the presence of clear positive symptoms, such as delusions or hallucinations, but for such brief periods of time that diagnostic criteria are not met; or the observation of precipitous deterioration in functioning in an individual for whom there is reason to suspect vulnerability as reflected by schizotypal personality features or a first-degree relative with schizophrenia [20]. In samples of individuals who have sought treatment and meet such criteria up to one-third develop a diagnosable psychotic disorder (usually schizophrenia spectrum) within 3 years [19]. Such findings can leave clinicians with conundrums about how to proceed when encountering someone in an apparent high-risk state, particularly if there are concerns about the psychological and social impact of formally identifying someone as being at risk for serious mental illness.

Recommendations for responding to such situations include the use of a consensus diagnostic criteria to improve reliability of case identification (e.g., attenuated psychotic syndrome included in the appendix of DSM-5) [4] and, if feasible, employing evidence-based, actuarial risk prediction tools (e.g., a risk calculator) that utilizes information on age, exposure to trauma, neurocognition, family history, and prodromal symptom severity (http://riskcalc.org:3838/napls/; [11]) to quantify the risk of transition to psychosis with some confidence. Periodic follow-up of these patients is warranted given the higher than usual risk of psychosis; such monitoring can be accomplished with the use of self-report scales, such as PQ-16 [28].

It is important to recognize that individuals who can be considered at risk for psychotic disorders generally have distressing symptoms and functional compromises that need to be addressed regardless of whether they convert to psychosis. Given the non-specific nature of prodromal symptoms, a key conundrum is the type and duration of intervention that can be offered. If the clinician is fortunate enough to have access to specialized early intervention services, then a referral is certainly indicated. Regardless of the availability of such dedicated resources, treatment relevant guidelines recommend that the at-risk state be first addressed by psychological interventions such as CBT with supplementation by low-dose second-generation antipsychotics only if necessary [36, 47]. It is also important that comorbid conditions such as depression, anxiety, and substance abuse as well as issues related to psychosocial functioning be treated as appropriate. In the example above, referring Rick to the EIP team at the time of starting antidepressants would have been appropriate.

10.3.2 Treatment Setting for First-Episode Psychosis

Once a psychotic episode is diagnosed, what is the best setting to treat the illness? Specialized EIP programs have been established in many countries. Such programs are intended to facilitate early identification of those with psychotic illness and provide state-of-the-art treatment including psychopharmacology, psychosocial intervention, and case management services for patients as well as support and educational interventions for families. In addition, EIP services should be designed to address the challenges of engagement with young people and have close liaisons with community agencies that can facilitate early detection efforts and support recovery with respect to housing, education, employment, and other domains. Standards for such programs are well established [9, 21].There is now strong evidence that EIP services can lead to better results from the treatment of first-episode psychosis [8, 13, 42].

It is very unlikely that a sole clinician can address all the challenges of engagement and treatment of a young person with first-episode psychosis and provide the types of comprehensive care and follow-up that will increase the likelihood of recovery. The EIP programs designed to meet these needs are likely to be located in urban areas. Efforts are underway in some jurisdictions to develop outreach programs and satellite services to less populated regions. It is important to note that even when EIP services are available, nonmental health clinicians play a key role in identification of those with psychotic disorders and provision of necessary services. For instance, family physicians and those working in student health services are often the first point of contact in pathways to EIP [5] and essential in the provision of follow-up care. Development of shared care protocols between EIP services and primary care providers may be

particularly important in determining long-term outcomes. In the absence of specialized EIP services, support from a community psychiatric nurse and access to social care is recommended as a minimum when managing first-episode psychosis.

10.3.3 Choosing the Appropriate Medication

This is a critical decision to be made at the start of the treatment by the clinician-patient dyad and one that raises several clinical challenges. Despite the several hundreds of double-blind randomized controlled studies reporting on the efficacy of several antipsychotics, most of these included patients with a relapsing disease course and not specifically first-episode patients. Most national and international guidelines have based the foundation for treatment recommendations in psychosis on the basis of the extrapolate evidence from "acute on chronic" schizophrenia to FEP. The largest available RCT with a head-to-head comparison of different antipsychotics in FEP (amisulpride, olanzapine, quetiapine, ziprasidone, and haloperidol) is the open-label EUFEST study [30], (n = 498; duration, 52 weeks; primary outcome, treatment discontinuation). Discontinuation for any reasons was higher in the haloperidol group compared to the other drugs (apart from quetiapine). However, symptomatic improvement and hospitalization rates were comparable between all drugs. Haloperidol showed significantly more motor side effects and olanzapine the most weight gain [30]. Specific evidence from 22 first-episode trials comparing 12 second-generation (SGA) vs first-generation (FGA) antipsychotic pairs (n = 2509) is available from one meta-analysis. This meta-analysis showed that SGAs as a group were as effective as FGAs with regard to several outcome dimensions [54]. However, SGAs were superior to FGAs in treatment discontinuation, negative symptom, and cognition change and in inducing less motor side effects. However, SGAs were associated with more metabolic side effects in terms of weight increase

[54].Thus the classification in SGAs and FGAs is from a clinical point of view not very useful and that differences in efficacy are lower than differences in side effects [12]. Moreover, there are only few head-to-head studies that allow a direct comparison of any two antipsychotics; the so-called multiple-treatment meta-analysis (MTMA) offers a proxy method that enables hierarchical ranking of treatments. For schizophrenia, MT meta-analyses are available for acute (both first and multi-episode) schizophrenia [35] and for treatment-resistant patients [45]. The MTMA conducted on acute schizophrenia trials confirms the current view on antipsychotic treatment that subtle efficacy differences can be found but that clearer hierarchies can be defined for side effect profiles [35]. In this MTMA, clozapine, olanzapine, and risperidone were the most effective antipsychotics compared to all other drugs. The translation of this knowledge needs to focus on several aspects that need to be considered in clinical practice:

- In FEP, there is a high likelihood (up to 75%) for response to *any* antipsychotic treatment. As a result, the tolerability of different agents becomes more important in guiding the treatment decision.
- Patients with FEP have a higher likelihood to develop antipsychotic-induced side effect than patients with a chronic disease course. Those patients are highly sensitive to motor and metabolic side effects. Therefore, choosing agents with lower propensity for motor and metabolic side effects is of paramount importance. Various national and international guidelines [27] recommend the following antipsychotics in FEP [amisulpride/aripiprazole/ quetiapine/risperidone/olanzapine/ziprasidone], although some do not recommend the first-line use of olanzapine [33], while others specifically recommend this agent (e.g., Swedish guidelines) due to the higher efficacy.
- Many other side effects (e.g., cardiovascular, hormonal/sexual) may impact the patient's quality of life and result in treatment complications. Therefore, a well-implemented monitoring plan for all side effects is a key element in the antipsychotic treatment of FEP.
- Finally, recovery, however defined, is firmly based on navigating psychosocial challenges. Therefore, psychosocial treatment, including fostering therapeutic alliance, psychoeducation, cognitive behavioral therapy, and family intervention, must be offered to every first-episode patient. A treatment plan must be formulated and implemented on the basis of a shared decision-making process, and, with the patient's permission, family members and significant others should be involved [25].

10.3.4 Treatment Continuation

While 60–75% of patients show at least 25% improvement in baseline PANSS [34] with the first treatment attempts (responders), nearly 25 to 40% do not (nonresponders). A pertinent issue is how long we should wait until switching antipsychotics. This question is clinically highly relevant, but controlled trials in first-episode and chronic schizophrenia patients are lacking. Guidelines vary in the recommended time interval before switching, and the defined ranges are from 2 to 8 weeks [25]. One meta-analysis supports the idea of an early switch, showing in an analysis of 34 studies with 9460 participants that a reduction in PANSS or BPRS below 20% at week 2 predicts a nonresponse at the respective endpoint with a specificity of 86% and a positive predictive value of 90% [46]. An early switch after a maximum of 3 to 4 weeks is increasingly supported in cases of nonresponse.

Interestingly, clozapine, often used as a third-line agent after other SGAs and FGAs, has been shown to be effective in first-episode patients [43]. While clozapine has not been recommended as the first-choice agent, there are no grounds to deny or delay clozapine use in first-episode patients, especially in those who develop treatment resistance.

Another relevant question is how long to treat patients such as Rick for the first episode of psychosis. For this question no clear evidence is available, and guidelines recommend 6 to 12 months of treatment after remission in first-episode patients [27]. It is important that after this period, medication should not be stopped immediately but tapered down slowly over 8 to 12 weeks with a continuous monitoring of psychotic symptoms. There are some concerns that long-term antipsychotic use can lead to loss of brain tissue, but evidence is inconclusive. A summary of structural brain changes seen in first-episode psychosis and chronic schizophrenia is shown in Fig. 10.1.

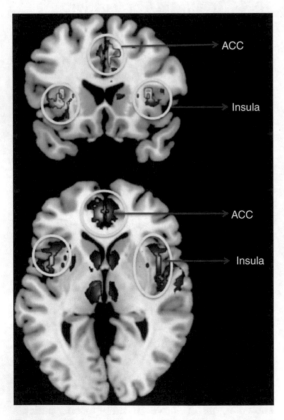

Fig. 10.1 Illustration of regions of significantly decreased gray matter derived from several meta-analyses of structural imaging studies of first-episode schizophrenia [axial view with red clusters] and chronic schizophrenia samples that included a range of episodes [coronal view with blue-green clusters]. All reported coordinates were included. The details of individual meta-analytic studies are published by Palaniyappan et al. [40]. Insula and anterior cingulate cortex (ACC) are the most affected regions that are encircled

10.3.5 Relapse Prevention

Although most patients will show remission of their initial psychotic symptoms, there is a substantial likelihood of relapse [3]. Such relapses, typically defined solely by positive symptoms, may increase the likelihood of a more chronic course of illness [51] and are disruptive of a patient's functional and social recovery. While every effort should be made to avoid relapses, it is also important not to catastrophize their occurrence, and for some patient's they can serve a function in developing acceptance of the nature of their illness and need for treatment [52]. Essential to relapse reduction is an understanding of the factors which increase the risk of their occurrence.

Identifying aspects of an individual's presentation, which may indicate that relapse is imminent or has started, could serve to reduce the negative consequences of a relapse. Such indicators, sometimes referred to as a "relapse signature," can include changes in mood, thought patterns, interaction style, or even simple mannerisms. These signs may be accessible by patients or those close to the person including perceptive clinicians [10, 17]. Relapse signature may sometimes reflect prodromes of the initial episode of psychosis but is challenging to investigate as they can be highly individualized to a patient [37]. There is also increasing interest in the possibility of identifying a risk signature based on biological observations [14, 50], though this has not reached fruition as of yet.

Premature treatment discontinuation is the main predictor of relapse in the first episode [3]. Other predictors of relapse include persistent substance use and higher expressed emotions in the family [3]. It is important to note that nearly 15% of patients with FEP will not have another episode of psychosis, irrespective of the period of antipsychotic treatment (PEPP data; [2]). Nevertheless, at present, there is no reliable method to predict the individuals who will have such a positive outcome. Follow-up studies suggest shorter DUP, and early response to antipsychotics are features that may point to this group, albeit with small predictive value [2].

Table 10.1 Principles of adherence training

Training professionals in medication management
Formulation of a midterm to long-term treatment plan
Optimization of the antipsychotic treatment regime (e.g., minimum required dose, LAI use, or using one pill a day)
Educating patients on treatment management (e.g., how do I get medication, is there someone to help me?)
Integration of persons of trust (e.g., family, friends)
Clearly laid out plans of cooperation of different sectors of the healthcare system

From Gray et al. [22] and Schulz et al. [49]

The overall aim of the maintenance treatment in first-episode schizophrenia is to prevent relapse but also to prevent the development of burdensome side effects that may result in both discontinuation and life-shortening complications. This balance between benefit and risk is the most important issue in the management of schizophrenia.

In this regard, long-acting injectables (LAIs) are beneficial, but the evidence for first-episode patients is low. It is important to note that RCT is an inherently flawed design to compare LAIs with oral drugs, due to extremely high adherence to oral drugs seen in RCTs [23]. A clear superiority emerges in pragmatic trials, supporting the view that LAIs should be offered to those patients who are at risk for discontinuation of treatment and those who prefer a LAI (Table 10.1).

Table 10.1 lists key measures to improve adherence to antipsychotic treatments. Most early intervention centers have implemented these strategies, but all professionals working with schizophrenia should adhere to those strategies.

10.3.6 Risk Assessment and Risk Management

10.3.6.1 Excess Mortality and Side Effects

First-episode schizophrenia is a severe mental illness, and patients are at a crossroad for their further individual development. Moreover, patients face several risks beyond the risks of relapse.

Schizophrenia patients are at high risk for excess mortality resulting in a life expectancy reduction of 15 to 25 years [15] and a 3.5-fold increased risk of dying [39]. Reasons for this excess mortality are somatic comorbidities (e.g., COPD, diabetes, heart diseases) and suicidality. The reasons for the increased risk for somatic comorbidities are manifold, including barriers to care, disease-associated factors, or treatment-associated factors [15]. Antipsychotic-induced weight gain or pathological QTc prolongations may contribute to the excess mortality, and thus, all patients treated with antipsychotics should be monitored regularly. Such programs include regular assessments of weight and BMI, waist circumference, blood pressure, fasting plasma glucose and lipid profiles, blood cell counts, and ECG [25]. If a patient gains more than 7% weight within the first few weeks of treatment, switching antipsychotics [16] has to be considered. There are other strategies to overcome antipsychotic-induced weight gain (e.g., adding metformin), but in first-episode patients, such strategies should be considered as second line. Apart from weight gain and metabolic side effects, sexual side effects (due to prolactin increase), sedation, or cardiac side effects (e.g., QTc prolongation, myocarditis, tachycardia) can impact the outcome of patients. Side effects that impair quality of life (e.g., sexual dysfunction, sedation) may lead to treatment discontinuation, whereas cardiac side effects may result in excess mortality. Motor side effects can occur with every antipsychotic and are related to dopaminergic antagonism. Motor side effects occur frequently in first-episode patients and should be intensively monitored as these effects are frequent and burdensome and remain underdiagnosed in clinical practice [25]. Five different groups of motor side effects can be distinguished comprising acute dystonic reactions, Parkinsonism, and akathisia as early complications, whereas tardive dyskinesia is a late-occurring motor side effect. Finally, neuroleptic malignant syndrome (NMS) is a dangerous condition that can occur with every antipsychotic and that is related to treatment initiation and to rapid dose escalation. From all motor side effects, akathisia is the most frequent side effect and is unfortunately significantly underdiagnosed. Akathisia, but also other motor side effects, area burdensome, are a major contributor to treatment discontinuation and can lead to suicidality. Parkinsonism and acute dystonia need a switch to an antipsychotic with fewer motor side effects and can be treated with anticholinergics. Akathisia can be also managed with an antipsychotic switch or with the application of propranolol.

Drug abuse Drug abuse occurs frequently in first-episode schizophrenia, and the highest prevalence rates are reported for tobacco and alcohol dependency. Tobacco abuse contributes to the excess mortality and, thus, evidence-based strategies for smoking cessation, including nicotine replacement treatment or the application of varenicline [7, 26, 44]. Another issue is cannabis abuse in first-episode schizophrenia, especially in the younger patients [32]. Cannabis abuse or dependency results in more severe symptoms and is a high-risk factor for relapse. One meta-analysis confirmed the relationship between cannabis use and hospitalization, relapse, and positive symptoms and showed that cannabis discontinuation can reduce this risk to the level of nonusers [48]. Therefore, encouraging cannabis-dependent FEP to enter a specific cannabis reduction/abstinence program is likely to be beneficial.

Suicidality Schizophrenia is associated with a high risk for suicide, and it is estimated that 5–15% commit suicide [26], with this risk being especially high in patients in early stages of the disorders [41] (Table 10.2).

Patients with first-episode schizophrenia should be screened for suicidality and depressive symptoms on a regular basis (see Table 10.2). To

Table 10.2 Risk factors for suicidality in first- episode psychosis

Modifiable factors	Static factors
Severe hallucinations	Male gender
Motor side effects (especially akathisia)	A high premorbid IQ
	Acute phase of the early onset illness
Depressive symptoms	
Lack of social support	Recent discharge from inpatient treatment

From Hasan et al. [26]

screen for and to quantify depressive symptoms, the Calgary Depression Scale for schizophrenia should be used. Optimization of treatment and hospitalization are main factors for the management of suicidality [26].

10.3.7 Non-pharmacological Options

As described before, antipsychotics are highly effective and should be offered to every patient with first-episode psychosis. However, just the prescription of antipsychotics does not fulfill the needs of the patients such as Rick. Every patient with a first-episode psychosis should have access to cognitive behavioral therapy (CBT) and family interventions. The effect sizes for CBT and family intervention are high, especially in terms of relapse prevention. The recently published "2-Year Outcomes From the NIMH RAISE Early Treatment Program" highlighted that patients with first-episode psychosis need guideline-based individualized antipsychotic treatment, family psychoeducation, resilience-focused individual therapy, as well as supported employment and education [31]. These five aspects provide a fully integrated care for first-episode psychosis.

10.4 Summary of Approach

One common theme to successfully mitigating the challenges raised above is the use of tools that allow us to quantify severity, monitor response, and measure side effect burden in psychosis. Measurement-based care (MBC) is a practice framework that enables clinical decisions to be based on routinely collected client data during treatment. MBC approaches have empirical support in many fields of medical practice. With the introduction of specific tools in DSM-5, a specific emphasis has been provided to the use of MBC in routine practice. Using MBC framework greatly enhances the overall outcomes in depressed subjects, compared to providing the same treatments but without periodic measurements. Analogous to pragmatic RCTs that purport to make trials close to real-world practice, MBC enables our clinical

Table 10.3 A toolkit measurement-based care in first-episode psychosis

PQ-16 for suspected prodrome
PANSS-8, Clinical Global Impression (severity), and Calgary Depression Scale in FEP
Metabolic monitoring protocol (3-monthly)
Recording weight and waistline (every month for first 3 months, then 3-monthly)
SOFAS along with weeks of full/part-time employment and independent living
Compliance rating for antipsychotics
Self-report checklist for adverse effects and substance use

practice to move closer to the trials, thus enabling patients to achieve the incremental benefits seen when they participate in trials.

The use of MBC in EIP can help clinicians and patients to make informed decisions about antipsychotic choice, dose changes, treatment switching, and compliance. In addition, it can also provide objective tools for patient and family education and provide a basis for evaluation of the clinical program. Most MBC initiatives, including the scales promoted by DSM working groups, focus on short instruments that can be used both at baseline and to assess change over the course, mostly based on self-report to reduce measurement burden [18]. We provide a minimal set toolkit (Table 10.3) that can be used for MBC in EIP practice, which can help us navigate a number of conundrums if used in conjunction with evidence-based recommendations discussed above.

Disclosure Statement Alkomiet Hasan has received paid speakership by Desitin, Otsuka and Janssen Cilag. He was a member of the Roche, Lundbeck and Janssen-Cilag Advisory Board. Lena Palaniyappan has received paid speakership by Otsuka / Lundbeck. Other authors declare no conflicts.

References

1. Addington D, Addington J, Maticka-Tyndale E. Assessing depression in schizophrenia: the Calgary Depression Scale. Br J Psychiatry Suppl. 1993;(22):39–44.
2. Alvarez-Jimenez M, Gleeson JF, Henry LP, Harrigan SM, Harris MG, Amminger GP, McGorry PD. Prediction of a single psychotic episode: a 7.5-year, prospective study in first-episode psychosis. Schizophr Res. 2011;125(2–3):236–46. https://doi.org/10.1016/j.schres. 2010.10.020. S0920-9964(10)01595-1 [pii].
3. Alvarez-Jimenez M, Priede A, Hetrick SE, Bendall S, Killackey E, Parker AG, McGorry PD, Gleeson JF. Risk factors for relapse following treatment for first episode psychosis: a systematic review and meta-analysis of longitudinal studies. Schizophr Res. 2012;139(1–3):116–28. https://doi.org/10.1016/j.schres.2012. 05.007. S0920-9964(12)00259-9 [pii].
4. American Psychiatric Association. Diagnostic and statistical manual of mental disorders. Washington, DC: American Psychiatric Association; 1994.
5. Anderson KK, Fuhrer R, Malla AK. The pathways to mental health care of first-episode psychosis patients: a systematic review. Psychol Med. 2010;40(10):1585–97. https://doi.org/10.1017/S0033291710000371. S0033291710000371 [pii].
6. Andreasen NC, Carpenter WT Jr, Kane JM, Lasser RA, Marder SR, Weinberger DR. Remission in schizophrenia: proposed criteria and rationale for consensus. Am J Psychiatry. 2005;162(3):441–9.
7. Anthenelli RM, Benowitz NL, West R, St Aubin L, McRae T, Lawrence D, Ascher J, Russ C, Krishen A, Evins AE. Neuropsychiatric safety and efficacy of varenicline, bupropion, and nicotine patch in smokers with and without psychiatric disorders (EAGLES): a double-blind, randomised, placebo-controlled clinical trial. Lancet. 2016;387(10037):2507–20. https://doi.org/10.1016/S0140-6736(16)30272-0. S0140-6736(16)30272-0 [pii].
8. Bertelsen M, Jeppesen P, Petersen L, Thorup A, Ohlenschlaeger J, le Quach P, Christensen TØ, Krarup G, Jørgensen P, Nordentoft M. Five-year follow-up of a randomized multicenter trial of intensive early intervention vs standard treatment for patients with a first episode of psychotic illness: the OPUS trial. Arch Gen Psychiatry. 2008;65(7):762–71.
9. Bertolote J, McGorry P. Early intervention and recovery for young people with early psychosis: consensus statement. Br J Psychiatry Suppl. 2005;48:s116–9. https://doi.org/10.1192/bjp.187.48. s116. 187/48/s116 [pii].
10. Birchwood M, Spencer E, McGovern D. Schizophrenia: early warning signs. Adv Psychiatr Treat. 2000;6:93–101.
11. Cannon TD, Yu C, Addington J, Bearden CE, Cadenhead KS, Cornblatt BA, Heinssen R, Jeffries CD, Mathalon DH, McGlashan TH, Perkins DO, Seidman LJ, Tsuang MT, Walker EF, Woods SW, Kattan MW. An individualized risk calculator for research in prodromal psychosis. Am J Psychiatry. 2016;173(10):980–8. https://doi.org/10.1176/appi. ajp.2016.15070890.
12. Correll CU, De Hert M. Antipsychotics for acute schizophrenia: making choices. Lancet. 2013;382(9896):919–20. https://doi.org/10.1016/S0140-6736(13)61032-6. S0140-6736(13)61032-6 [pii].
13. Craig TK, Garety P, Power P, Rahaman N, Colbert S, Fornells-Ambrojo M, Dunn G. The Lambeth early

onset (LEO) team: randomized controlled trial of the effectiveness of specialized care for early psychosis. Br Med J. 2004;329(7474):1067.

14. Cropley VL, Pantelis C. Using longitudinal imaging to map the 'relapse signature' of schizophrenia and other psychoses. Epidemiol Psychiatr Sci. 2014;23(3):219–25. https://doi.org/10.1017/S2045796014000341. S2045796014000341 [pii].

15. De Hert M, Correll CU, Bobes J, Cetkovich-Bakmas M, Cohen D, Asai I, Detraux J, Gautam S, Möller HJ, Ndetei DM, Newcomer JW, Uwakwe R, Leucht S. Physical illness in patients with severe mental disorders. I. Prevalence, impact of medications and disparities in health care. World Psychiatry. 2011;10(1):52–77.

16. De Hert M, Dekker JM, Wood D, Kahl KG, Holt RI, Moller HJ. Cardiovascular disease and diabetes in people with severe mental illness position statement from the European Psychiatric Association (EPA), supported by the European Association for the Study of Diabetes (EASD) and the European Society of Cardiology (ESC). Eur Psychiatry. 2009;24(6):412–24. https://doi.org/10.1016/j.eurpsy.2009.01.005. S0924-9338(09)00017-0 [pii].

17. Early Psychosis Guidelines Writing Group, & and EPPIC National Support Program. Australian clinical guidelines for early psychosis. 2nd ed. Melbourne: Orygen, The National Centre of Excellence in Mental Health; 2016.

18. Fortney JC, Unutzer J, Wrenn G, Pyne JM, Smith GR, Schoenbaum M, Harbin HT. A tipping point for measurement-based care. Psychiatr Serv. 2017;68(2):179–88. https://doi.org/10.1176/appi.ps.201500439.

19. Fusar-Poli P, Bonoldi I, Yung AR, Borgwardt S, Kempton MJ, Valmaggia L, Barale F, Caverzasi E, McGuire P. Predicting psychosis: meta-analysis of transition outcomes in individuals at high clinical risk. Arch Gen Psychiatry. 2012;69(3):220–9. https://doi.org/10.1001/archgenpsychiatry.2011.1472. 69/3/220 [pii].

20. Fusar-Poli P, Borgwardt S, Bechdolf A, Addington J, Riecher-Rossler A, Schultze-Lutter F, Keshavan M, Wood S, Ruhrmann S, Seidman LJ, Valmaggia L, Cannon T, Velthorst E, De Haan L, Cornblatt B, Bonoldi I, Birchwood M, McGlashan T, Carpenter W, McGorry P, Klosterkötter J, McGuire P, Yung A. The psychosis high-risk state: a comprehensive state-of-the-art review. JAMA Psychiat. 2013;70(1):107–20. https://doi.org/10.1001/jamapsychiatry.2013.269. 1392281 [pii].

21. Government of Ontario. Early psychosis intervention program standards. Toronto: Services Ontario; 2011.

22. Gray R, Wykes T, Edmonds M, Leese M, Gournay K. Effect of a medication management training package for nurses on clinical outcomes for patients with schizophrenia: cluster randomised controlled trial. Br J Psychiatry. 2004;185:157–62. https://doi.org/10.1192/bjp.185.2.157. 185/2/157 [pii].

23. Haddad PM, Kishimoto T, Correll CU, Kane JM. Ambiguous findings concerning potential advan-tages of depot antipsychotics: in search of clinical relevance. Curr Opin Psychiatry. 2015;28(3):216–21. https://doi.org/10.1097/YCO.0000000000000160.

24. Haro JM, Kamath SA, Ochoa S, Novick D, Rele K, Fargas A, Rodríguez MJ, Rele R, Orta J, Kharbeng A, Araya S, Gervin M, Alonso J, Mavreas V, Lavrentzou E, Liontos N, Gregor K Jones PB. (2003). The clinical global impression-schizophrenia scale: a simple instrument to measure the diversity of symptoms present in schizo-phrenia. Acta Psychiatr Scand Suppl. 2003;416:16–23. https://doi.org/10.1034/j.1600-0447.107.s416.5.x.

25. Hasan A, Falkai P, Wobrock T, Lieberman J, Glenthoj B, Gattaz WF, Thibaut F, Moller HJ. World Federation of Societies of biological psychiatry (WFSBP) guide-lines for biological treatment of schizophrenia, part 1: update 2012 on the acute treatment of schizophrenia and the management of treatment resistance. World J Biol Psychiatry. 2012;13(5):318–78. https://doi.org/10.3109/15622975.2012.696143.

26. Hasan A, Falkai P, Wobrock T, Lieberman J, Glenthoj B, Gattaz WF, Thibaut F, Moller HJ, World Federation of Societies of Biological Psychiatry (WFSBP) Guidelines for Biological Treatment of Schizophrenia. Part 3: Update 2015 Management of special circumstances: Depression, Suicidality, sub-stance use disorders and pregnancy and lactation. World J Biol Psychiatry. 2015;16(3):142–70. https://doi.org/10.3109/15622975.2015.1009163.

27. Hasan A, Wobrock T, Gaebel W, Janssen B, Zielasek J, Falkai P. [National and international schizophrenia guidelines. Update 2013 regarding recommendations about antipsychotic pharmacotherapy]. Nervenarzt. 2013;84(11):1359–60, 1362–54, 1366–58. https://doi.org/10.1007/s00115-013-3913-6.

28. Ising HK, Veling W, Loewy RL, Rietveld MW, Rietdijk J, Dragt S, Klaassen RM, Nieman DH, Wunderink L, Linszen DH, van der Gaag M. The validity of the 16-item version of the Prodromal Questionnaire (PQ-16) to screen for ultra high risk of developing psychosis in the general help-seeking population. Schizophr Bull. 2012;38(6):1288–96. https://doi.org/10.1093/schbul/sbs068. sbs068 [pii].

29. Jaaskelainen E, Juola P, Hirvonen N, McGrath JJ, Saha S, Isohanni M, Veijola J, Miettunen J. A sys-tematic review and meta-analysis of recovery in schizophrenia. Schizophr Bull. 2013;39(6):1296–306. https://doi.org/10.1093/schbul/sbs130. sbs130 [pii].

30. Kahn RS, Fleischhacker WW, Boter H, Davidson M, Vergouwe Y, Keet IP, Gheorghe MD, Rybakowski JK, Galderisi S, Libiger J, Hummer M, Dollfus S, López-Ibor JJ, Hranov LG, Gaebel W, Peuskens J, Lindefors N, Riecher-Rössler A, Grobbee DE. Effectiveness of antipsychotic drugs in first-episode schizophrenia and schizophreniform disorder: an open randomised clini-cal trial. Lancet. 2008;371(9618):1085–97. https://doi.org/10.1016/S0140-6736(08)60486-9. S0140-6736(08)60486-9 [pii].

31. Kane JM, Robinson DG, Schooler NR, Mueser KT, Penn DL, Rosenheck RA, Addington J, Brunette

MF, Correll CU, Estroff SE, Marcy P, Robinson J, Meyer-Kalos PS, Gottlieb JD, Glynn SM, Lynde DW, Pipes R, Kurian BT, Miller AL, Azrin ST, Goldstein AB, Severe JB, Lin H, Sint KJ, John M, Heinssen RK. Comprehensive Versus Usual Community Care for First-Episode Psychosis: 2-year outcomes from the NIMH RAISE early treatment program. Am J Psychiatry. 2016;173(4):362–72. https://doi.org/10.1176/appi.ajp.2015.15050632.

32. Koskinen J, Lohonen J, Koponen H, Isohanni M, Miettunen J. Rate of cannabis use disorders in clinical samples of patients with schizophrenia: a meta-analysis. Schizophr Bull. 2010;36(6):1115–30. https://doi.org/10.1093/schbul/sbp031. sbp031 [pii].

33. Kreyenbuhl J, Buchanan RW, Dickerson FB, Dixon LB. The schizophrenia patient outcomes research team (PORT): updated treatment recommendations 2009. Schizophr Bull. 2010;36(1):94–103. https://doi.org/10.1093/schbul/sbp130. sbp130 [pii].

34. Leucht S. Measurements of response, remission, and recovery in schizophrenia and examples for their clinical application. J Clin Psychiatry. 2014;75(Suppl 1):8–14. https://doi.org/10.4088/JCP.13049su1c.02.

35. Leucht S, Cipriani A, Spineli L, Mavridis D, Orey D, Richter F, Samara M, Barbui C, Engel RR, Geddes JR, Kissling W, Stapf MP, Lässig B, Salanti G, Davis JM. Comparative efficacy and tolerability of 15 antipsychotic drugs in schizophrenia: a multiple-treatments meta-analysis. Lancet. 2013;382(9896):951–62. https://doi.org/10.1016/S0140-6736(13)60733-3. S0140-6736(13)60733-3 [pii].

36. National Collaborating Centre for Mental Health. Psychosis and schizophrenia in adults: the NICE guideline on treatment and management. London: National Institute for Health and Care Excellent; 2014.

37. Norman RM, Malla AK. Prodromal symptoms of relapse in schizophrenia: a review. Schizophr Bull. 1995;21(4):527–39.

38. Norman RM, Manchanda R, Malla AK, Windell D, Harricharan R, Northcott S. Symptom and functional outcomes for a 5 year early intervention program for psychoses. Schizophr Res. 2011;129(2–3):111–5. https://doi.org/10.1016/j.schres.2011.04.006. S0920-9964(11)00212-X [pii].

39. Olfson M, Gerhard T, Huang C, Crystal S, Stroup TS. Premature mortality among adults with schizophrenia in the United States. JAMA Psychiat. 2015;72(12):1172–81. https://doi.org/10.1001/jamapsychiatry.2015.1737. 2466831 [pii].

40. Palaniyappan L, White TP, Liddle PF. The concept of salience network dysfunction in schizophrenia: from neuroimaging observations to therapeutic opportunities. Curr Top Med Chem. 2012;12(21):2324–38.

41. Palmer BA, Pankratz VS, Bostwick JM. The lifetime risk of suicide in schizophrenia: a reexamination. Arch Gen Psychiatry. 2005;62(3):247–53. https://doi.org/10.1001/archpsyc.62.3.247. 62/3/247 [pii].

42. Petersen L, Jeppesen P, Thorup A, Abel MB, Ohlenschlaeger J, Christensen TO, Krarup G, Jørgensen P, Nordentoft M. A randomised multicentre trial of integrated versus standard treatment for patients with a first episode of psychotic illness. Br Med J. 2005;331(7517):602.

43. Remington G, Agid O, Foussias G, Hahn M, Rao N, Sinyor M. Clozapine's role in the treatment of first-episode schizophrenia. Am J Psychiatry. 2013;170(2):146–51. https://doi.org/10.1176/appi.ajp.2012.12060778. 1566895 [pii].

44. Ruther T, Bobes J, De Hert M, Svensson TH, Mann K, Batra A, Gorwood P, Moller HJ. EPA guidance on tobacco dependence and strategies for smoking cessation in people with mental illness. Eur Psychiatry. 2014;29(2):65–82. https://doi.org/10.1016/j.eurpsy.2013.11.002. S0924-9338(13)00443-4 [pii].

45. Samara MT, Dold M, Gianatsi M, Nikolakopoulou A, Helfer B, Salanti G, Leucht S. Efficacy, acceptability, and tolerability of antipsychotics in treatment-resistant schizophrenia: a network meta-analysis. JAMA Psychiat. 2016;73(3):199–210. https://doi.org/10.1001/jamapsychiatry.2015.2955. 2488040 [pii].

46. Samara MT, Leucht C, Leeflang MM, Anghelescu IG, Chung YC, Crespo-Facorro B, Elkis H, Hatta K, Giegling I, Kane JM, Kayo M, Lambert M, Lin CH, Möller HJ, Pelayo-Terán JM, Riedel M, Rujescu D, Schimmelmann BG, Serretti A, Correll CU, Leucht S. Early improvement as a predictor of later response to antipsychotics in schizophrenia: a diagnostic test review. Am J Psychiatry. 2015;172(7):617–29. https://doi.org/10.1176/appi.ajp.2015.14101329. 10.1176/appi.ajp.2015.14101329.

47. Schmidt SJ, Schultze-Lutter F, Schimmelmann BG, Maric NP, Salokangas RK, Riecher-Rossler A, van der Gaag M, Meneghelli A, Nordentoft M, Marshall M, Morrison A, Raballo A, Klosterkötter J, Ruhrmann S. EPA guidance on the early intervention in clinical high risk states of psychoses. Eur Psychiatry. 2015;30(3):388–404. https://doi.org/10.1016/j.eurpsy.2015.01.013. S0924-9338(15)00057-7 [pii].

48. Schoeler T, Monk A, Sami MB, Klamerus E, Foglia E, Brown R, Camuri G, Altamura AC, Murray R, Bhattacharyya S. Continued versus discontinued cannabis use in patients with psychosis: a systematic review and meta-analysis. Lancet Psychiatry. 2016;3(3):215–25. https://doi.org/10.1016/S2215-0366(15)00363-6. S2215-0366(15)00363-6 [pii].

49. Schulz M, Gray R, Spiekermann A, Abderhalden C, Behrens J, Driessen M. Adherence therapy following an acute episode of schizophrenia: a multi-centre randomised controlled trial. Schizophr Res. 2013;146(1–3):59–63. https://doi.org/10.1016/j.schres.2013.01.028. S0920-9964(13)00066-2 [pii].

50. Schwarz E, Guest PC, Steiner J, Bogerts B, Bahn S. Identification of blood-based molecular signatures for prediction of response and relapse in schizophrenia patients. Transl Psychiatry. 2012;2:e82. https://doi.org/10.1038/tp.2012.3. tp20123 [pii].

51. Wiersma D, Nienhuis FJ, Slooff CJ, Giel R. Natural course of schizophrenic disorders: a 15-year followup of a Dutch incidence cohort. Schizophr Bull. 1998;24(1):75–85.
52. Windell DL, Norman R, Lal S, Malla A. Subjective experiences of illness recovery in individuals treated for first-episode psychosis. Soc Psychiatry Psychiatr Epidemiol. 2015;50(7):1069–77. https://doi.org/10.1007/s00127-014-1006-x.
53. Young RC, Biggs JT, Ziegler VE, Meyer DA. A rating scale for mania: reliability, validity and sensitivity. Br J Psychiatry. 1978;133:429–35.
54. Zhang JP, Gallego JA, Robinson DG, Malhotra AK, Kane JM, Correll CU. Efficacy and safety of individual second-generation vs. first-generation antipsychotics in first-episode psychosis: a systematic review and meta-analysis. Int J Neuropsychopharmacol. 2013;16(6):1205–18. https://doi.org/10.1017/S1461145712001277. S1461145712001277 [pii].

The Role of Clozapine in Treatment-Resistant Schizophrenia

Kuppuswami Shivakumar, Shabbir Amanullah, Ranga Shivakumar, Kevin Saroka, Nicolas Rouleau, and Nirosha J. Murugan

11.1 Case History

Mr. X is a 35-year-old male with a DSM-5 diagnosis schizophrenia. During his first episode of psychosis which started at the age of 18, he exhibited positive symptoms including disordered thought process, disorganization, bizarre behavior, and agitation. During his initial assessment,

K. Shivakumar, MD, MPH, MRCPsych(UK), FRCPC (✉) • R. Shivakumar, MD, MRCP, FRCPC, ABIM • K. Saroka, BSc, MA, PhD
Department of Psychiatry, Northern Ontario School of Medicine Psychiatry Department,
Sudbury, ON, Canada
e-mail: kshivakumar@hsnsudbury.ca; rshivakumar@hsnsudbury.ca; ks.saroka@hsnsudbury.ca

S. Amanullah, MD, DPM, FRCPsych(UK), CCT,FRCPC
University of Western Ontario, Woodstock General Hospital University of Western Ontario, Woodstock, ON, Canada

N. Rouleau, Ph.D
Department of Biomedical Engineering, Initiative for Neural Science, Disease and Engineering (INScide) at Tufts University, Science and Engineering Complex (SEC), Medford, MA, USA
e-mail: nicolas.rouleau@tufts.edu

N. J. Murugan, Ph.D
Allen Discovery Center at Tufts; Tufts Center for Regenerative and Developmental Biology,
Science and Engineering Complex (SEC),
Medford, MA, USA
e-mail: nirosha.murugan@tufts.edu

his baseline symptom severity was assessed using PANSS (Positive and Negative Symptom Scale) on which he scored 115 indicating severe psychosis. In addition to his positive symptoms, he also exhibited some negative symptoms including apathy, amotivation, and lack of interest. He was admitted to a psychiatric hospital and treated with a trial of second-generation antipsychotic agent. He responded well to the medication trial, and after his symptom resolution, he was discharged back to the community with a follow-up through the First-Episode Psychosis Program. For the first 18 months of his treatment, he engaged poorly with the team and had a relapse of his symptoms which were only secured following an involuntary admission to the local hospital. During this admission he showed almost similar symptoms to his first presentation. During his second cause of admission, he was commenced on a trial of second-generation atypical long-acting injection. He also received to have relapse prevention work and medication monitoring support; however his symptoms were not adequately controlled. Despite being on the long-acting injection, he experienced symptoms including paranoia, suspiciousness, positive symptoms, and some negative symptoms. After discussion with the patient, family, and the team, it was agreed that he would be a suitable candidate for a trial of clozapine. Treatment was initiated at 25 mg per day and gradually titrated up to 450 mg for which he

© Springer International Publishing AG, part of Springer Nature 2018
K. Shivakumar, S. Amanullah (eds.), *Complex Clinical Conundrums in Psychiatry*,
https://doi.org/10.1007/978-3-319-70311-4_11

showed marked improvement in his psychotic symptoms and became calm and cooperative.

11.2 Questions

11.2.1 What Are the Current National Guidelines Available in the Treatment of Schizophrenia?

There are five clinical guidelines available in the management of schizophrenia including (1) Canadian Clinical Guidelines for Schizophrenia developed in 2017, (2) American Practice Guideline for the Treatment of Patients with Schizophrenia, (3) The UK Guidelines (National Collaborating Centre for Mental Health), and (4) National Institute of Clinical Guidelines (Table 11.1).

11.2.2 What Is the History of Clozapine?

In 1959 a Swiss pharmaceutical company Wander Laboratories first identified clozapine, and in 1971 clozapine became available in Europe. However, in 1975 clozapine was withdrawn by the pharmaceutical company due to serious side effects in a Finnish population. The first case of agranulocytosis was in Finland in 1975 followed by several cases of clozapine-induced agranulocytosis. But later clozapine was gradually reintroduced with strict monitoring guidelines. In early to mid-1980s after the approval of FDA, 1990 clozapine became available in the USA followed by the rest of the world. Now almost 50 years gone, clozaril remains a drug of choice for treatment-resistant schizophrenia.

11.2.3 What Is the Psychopharmacology and the Mechanism of Action of Clozapine?

Clozapine belongs to the group of tricyclic antipsychotics known as the dibenzodiazepines. The actual chemical structure is quite similar to a typical antipsychotic loxapine with some minor differences. Clozapine's mechanism of action is described in Table 11.2.

A number of hypotheses have been proposed to explain how clozapine can reduce positive

Table 11.1 Currently available National Clinical Guidelines

Country	
Canadian Guidelines	Developed by the Canadian Psychiatric Association in 2017 and provides evidence-based recommendations for the treatment of schizophrenia and schizophrenia spectrum disorders Focuses on assessment for all phases, psychotherapy, pharmacotherapy, psychosocial interventions, and service delivery. Recommendations are also provided as guidance to physicians and patients
American Guidelines	Developed by the American Psychiatric Association Focuses on treatment formulation, therapeutic alliances, treatment setting and housing options, social issues in treating schizophrenia
United Kingdom Guidelines	Developed by the National Collaborating Centre for mental health Focuses on recommendations for prevention and promoting recovery as well Includes recommendations for research topics to guide future guidelines and improve patient care
Australian Guidelines.	Developed by Royal Australian new Zealand College of Psychiatrists in 2016. The guideline provides recommendations for the clinical management of schizophrenia and related disorders. It takes a holistic approach in providing care for people with schizophrenia focusing on diagnosis, symptom relief, and optimal recovery of social functioning

symptoms. Although clozapine has been used for the last 50 years since it was discovered, its exact mechanism of action is unknown; however there are several hypotheses that have been proposed to explain how clozapine can reduce psychotic symptoms without producing extrapyramidal symptoms:

1. It has low propensity to cause extrapyramidal side effects (EPS).
2. Low percentage of D2 receptor occupancy may explain its low rate of EPS.
3. It has fast off D2 receptor dissociation from the D2 receptors which could give rise to its low occurrence of EPS and efficacy for severe psychosis.
4. High binding affinity to the 5-HT2A receptors.

11.2.4 What Are Some Known Side Effects Associated with Clozapine?

11.2.4.1 Side Effects of Clozapine
The most common drug aversive effects are sedation, dizziness, syncope, tachycardia, ECG changes, nausea, and vomiting. Other common adverse effects include fatigue, weight gain, constipation, various anticholinergic effects, and muscle weakness.

11.2.5 What Are the Hematological Side Effects Associated with Clozapine Therapy?

11.2.5.1 Agranulocytosis
Although it is a rare side effect, it is of a serious concern. Patients on clozaril can have either granulocytopenia or agranulocytosis. Granulocytopenia is defined as a granulocyte count less than $<1.5 \times 10^9$/L. Agranulocytosis is defined as less than $<0.5 \times 10^9$/L. Approximately 88% of agranulocytosis occurs during the first 26 weeks of therapy, but some have occurred years after clozapine use. Age can be an impor-

Table 11.2 Clozapine mechanism of action

Clozapine mechanism of action
Dopamine receptors – D2 antagonists bind to D2 receptors approximately 100 times less than haloperidol. At the normal therapeutic doses, it occupies only 40–60% of D2 receptors
Serotonin receptors – Binds to 5-HT2A, B, and C receptors an d has high affinity for 5-HT5 receptors and also acts as a partial agonist at 5-HT1A receptors
Muscarinic receptors – Strongly binds to M1 receptors and causes well-known side effects such as sedation, constipation, and drowsiness
Adrenergic receptors – Strongly binds to α 1 adrenergic receptors and likely to contributes it's sedative, cardiac side effects including orthostatic hypotension
Histamine receptors – Very strong binding capacity to H1 histamine receptors and likely to contribute to its side effects including increase in appetite, weight gain, possibly metabolic side effects
Glutamate receptors – Does not bind directly, but clozapine main metabolite (nor clozapine) is an M1 agonist
GABA receptors – Low affinity toward GABA receptors

tant factor as the risk of neutropenia and agranulocytosis increases with age. It is important to note that the development of agranulocytosis and granulocytopenia does not seem to be dose-dependent. The exact mechanism of clozapine-induced agranulocytosis is not clear. There is no convincing evidence to suggest direct toxicity of clozapine or its metabolite, n-dimethyl clozapine. The exact mechanism ofclozapine-induced agranulocytosis is unknown, but several theories have been proposed including genetic and some complex multistep immunological phenomenon involving HLA (human leukocyte antigen class I and II). Unlike individuals who are younger in age, agranulocytosis is about 10–16 times more likely to develop in individuals who are older [1].

Given its severe risk of causing a medical emergency, it should be stopped immediately if these symptoms occur. The following chart summarizes the course of action during clozapine therapy; however it may vary according to the jurisdiction.

Treatment	Course of Action
BASELINE Hematological requirements for initiation of treatment: • WBC >= 3.5x10^9/L • ANC >= 2.0x10^9	• Begin treatment with C lozapine
GREEN If WBC >= 3.5x10^9/L and >= 2.0x10^9.L	• Continue treatment with Clozapine • Monitor patient as follows: • Weekly for the first 26 weeks • Every 2 weeks for the next 26 weeks • Every 4 weeks therafter
FLASHING YELLOW • A single fall or sum of falls in WBC count of 3.0x10^9/L or more is measured in the last four weeks, reaching a value of <4.0x10^9 • A single fall or sum of falls in ANC of 1.5 x10^9/L or more is measured in the last four weeks, reaching a value of '2.5 x10^9/L	• Patient should be evaluated immediately • Check WBC count and ANC twice weekly • Continue treatment with Clozapine
YELLOW If any of the following: • WBC count falls to between 2.0 x10^9/L and 3.5 x10^9/L • ANC falls to between 1.5 x10^9/L and 2.0 x10^9/L	• Patient should be evaluated immediately • Check WBC count and ANC twice weekly • Continue treatment with Clozapine
RED If any of the following: • Total WBC count falls to below 2.0 x10^9/L • ANC falls to below 1.5 x10^9/L	• Immediately stop treatment with Clozapine and confirm results within 24 hours • Patient must be closely monitored • Attention must be paid to any flu-like symptoms or other symptoms which might suggest infection • Clozapine therapy must NOT be resumed if results are confirmed and the patient should be assigned a non-challengeable status
CRITICAL If any of the following: • WBC count continues to fall below 1.0 x10^9/L • ANC drops below 0.5 x10^9/L	• Place the patient in protective isolation with close observation • Physician must watch for signs of infection

Modified from AA Pharma [2]

11.2.6 What Are the Cardiovascular Side Effects Associated with Clozapine Therapy?

The most common cardiovascular side effects include myocarditis, cardiomyopathy, pericarditis, myocardial effusion, heart failure, myocardial infarction, and mitral valve insufficiency.

11.2.6.1 Myocarditis

The association between clozapine and myocarditis was first studied by Kilian et al. in 1999 [3]. Myocarditis is a rare but fatal side effect with an incidence rate of ~0.06%. But some other studies have shown different estimates, for example, some Canadian studies have shown that fatal myocarditis was estimated to be 1 in 12,500 and in the USA 1 in 67,000 [4]. It can be fatal particularly during the first month of therapy but extending up to 60 days. It is an inflammatory disease of the myocardium with a wide range of clinical presentation [5]. It is believed to be a hypersensitivity reaction also unrelated to dose. Table 11.3 describes the monitoring protocol and the symptoms of clozapine-induced myocarditis (Table 11.4).

It is important to note that many of these symptoms occur in patients on clozapine not developing myocarditis; however the absence

Table 11.3 Monitoring protocol for clozapine-induced myocarditis

Time/condition	Signs/symptoms to monitor
Baseline	Pulse, blood pressure, temperature, respiratory rate Full blood count (FBC) C-reactive protein (CRP) Troponin Echocardiography
Daily	Pulse, blood pressure, temperature, respiratory rate Ask about: Chest pain, fever, cough, shortness of breath, exercise capacity
Ask patients for	Chest pain, fever, cough, shortness of breath, vomiting, nausea, myalgia, headache, sweatiness, urinary discomfort or frequency
On days 7, 14, 21, and 28	C-reactive protein (CRP) Troponin I or T Full blood count (FBC) Electrocardiogram (ECG)
If patient develops signs and symptoms of unidentified illness OR HR > = 120 bpm or increased by >30 bpm OR CRP 50–100 mg/L OR mild elevation in troponin (<= 2 ULN)	Continue clozapine with increased monitoring Check troponin and CRP daily and monitor patient for developing illness until features normalize
If the patient shows troponin >2 ULN OR CRP > 100 mg/L	Cease clozapine and repeat echocardiography Consult a cardiologist or an internist

Table adapted from Refs. [6, 7]

Table 11.4 Clinical symptoms of clozapine-induced myocarditis

Clinical symptoms of clozapine-related myocarditis:
1. Malaise and fatigue
2. Dyspnea with increased respiratory rate
3. Chest pain
4. Flu-like symptoms
5. Fever
6. Peripheral eosinophilia
7. Sinus tachycardia
8. Drug rash [8]
9. Hypotension
10. ECG changes including ST depression
11. Enlarged heart on radiography or echo
12. Eosinophilia

of these symptoms does not rule out myocarditis. The suggested monitoring protocol for clozapine-induced myocarditis was proposed by Ronaldson et al. [6].

If patients develop tachycardia at rest, chest pain, shortness of breath, or arrhythmia, the patient should be investigated, and clozapine should be discontinued. Studies have shown that re-challenge can be successfully completed using beta-blockers and angiotensin-converting enzymes, but recurrence is possible [9, 10, 11, 12, 13, 14].

11.2.6.2   Cardiomyopathy

Clozapine-induced cardiomyopathies are very rare, but nonetheless dangerous side effects with an incidence rate of 0.02–0.1% have been reported [15]. Cardiomyopathy should be suspected in patients if they show symptoms of palpitation, chest pain, syncope, sweating, decreased exercise capacity, or breathing difficulties. Because the mortality rate is up to 17.9% and there is an increased risk of sudden death, clozapine should be ceased, and the patient should be given a referred for further assessment [3].

11.2.7 What Are Some Other Side Effects Associated with Clozapine Therapy?

11.2.7.1 Sialorrhea or Hypersalivation

Sialorrhea, or hypersalivation, is a most troublesome side effect in clozapine-treated patients. It is a very common (up to 31% of patients). The pathophysiology of clozapine-induced hypersalivation is not clear; however suggested mechanisms include M4 agonism, adrenergic alpha-2 antagonism, and inhibition of the swallowing reflex [16].

11.2.7.2 Seizures

A clozapine-induced seizure is a known risk, and it may occur at any time [17]. It depends on the total daily dose (traditionally more than 600 mg/day), plasma levels of clozapine above 1000 ng/ml, concurrent medication administration, and a rapid dose escalation. Several studies have shown different rates of clozapine-induced seizures, and it occurs in 0.6% of patients treated with clozapine. The tonic-clonic seizure is the most frequently described type of seizure; however other myoclonic-atonic, simple, and partial seizures and absence seizures are also seen [18]. The exact mechanism of clozapine-induced seizures is not well studied, but studies have shown that it may be associated with the selectivity of clozapine toward mesolimbic and cortical dopamine D 4 receptors.

Management Principles of Clozapine-Induced Seizure [19].

A thorough evaluation of the patient:

1. Investigate the possible triggering factors.
2. Discontinue the clozapine for 24 h and restart at half of the seizure-initiating dose.
3. Order clozapine serum concentrations.
4. Continue on prophylactic antiepileptic drugs such as sodium valproate, gabapentin, lamotrigine, or topiramate.

If an antiepileptic drug is considered, it is important to consider the pharmacokinetic drug interactions that accompany many antiepileptic drugs and the other hematological side effects which could occur with the antiepileptic drugs.

11.2.7.3 Stuttering

Numerous case studies have been shown that clozapine is associated with stuttering in 0.92% of individuals treated with clozapine. It is associated with an increase in treatment dose or with dose titration. The exact mechanism of clozapine-associated stuttering is not known, but it can be associated with further social isolation and withdrawal of the patients.

11.2.7.4 Venous Thromboembolism and Pulmonary Embolism

The connection between clozapine to cause venous thromboembolism has been shown, and studies based on Hagg [20] estimated the incidence of venous thromboembolism to be between 1/2000 and 6000 individuals that were just treated with clozapine for 1 year. Several theories have been proposed to explain the mechanism leading to thromboembolism during clozapine therapy (Table 11.5).

There are several other risk factors which are commonly seen in psychiatric patients treated with clozapine and may predispose to venous thromboembolism and pulmonary embolism. Some risk factors include long-term hospitalization, immobilization due to physical restraints, dehydration, concurrent administration of other medications such as benzodiazepines and other antipsychotic medication, hyperprolactinemia associated with co-prescribing hyperhomocysteinemia, and diagnosis of schizophrenia.

11.2.7.5 Sedation

Sedation and fatigue is common especially during the first 2 weeks of therapy, and it is a result of antagonism at H1, Ach, dopamine, and alpha-1 receptors. It is generally mild and usually settles as the treatment continues.

Table 11.5 Possible biological mechanism of action of clozapine in relation to venous thrombosis and pulmonary embolism

Sedation and obesity associated with clozapine which reduces movement and activities
Sedation and obesity associated with clozapine which reduces movement and activities
Clozapine has the high affinity for the 5-HT2A receptors which can contribute to serotonin-induced platelet aggregation [21]
Some in vitro studies have shown an increase in platelet adhesion and aggregation which can predispose to venous thromboembolism
Clozapine can increase the creation of antiphospholipid antibodies and the increase of the C-reactive protein [22]
Hypotension-associated with clozapine therapy may contribute to post-thrombogenic mechanism

11.2.7.6 Weight Gain

Weight gain tends to occur in the first 6–12 weeks of treatment with clozapine [23]. Because of its propensity to raise insulin levels, there have been reports of ketoacidosis in some patients. Weight should be routinely monitored, and behavioral interventions, such as diet modification and increasing level of exercise, should be recommended if the patients gain weight on clozapine. Some studies have shown that metformin can be used to blunt antipsychotic-induced weight gain and also improve insulin sensitivity [24].

11.2.7.7 Urinary Incontinence

Urinary incontinence is a rare side effect caused by clozapine's anti-alpha adrenergic effects leading to bladder neck sphincter relaxation [23]. An open trial of 16 patients suggested that ephedrine, which is an alpha-adrenergic agonist, may be effective in treating clozapine-induced urinary incontinence. A dose of 25 mg ephedrine at night or 25 mg twice daily is usually sufficient [25, 26]. Some other simple measures such as reducing the dose or manipulating dose schedule to avoid periods of deep sedation or avoiding fluids before bedtime may be helpful; however some cases of urinary incontinence may resolve spontaneously but also may persist for many months or years.

Overall clozapine remains an important medication in the treatment of severe psychosis. Some of the side effects are most difficult; however with careful selection and monitoring, it remains an excellent medication for severe psychosis and several other conditions.

Disclosure Statement "The authors have nothing to disclose".

References

1. Herst L, Powell GI. Clozapine safe in the elderly? Aust N Z J Psychiatry. 1997;31:411–7.
2. AA Pharma. Starting Patients on AA Clozapine. 2017.
3. Kilian JG, Kerr K, Lawrence C, Celermajer DS. Myocarditis and cardiomyopathy associated with clozapine. Lancet. 1999;354:1841–5.
4. Warner B, et al. Clozapine and sudden death. Lancet. 2000;355:842.
5. Haas SJ, et al. Clozapine-associated myocarditis. Drug Saf. 2007;30(1):47–57.
6. Ronaldson KJ, et al. A new monitoring protocol for clozapine-induced myocarditis based on an analysis of 75 cases and 94 controls. Aust N Z J Psychiatry. 2011;45:458–65.
7. Taylor D, Paton C, Shitij K. Prescribing guidelines in psychiatry: 12th edition. Wiley Blackwell: Oxford; 2015.
8. Magnani JW, Dec GW. Myocarditis. Circulation. 2006;113(6):876–90.
9. Reinders J, et al. Clozapine-related myocarditis and cardiomyopathy in an Australian metropolitan psychiatric service. Aust N Z Psychiatry. 2004;38:915–22.
10. Rostagno C, et al. Beta-blocker and angiotensin-converting enzyme inhibitor may limit certain cardiac adverse effects of clozapine. Gen Hosp Psychiatry. 2008;30:280–32.
11. Floreani J, et al. Successful re-challenge with clozapine following development of clozapine-induced cardiomyopathy. Aust N Z J Psychiatry. 2008;42:747–849.
12. Roh S, et al. Cardiomyopathy associated with clozapine. Exp Clin Psychopharmacol. 2006;14:94–8.
13. Masopust J, et al. Repeated occurrence of clozapine-induced myocarditis in a patient with schizoaffective disorder and comorbid Parkinson's disease. Neuro Endocrinol Lett. 2009;30:19–21.

14. Roaldson KJ, et al. Observations from 8 cases of clozapine rechallenge after development of myocarditis. J Clin Psychiatry. 2012;73:252–4.
15. Fontana PG, Sumegi B. Association of Clozaril (clozapine) with cardiovascular toxicity. Novartis Pharmaceuticals Canada Inc. 2002.
16. Praharaj SK, Arora M, Gandotra S. Clozapine-induced sialorrhea: pathophysiology and management strategies. Psychopharmacology. 2006;185:265–73.
17. Pacia SV, Devinsky O. Clozapine-related seizures: experience with 5629 patients. Neurology. 1994;44(12):2247–9.
18. Varma S. Clozapine– related EEG changes and seizures: dose and plasma level relationships. Ther Adv Psychopharmacol. 2011;1(2):47–66.
19. Williams AM, Park SH. Seizure associated with clozapine: incidence, etiology, and management. CNS Drugs. 2015;29:101–11.
20. Hägg S, Spigset O, Söderström T. Association of venous thromboembolism and clozapine. Lancet. 2000;355:1155–6.
21. Axelsson S, Hägg S, Eriksson A, Lindahl T, Whiss P. In vitro effects of antipsychotics of human platelet adhesion and aggregation and plasma coagulation. Clin Exp Pharmacol Physiol. 2007;34:775–80.
22. Hägg S, Jönsson A, Spigset O. Risk of venous thromboembolism due to antipsychotic drug therapy. Expert Opin Drug Saf. 2009;8:537–47.
23. AA Pharma. Using clozapine today: treating schizophrenia from tertiary care to community care. 2017;1(1).
24. Carrizo E, Fernandez V, Connell L, Sandia I, Prieto D, Mogollon J, Valbuena D, et al. Extended release metformin for metabolic control assistance during prolonged clozapine administration: a 14 week, double-blind, parallel group, placebo-controlled study. Schizophr Res. 2009;113(1):19–26.
25. Fuller MA, Borovicka MC, Jaskiw GE, Simon MR, Kown K, Konicki PE. Clozapine-induced urinary incontinence: incidence and treatment with ephedrine. J Clin Psychiatry. 1996;57(11):514.
26. Freudenreich O, McEvoy J. Guidelines for prescribing clozapine in schizophrenia. UpToDate. Retrieved from: https://www.uptodate.com/contents/guidelines-for-prescribing-clozapine-in-schizophrenia.

Complementary and Alternative Therapies for Treatment-Resistant Depression: A Clinical Perspective

Rosalia Sun Young Yoon, Nisha Ravindran, and Arun Ravindran

12.1 Case Report

Mary G is a 49-year-old woman, separated for the past year and a half, with two adult children. She is on a long-term disability from her job as a government clerk.

Ms. G experienced her first episode of depression at 22, thought to have been triggered by her move from a small town to living in university residence. Her symptoms at that time consisted of low mood persistent throughout the day, social isolation, late insomnia, decreased appetite, and weight loss of 15 lbs.

She sought help from her university health service and received supportive therapy from a social worker and was started on a course of fluoxetine. After 1 week, she complained of feeling restless and agitated, and treatment was switched to paroxetine, which was titrated to 40 mg over a period of 1 month. She gradually began to feel better and would at times be nonadherent to treatment, leading to discontinuation of symptoms, and eventually decided to stop pharmacological treatment. However, she continued with supportive therapy and was able to maintain her improvements, but noted that it took 3 years for her to achieve full remission.

After completion of her degree, Ms. G sought employment with the government and has maintained steady work in various departments. She married at the age of 27 and had two children. There are no significant issues in her medical history, and she functioned well in her career and was able to balance family life with a number of close friendships.

Two years ago, Ms. G experienced significant interpersonal conflict with a manager at work. She began to ruminate at night, developing initial insomnia and decreased appetite. She became unable to concentrate on her work. She saw her family physician and was started on escitalopram after being diagnosed with her second episode of major depression, which was eventually optimized to 20 mg. She had a partial response to this treatment, achieving a 40% reduction in her symptoms as measured on the PHQ-9. However, her depression was affecting the marital relationship, and Ms. G separated from her husband, with further deterioration in her depressive symptoms. During this period, she received two other antidepressants of desvenlafaxine 50–100 mg and sertraline 150 mg p.o. daily with each trial over 12 weeks. With both agents she had similar degrees of benefits as escitalopram. Subsequently, sertraline was augmented with 900 mg of lithium, which she tolerated well, apart from development

R.S.Y. Yoon, MSc, PhD • N. Ravindran, MD, FRCPC
A. Ravindran, MB, PhD (✉)
Department of Psychiatry, University of Toronto, Toronto, ON, Canada

Centre for Addiction and Mental Health, Mood and Anxiety, Toronto, ON, Canada
e-mail: Rosalia.Yoon@camh.ca;
Nisha.ravindran@camh.ca; Arun.ravindran@camh.ca

of facial acne, but with no additional benefits. She then received an augmentation trial of aripiprazole, starting at 2 mg, and titrated to 5 mg daily. However, it caused severe akathisia, and Ms. G stopped it abruptly. She was offered the option of adding olanzapine or quetiapine but was reluctant because of the possibility of weight gain.

12.2   Introduction

Major depressive disorder (MDD) is a common illness that often follows a chronic and recurrent course. Associated with significant morbidity and mortality, it is a leading cause of disability worldwide [105]. Despite extensive research on its pathophysiology and treatment, MDD remains a difficult illness to treat in a significant proportion of patients. Current first-line treatments for MDD include pharmacological agents and psychological therapies. Among the pharmacological agents, selective serotonin reuptake inhibitors (SSRIs) and serotonin-norepinephrine reuptake inhibitors (SNRIs) have been established as first-line treatment options [43]. However, as with many pharmacological agents, antidepressant medications are not without problems. Studies have shown that only 30–50% of patients with MDD exhibit response to the initial antidepressant [30, 62], and less than half attain remission even with optimal treatment, indicating that issues of partial response and nonresponse to medications are common in depression.

The term treatment-resistant depression (TRD) is often used to describe patients who do not respond to antidepressant treatment. Several operational definitions have been proposed for TRD since the term first appeared in the literature in the 1970s, but without a clear consensus on it. A commonly used definition for TRD is failure to respond to two or more optimal trials of antidepressants of different classes [51, 55]. Response is conventionally defined as a ≥ 50% reduction in symptoms as measured by a standard rating scale, such as the Hamilton Depression Rating Scale (HAM-D) or the Montgomery-Åsberg Depression Rating Scale (MADRS) [51]. Those who show

25–50% response are frequently referred to as partial responders and, as such, are often included in the TRD rubric [51].

It has been estimated that 12–20% of patients with depression will fulfill criteria for TRD [60]. The socioeconomic impacts of TRD for the individual, family, and society are significant, as TRD is often associated with higher rates of medical and psychiatric comorbidities, lower quality of life, and significant functional impairment. Moreover, health economic studies confirm its significant economic impact due to higher healthcare costs and lost productivity [60].

The pathophysiological mechanisms underlying TRD remain poorly understood, but it is generally accepted that multiple factors are contributory. There are currently no neurobiological markers for diagnosing and/or predicting TRD, but some possible physiological correlates have been identified, including abnormal neural connectivity and altered function in specific brain areas (e.g., caudate, insula, anterior cingulate cortices, etc.) [11, 73, 106] and genetic contributors (e.g., polymorphisms of monoamine genes) [41, 42].

Similarly, demographic factors, including female gender, older age, and lower education level and economic status, as well as the presence of life stressors, have been proposed to be associated with poor treatment response [57, 99]. As well, comorbid medical and psychiatric conditions are noted to increase the likelihood of non response [68, 92].

12.2.1 Clinical Conundrums in the Management of TRD

There is consistent evidence that the presence of residual depressive symptoms following pharmacotherapy is associated with greater likelihood of relapse [78]. In addition, remission rates are noted to be inversely proportional to number of failed acute therapies and subsequent relapse rates [55]. As such, the goal in treating an acute episode of depression is for the patient to achieve remission with minimal to no residual symptoms.

When presented with a case of treatment resistance, the suggested first step is to carefully review the psychiatric and medical diagnoses to identify any factors contributing to resistance and to avoid misdiagnosis. Antidepressant medication history also needs to be reviewed to determine adequacy of past trials, as there is evidence that many MDD patients do not receive adequate treatment [21]. An adequate trial is often described as medication taken at an effective therapeutic dose, for a minimum of 6–12 weeks [69]. The Antidepressant Treatment History Form (ATHF) and the Massachusetts General Hospital Antidepressant Treatment Response Questionnaire (MGH ATRQ) are useful instruments to evaluate adequacy of prior antidepressant trials. Another important factor to take into consideration is treatment adherence. Although nonresponse due to poor adherence does not, by definition, constitute treatment resistance, nonadherence occurs in up to 50% of patients prescribed with antidepressants and is likely to contribute substantially to cases of pseudo-resistance [9].

Once medical and psychiatric conditions and other confounding factors have been ruled out and treatment resistance has been established, commonly used pharmacotherapy strategies for TRD include switching to another antidepressant class or augmenting current antidepressant treatment with another pharmacological agent. These strategies have been reviewed elsewhere [43, 55, 69]. Briefly, there is some evidence that switching from an initial failed SSRI trial to an antidepressant, such as venlafaxine [33] or bupropion [86], can be beneficial for some patients. While such strategies are helpful for many patients, in others, the benefit is only modest, as evidenced by remission rates of 30–50% following switch or augmentation [5, 101]. Moreover, certain pharmacologic strategies may not be appropriate for some patients due to issues of medication tolerance, drug-drug interactions, and safety. Further, the high price of antidepressant medications can be problematic for some patients, particularly for those who do not have insurance to cover such costs. Finally, some patients are simply not open to the idea of taking psychotropic

Table 12.1 Common reasons for nonadherence

Common reasons for nonadherence		
Nonresponse Adverse drug reactions Fear of developing drug reaction Cost of medications	Complicated treatment regimens Poor mental health literacy Stigma	Negative attitudes toward antidepressant medications Religious and/or cultural beliefs

Sundborn and Bingefors [98]; Ho et al. [40]

medications for personal reasons. The table below lists some of the common reasons for antidepressant nonadherence. Taken together, there is a wide range of limitations in currently available pharmacotherapy options for TRD, highlighting the need for alternative options for the management of TRD (Table 12.1).

12.3 Is There a Place for Complementary and Alternative Medicine Therapies in TRD?

Complementary and alternative medicine (CAM) therapies are often defined as "a group of diverse medical and health systems, practices, and products that are not currently considered to be part of conventional medicine" [61]. There are currently more than 120 CAM therapies available, including physical therapies, herbal remedies and nutraceuticals, and mindfulness-based interventions [79].

CAM therapies tend to be more cost-effective and available without a prescription, and they are often perceived to be safer alternatives without many of the adverse effects commonly associated with pharmacotherapy. In the past few years, many studies have investigated efficacy of CAMs in different medical and psychiatric illnesses, with some promising results. This, in conjunction with patients' preference for self-directed over practitioner-directed therapies and a belief that "natural is better" has resulted in a steady rise in the popularity of CAMs [100]. A national US survey noted a 47% increase in visits to CAM practitioners between 1990 and 1997 [27]. In

Table 12.2 CAM therapy recommendations for major depressive disorder [80]

Intervention	Indication	Recommendation	Evidence	Monotherapy or adjunctive therapy
Physical and meditative treatments				
Exercise	Mild to moderate	First line	Level 1	Monotherapy
	Moderate to severe	Second line	Level 1	Adjunctive
Light therapy	Seasonal (winter)	First line	Level 1	Monotherapy
	Mild to moderate nonseasonal	Second line	Level 2	Monotherapy or adjunctive
Yoga	Mild to moderate	Second line	Level 2	Adjunctive
Natural health products				
St. John's wort	Mild to moderate	First line	Level 1	Monotherapy
	Moderate to severe	Second line	Level 2	Adjunctive
Omega-3	Mild to moderate	Second line	Level 1	Monotherapy or adjunctive
	Moderate to severe	Second line	Level 2	Adjunctive
SAMe	Mild to moderate	Second line	Level 1	Adjunctive
	Moderate to severe	Second line	Level 2	Adjunctive

Adapted from [80]

depression, national self-report surveys indicate that CAM techniques are used by up to 54% of patients, suggesting substantial demand [27] (Table 12.2).

There is great potential in integrating CAM therapies in the management of TRD [80]. For instance, CAM therapies that work through mechanisms other than those targeted by antidepressant medications may be viable options for patients who have failed to achieve remission with pharmacotherapy. Moreover, augmentation of pharmacotherapy with CAMs can be a practical option for partial responders for whom antidepressant medication doses cannot be increased due to issues of safety and tolerability. However, the evidence on efficacy and safety of different CAM interventions in TRD is limited. Reported studies are sparse and varying in quality, often with equivocal results. Given the potential utility of CAMs and the growing popularity among patients, it is important to evaluate the benefits and risks of use. The aim of this chapter is to present the available evidence on CAM therapies for TRD to serve as a guide for the clinician to tailor an alternate therapeutic approach for patients with treatment resistance.

It is important to note that while there are over 120 CAM modalities available, only a small number has sufficient published evidence to warrant evaluation. As a result, this chapter covers

Table 12.3 CAM therapies reviewed in this chapter

Physical and meditative treatments	Natural health products
Exercise Light therapy Sleep deprivation Yoga Mindfulness-based cognitive therapy	Omega-3 fatty acids S-adenosylmethionine (SAMe)

some physical and meditative treatments (exercise, light therapy, yoga, mindfulness-based cognitive therapy) and natural health products (omega-3 fatty acids and S-adenosyl-L-methionine). Several other CAM therapies, such as sleep deprivation, acupuncture, St. John's wort, dehydroepiandrosterone (DHEA), tryptophan, and other herbal/natural supplements, have evidence for benefit in MDD, but are not reviewed here, as their use has not been systematically evaluated in TRD (Table 12.3).

12.3.1 What Are the Physical and Meditative Treatments That May Benefit TRD?

12.3.1.1 Exercise

Exercise is a structured physical activity undertaken to maintain or improve physical fitness and health [17]. Exercise is also known to promote mental health and psychological well-being, including antidepressant effects [32]. The positive effects of exercise on mood are believed to be partly mediated by improvements in brain efficiency, plasticity, and adaptability via modulation of neuronal signaling and synapse connectivity [46].

Several randomized controlled trials (RCTs) and meta-analyses have shown that physical activities, such as aerobic exercise and strengthening, have moderate antidepressant effect when used alone or as adjunct to usual treatment, when compared to controls or active comparators, and in both clinical and non-clinical depressed populations [17, 38, 85, 91]. The benefits have been shown to be comparable to that of traditional treatments, such as medications and psychotherapy, and studies confirm that exercise is well-tolerated [17, 80]. As such, many guidelines include exercise as a treatment option for MDD, either as monotherapy or as an adjunctive [80].

Less is known about the benefit of exercise specifically for TRD. However, there is preliminary evidence to support its use to augment the effects of pharmacotherapy in partial and nonresponders (see Table 12.4). In the open-label pilot study by Trivedi et al. [102], partial responders who underwent a 12-week exercise program adjunctive to antidepressant medications exhibited significant improvements in depressive symptoms at the end of the study. Moreover, two RCTs evaluating exercise programs as add-on to ongoing pharmacotherapy reported significant improvements in depressive symptoms, as well as in social and physical functioning compared to baseline and controls [58, 59, 76]. Efficacy of exercise as augmentation in TRD has also been demonstrated in an elderly population. In the study by Mather et al. [54], subjects aged 53 years or older were randomly assigned to exercise classes or health education for 10 weeks. Modest improvements in depressive symptoms were observed in both groups, but the exercise group had a significantly higher proportion of subjects with ≥30% reduction in HAM-D17 score than the health education group [54].

Although more research is needed to confirm benefits of exercise in TRD, these studies suggest that exercise as an adjunct to ongoing pharmacotherapy effects improvements in symptomatology and psychosocial functioning in TRD. Moreover, the exercise programs evaluated in these studies were well tolerated, as evidenced by no reports of adverse effects; and well accepted, as evidenced by adherence rates of 75–90% [54, 58, 102]. Due to the limited number of studies in this population, there are no practice guidelines for use in TRD, and the parameters for optimal results are likely to vary among patients. However, based on the published data, it would be reasonable to recommend 30–60 min of moderate aerobic exercise, 2–5 times per week, as an adjunct to pharmacotherapy in patients with TRD. This is in line with current recommendations in practice guidelines for treatment of MDD [66, 80].

12.3.1.2 Light Therapy

Light therapy (LT) is an intervention in which subjects are exposed daily to an artificial source of bright light that has been shown in several studies to have antidepressant effects when used at carefully timed doses [80]. The antidepressant effects of LT are purported to be mediated by modulation of neurophysiological and biochemical processes governed by the suprachiasmatic nuclei (SCN), including circadian cycle phase shifts, increases in daytime serum serotonin, and suppression of daytime melatonin secretion [67].

Light therapy has been shown to be effective in the treatment of seasonal affective disorder (SAD) [35, 52], with acute effects comparable to fluoxetine [47] and cognitive behavioral therapy (CBT) [83]. Efficacy has also been demonstrated in nonseasonal depression when used as monotherapy, though the evidence is limited by study design flaws, such as small sample size and inadequate controls [35, 74, 103]. Efficacy when used as an adjunct to antidepressant medications is less clear. Two meta-analyses concluded that adjunctive LT is not superior to pharmacotherapy alone [35, 103]. However, more recent RCTs have demonstrated significantly stronger therapeutic effects for combinations of LT and

Table 12.4 Exercise in TRD

Author	Study design	Sample size	Definition of resistance	Intervention	Control	Key findings
Trivedi et al. [102]	Open label Adjunct to ongoing pharmacotherapy (SSRIs or venlafaxine) 8 weeks	17 subjects with MDD	SSRI or venlafaxine at minimum therapeutic dose for ≥6 weeks	3–5 days aerobic exercise (walking, cycling, or treadmill)	None	8 subjects completed study, 10 subjects completed at least 4 weeks ITT analyses revealed significant** reductions in $HAMD_{17}$ and $IDS\text{-}SR_{30}$
Pilu et al. [76]	RCT Adjunct to ongoing pharmacotherapy (SSRI, SNRI, NRI, or TCA) 8 months	30 female subjects with MDD	No response (HAMD >13) to at least 1 antidepressant at adequate doses for at least 8 weeks	2 × 60 min physiological strengthening per week	Pharmacotherapy only	Significant reductions*** in HAMD, CGI, and GAF at 8 months follow-up in intervention but not control group
Mota-Pereira et al. [58]	RCT Adjunct to ongoing pharmacotherapy (TCA, SSRI, or SNRI) 12 weeks	33 subjects with treatment-resistant MDD	Combined pharmacotherapy for 9–15 months, without showing remission	30–45-min walks per day, 5 days per week	Pharmacotherapy only	6% dropout and 91% compliance rates Significant improvements* in BDI-II, $HAMD_{17}$, CGI, and GAF compared to baseline and control group
Mota-Pereira et al. [59]	Post hoc analysis of [58]					Significant improvements in WHOQOL-Bref social domain** and SF-36 physical functioning domain***
Mather et al. [54]	RCT Adjunct to ongoing pharmacotherapy (antidepressant therapy not specified) 10 weeks	85 elder subjects (53 years or older) with poor response	Pharmacotherapy for at least 6 weeks without evidence of sustained response	2 × 45-min weight-bearing exercises per week	Health education classes (2 × 30–40-min per week)	No dropout, attendant rates of 67% and 85% for intervention and control groups, respectively Both intervention groups demonstrated improvements, but exercise group had significantly higher proportion of subjects with ≥30% reduction in $HAMD_{17}$

BDI-II Beck Depression Inventory, *CGI* Clinical Global Impression, *GAF* Global Assessment of Functioning, *HAMD* Hamilton Rating Scale for Depression, *IDS-SR30* Inventory of Depressive Symptomatology-Self-Report, *ITT* intention-to-treat, *NRI* norepinephrine reuptake inhibitor, *RCT* randomized controlled trial, *SF-36* short form 36 items, *SNRI* serotonin and norepinephrine reuptake inhibitor, *SSRI* selective serotonin reuptake inhibitor, *TCA* tricyclic antidepressant, *WHOQOL-Bref* WHO quality of life

$*p < 0.05, **p < 0.01, ***p < 0.001$

antidepressants (fluoxetine or venlafaxine) compared to medication alone [37, 50]. Given the evidence in MDD, LT is currently recommended as a second-line monotherapy or adjunctive therapy in CAM treatment guidelines for MDD [80].

There is some evidence to suggest LT may be beneficial in TRD (see Table 12.5). The study by Wirz-Justice et al. [104], which evaluated efficacy of LT in women with antepartum depression, included four subjects who were on antidepressant medications with poor response at the time of the study. All four subjects were assigned to LT for 5 weeks, and all were reported to improve. Further details on these subjects, such as the degree of improvement, were not provided [104]. Moreover, two open-label studies evaluated LT as add-on to ongoing medication in treatment-resistant patients and reported significant improvements in depression scores [26, 77]. Efficacy of LT as adjunct to ongoing medications was also evaluated in RCTs using low-intensity (50 lux) light [64] and negative ion generator [15] as controls, and significant improvements in response and remission rates were observed.

Thus, there is preliminary evidence that LT may be a viable augmentation option for some patients with TRD, though further research is needed for confirmation in this population. The LT parameters used in the studies discussed herein (5000 to 10,000 lux, 0.5 to 2 h in the morning, for 2–6 weeks) are more or less in line with the standard protocol used in MDD (10,000 lux, 0.5 h in the morning, for 6 weeks) [52]. These parameters were associated with good adherence, as evidenced by high study completion rates (74% in Prasko et al. [77] and 87% in Chojnacka et al. [15]); and were well tolerated, as evidenced by the absence of serious adverse effects in the studies. In line with what has been reported in the MDD population, common adverse effects included mild and transient agitation and headaches [15].

12.3.1.3   Sleep Deprivation
Sleep deprivation (SD) is an intervention in which subjects are kept awake for approximately 36 h, which has been shown to effectively reduce depressive symptoms [6]. The antidepressant effects have been proposed to involve potentia-

tion of monoamine signaling, as well as functional and metabolic changes in the ventral/anterior cingulate cortex, and increased fronto-limbic connectivity [6].

Although it has not been specifically evaluated in TRD, there is substantial evidence that SD exerts benefits in depressive disorders [34, 53, 81]. Of note, although the onset of antidepressant effects is rapid, relapse after discontinuation is also rapid. As such, a practical limitation is maintaining SD for longer than a few weeks [80]. Daytime sleepiness is one of the most commonly reported adverse effects [80]. Recurrence of panic attacks and risk of SD-induced mania have also been noted, and, as such, caution is recommended for use in vulnerable populations [20]. Moreover, SD is contraindicated for epilepsy due to the high risk of seizure induction with sleep reduction [20].

Despite issues of practicality and potential risks, the rapid benefits of SD in MDD suggest that it could be beneficial in TRD, and more research in this population is warranted. In the absence of practice guidelines specifically for TRD, the parameters of use in MDD studies (total SD for up to 40 h or partial SD allowing 3–4 h of sleep per night, employed 2 to 4 times per week over the course of 1 week) may be applied to TRD [80]. Currently, there is level 2 evidence to support use in MDD, and guidelines recommend sleep deprivation as a third-line adjunctive treatment for more severe and refractory forms of MDD [80].

12.3.1.4   Yoga
Yoga is a system of integrated physical movements, breathing practices, and meditation that originated in India more than 4000 years ago. It exemplifies the principle that mental and physical health is achieved through unity of mind, body, and spirit [82]. It is often practiced to promote health and wellness, and, more recently, there has been interest in its utility as an intervention for physical and mental illnesses, including depression.

The mechanisms by which yoga exerts antidepressant effects are not yet fully understood. Studies have shown that yoga attenuates

Table 12.5 Light therapy in TRD

Author	Study design	Sample size	Definition of resistance	Intervention	Control	Key findings
Justice et al. [104]	RCT Monotherapy for all, except 4 subjects with ongoing pharmacotherapy (paroxetine, fluoxetine, or citalopram) 5 weeks	27 pregnant women with nonseasonal MDD	Not a study of efficacy in treatment resistance, per se, but sample included 4 women with depression despite pharmacotherapy	7000 lux, 1 h upon awakening	70 lux under same conditions as intervention group	All 4 medicated subjects were assigned to intervention group and all demonstrated improvement, though no other details on these subjects were provided
Prasko et al. [77]	Open label Adjunct (SSRIs) 6 weeks	17 female subjects with depression and comorbid BPD	SSRI treatment for at least 6 weeks without improvement	10,000 lux, 6:30–7:30 am	None	16 subjects completed the study Significant*** improvements in CGI-I, HAMD, MADRS, and BDI scores
Niederhofer and von Klitzing [64]	RCT Adjunct (fluoxetine) 4 weeks	28 adolescent inpatients	Significant depressive complaints despite fluoxetine treatment since 1 month prior to study start	1 week of LT at 2500 lux, 60 min in the AM; then 1 week of placebo at 50 lux under same conditions as week 1	1 week of placebo at 50 lux, 60 min in the AM; then 1 week of LT at 2500 lux under same conditions as week 1	Significant* improvements in BDI scores
Echizenya et al. [26]	Open label Adjunct (SSRI, SNRI, TCA, atypical antidepressant, benzodiazepines)	13 subjects with treatment resistance	Antidepressant treatment for at least 4 weeks without response	1 night total sleep deprivation, followed by 3 days sleep phase advance and 5 days LT at 5000 lux, 2 h in the AM	None	No dropouts Significant*** improvements in HAMD17 and SDS
Chojnacka et al. [15]	RCT Adjunct (antidepressants plus mood stabilizers and/ or antipsychotics) 2 weeks	50 with bipolar and 45 with unipolar depression)	At least 4 weeks of treatment	LT at 10,000 lux, 30 min in AM	Negative ion generator, 30 min in the AM	12 and 7 dropouts in the LT and control groups, respectively Significant*** improvements in both groups, but significantly** higher response and remission rates in LT group

BDI Beck Depression Inventory, *BPD* borderline personality disorder, *CGI* Clinical Global Impression, *HAMD* Hamilton Rating Scale for Depression, *LT* light therapy, *NRI* norepinephrine reuptake inhibitor, *RCT* randomized controlled trial, *SDS* Zung Self-Rating Depression Scale, *SNRI* serotonin and norepinephrine reuptake inhibitor, *SSRI* selective serotonin reuptake inhibitor, *TCA* tricyclic antidepressant
$*p < 0.05$, $**p < 0.01$, $***p < 0.001$

physiological imbalances commonly seen in depression, such as over-activation of the hypothalamic-pituitary-adrenal (HPA) axis and under-activation of the parasympathetic nervous system, thereby enhancing the adaptive stress response [93, 95]. Moreover, recent research has demonstrated maladaptive inflammatory response in the pathophysiology of depression, and the practice of yoga has been shown to reduce pro-inflammatory cytokines normally elevated in depression, such as IL-1, IL-6, and TNF-α [82, 93]. The practice of yoga also appears to effect long-term changes in the brain, as evidenced by studies reporting volumetric increases in brain areas involved in emotional regulation and executive functioning, such as the ventromedial prefrontal cortex; and diminished activity in brain areas associated with anxious states, such as the amygdala [25, 93].

The efficacy of yoga in depression has been evaluated in several clinical trials and meta-analyses, with mostly positive results. Yoga has been shown to be associated with improvements in symptoms of depression when used as monotherapy or as an adjunctive, and benefits have been shown to be comparable to that of medications, group therapy, and exercise [18, 19]. Given the evidence, yoga is currently recommended as a second-line adjunctive therapy in CAM guidelines for the treatment of MDD [80].

However, evidence on benefits of yoga specifically for TRD is limited (see Table 12.6). Butler et al. [10] evaluated the effects of 8 weeks of hatha yoga meditation in subjects with long-term depressive disorders. Follow-up analyses at 9 months revealed significantly more remissions in the intervention than in the control group. Although this was not a study on the efficacy of yoga in TRD, per se, about 20% of recruited subject were non/poor responders. Authors found that remission at 9-months follow-up was not associated with antidepressant use [10], suggesting benefit of yoga beyond that of combination with antidepressants. In the study by Shapiro et al. [89], subjects with unipolar depression in partial remission participated in an open-label 20-session Iyengar yoga intervention adjunct to ongoing pharmacother-

apy. Significant improvements in symptoms of depression, anxiety, and neuroticism, as well as in heart rate variability, were observed among study completers, and 11 subjects achieved remission [89]. Finally, a recent RCT by Sharma et al. [90] evaluated efficacy of an 8-week Sudarshan Kriya yoga (SKY) program in MDD patients with poor treatment response and reported significant improvements in symptoms of depression and anxiety.

Given the paucity of studies in TRD and the variety of yoga types and methodologies used in the published studies, it is difficult to ascertain whether yoga confers any benefit specifically to patients with TRD. Nevertheless, given the good safety profile (adverse effects are very rare), low cost, and added physical benefits, it is reasonable to infer that the adoption of yoga practice in TRD would yield more benefits than harm in TRD. In the absence of practice guidelines specifically for TRD, evidence from the MDD population may be used, where interventions averaging 2–4 sessions per week over the course of 2–3 months have yielded positive results [18].

12.3.1.5 Mindfulness-Based Cognitive Therapy

Mindfulness-based cognitive therapy (MBCT) is an intervention that was developed for relapse prevention of recurrent MDD [88]. It integrates elements of mindfulness meditation (to become more aware of and to take a nonjudgmental attitude toward incoming thoughts, feelings, and bodily sensations) and elements of CBT (to recognize own maladaptive thought patterns and deliberately disengage from them) [14, 16]. MCBT usually consists of eight weekly 2.5 h structured sessions and it can be used as monotherapy or adjunctive. Its benefits are reported to be comparable to traditional CBT, as well as pharmacological treatments [13, 45, 75, 94], though the evidence is limited by methodological shortcomings of the investigations, such as small sample size, lack of randomization and adequate control conditions, and heterogeneity of studies.

Given MBCT's efficacy in chronic depression, several recent investigations have focused on its

Table 12.6 Yoga in TRD

Author	Study design	Sample size	Definition of resistance	Intervention	Control	Key findings
Butler et al. [10]	RCT Monotherapy or adjunct (antidepressant medications and/or psychotherapy) 9 months	46 subjects with long-term depression	Not a study of efficacy in TRD, per se, but 20% of patients were non-/poor responders	Psychoeducation plus 8 times weekly 2-h supervised meditation and hatha yoga, plus 6 times 30-min self-directed practice per week, plus one booster session at week 12	Psychoeducation only	Significantly* higher remission rates in meditation than control group at 9-month follow-up
Shapiro et al. [89]	Open label Adjunct (SSRI, SNRI, and/or dopaminergic) 20 sessions	27 subjects with unipolar depression in partial remission	Residual symptoms despite treatment for at least 3 months	3 × 60–90-min Iyengar yoga sessions per week, for a total of 20 sessions	None	16 subjects attended up to 5 sessions, 4 attended 10–17 sessions, and 17 attended all sessions ITT analyses revealed significant*** improvements in HAMD scores Among study completers, significant* improvements in anxiety, neuroticism, and HRV 11 out of the 17 study completers achieved remission
Sharma et al. [90]	RCT Adjunct (antidepressant medications) 8 weeks	13 MDD subjects with poor treatment response	$HAMD_{17} \geq 17$ despite treatment for at least 8 weeks	*Week 1:* 6 × 3.5 h SKY sessions *Weeks 2–8:* 1.5 h SKY sessions per week plus daily 20-min home-based practice	Wait list	3 subjects dropped out ITT analyses revealed significant** improvements in HAMD, BDI, and BAI scores

AI Beck Anxiety Inventory, *BDI* Beck Depression Inventory, *HAMD* Hamilton Rating Scale for Depression, *HRV* heart rate variability, *ITT* intention-to-treat, *RCT* randomized controlled trial, *SKY* Sudarshan Kriya yoga, *SNRI* serotonin and norepinephrine reuptake inhibitor, *SSRI* selective serotonin reuptake inhibitor
*$p < 0.05$, **$p < 0.01$, ***$p < 0.001$

utility in TRD (see Table 12.7). Two open-label trials evaluated MBCT in TRD subjects and both found significant improvements in BDI scores and relapse rates [28, 44]. These positive findings were replicated in two recent RCTs. In the study by Chiesa et al. [14], subjects with TRD were randomized to receive MBCT or psychoeducation in addition to current treatment. Significant improvements in measures of depression and quality of life were observed in the MBCT group in both short- and long-terms [14]. In the study by Eisendrath et al. [29], TRD subjects were randomized to MBCT or to a Health Enhancement Program (HEP), which served to control such factors as group support and morale, facilitator attention, and treatment duration. The MBCT group exhibited significant improvements in depression scores and remission rates and was superior to HEP at posttreatment [29].

The results of these studies suggest efficacy of MCBT in the management of TRD. No adverse events were reported in either Chiesa et al. [14] or Eisendrath et al. [29], and dropout rates were similar (12–15%) in both studies, suggesting good safety and adherence profiles [14, 29]. Though the evidence is preliminary, the findings are promising and warrant further research to confirm utility in TRD.

12.3.2 What Natural Health Products May Help Clinicians to Treat TRD?

12.3.2.1 Omega-3 Fatty Acids

Omega-3 fatty acids (ω-3 FAs) are essential dietary polyunsaturated fatty acid (PUFA) compounds found in fish oil, seafood, and some vegetables. These fatty acids have important roles in human physiology, including brain development and function. Dietary deficiencies in long-chain ω-3 FA compounds, including eicosapentaenoic acid (EPA) and docosahexaenoic acid (DHA), are speculated to be risk factors for mood disorders, including MDD [56]. In line with this, studies have shown that cultures with diets rich in fish oil have lower rates of depressive disorders [39, 65], suggesting preventative and therapeutic roles in

depression. Proposed mechanisms for the antidepressant effects of ω-3 FAs include improvements in serotonergic and dopaminergic neurotransmission through normalization of cell membrane microstructure and signal transduction [23, 24, 56].

Several clinical trials and meta-analyses on the efficacy of ω-3 FAs in depressive disorders have been conducted, with somewhat variable results. At least two meta-analyses reported positive results for ω-3 FA when used as monotherapy or adjunct to antidepressants [31, 49], one reported positive results for trials of ω-3 FA supplements with at least 60% EPA composition [97], one found benefits mainly in EPA supplements used as adjunctive therapy [36], one reported small to moderate benefits unlikely to be of clinical significance [3], and two meta-analyses found no benefits compared to placebo [2, 7]. The variability of results has been attributed to the heterogeneity of included studies with respect to study design, study population (e.g., inclusion of MDD, BD, comorbidities), sample size, and supplement dose and composition (e.g., different ratios of EPA to DHA), among other factors. In general, ω-3 FAs are recommended as second-line monotherapy for mild to moderate MDD, and as adjunctive for moderate to severe MDD [80].

The evidence for benefit of ω-3 FAs in TRD is promising (see Table 12.8). Two RCTs evaluated efficacy of adjunct EPA (albeit at different doses and durations of treatment) in medicated subjects with persistent depression, and reported significant improvements in depressive symptoms compared to baseline and controls [63, 72]. Another RCT evaluated the effect of adjunct ω-3 FA supplements in an 8-week trial in medicated subjects with depression, and found significant improvement in HAM-D score [96]. More recently, an open-label study evaluated the effect of a 10-week adjunctive treatment with low- and high-dose ω-3 FA supplements in SSRI-resistant adolescents [56]. Significant improvements in depression scores and higher remission were observed in the high-dose group [56].

The above findings suggest benefits of ω-3 FA supplements as add-on to ongoing pharmacother-

Table 12.7 MCBT in TRD

Author	Study Design	Sample Size	Definition of Resistance	Intervention	Control	Key findings
Kenny and Williams [44]	Open label Monotherapy or adjunct 8 weeks	50 subjects with treatment-resistant depressive disorders	Three or more episodes of depression or chronic course greater than 1 year	8 times 2 h weekly sessions plus 1 h per day of self-directed meditation or yoga	None	Significant reductions in BDI score***
Eisendrath et al. [28]	Open label Adjunctive 8 weeks	55 subjects with TRD	Failure to remit with at least 2 antidepressant treatments	8 times 2-hr. weekly sessions	None	51 completers Significant reduction in BDI score*** and 16 subjects (29%) went into remission
Chiesa et al. [14]	RCT Adjunctive (SSRIs, SNRIs, other antidepressants 8 weeks	43 subjects with TRD	Failure to remit with antidepressant trial for minimum 8 weeks	8 times 2 h weekly sessions	Psychoeducation	19/26 completers in MCBT and 18/26 completers in control group Significant improvements in $HAMD_{21}$** and quality of life** in short term (8 weeks) and long term (26 weeks) compared to baseline and control group
Eisendrath et al. [29]	RCT Adjunctive to ongoing medications, changes allowed 8 weeks	173 subjects with TRD	Failure to remit with 2 or more antidepressant trials of at least 4 weeks each	8 times 2 h weekly sessions plus 6 times self-directed 45-min sessions per week	Health enhancement program	Completion rates of 87% and 83% in MBCT and control groups, respectively Significant improvements in $HAMD_{17}$**, CGI***, and response rates* compared to baseline and controls

BDI Beck Depression Inventory, *CGI* Clinical Global Impression, *HAMD* Hamilton Rating Scale for Depression, *MBCT* mindfulness-based cognitive therapy, *RCT* randomized controlled trial

$*p < 0.05$, $**p < 0.01$, $***p < 0.001$

Table 12.8 Omega-3 fatty acids in TRD

Author	Study Design	Sample size	Definition of resistance	Intervention	Control	Key findings
Peet and Horrobin [72]	RCT Adjunct (TCA, SSRI, or other norepinephrine or mixed reuptake inhibitor) 12 weeks	70 subjects with persistent depression	$HAMD_{17} \geq 15$ despite ongoing treatment with standard antidepressants at adequate dose	1 g/day EPA Vs 2 g/day EPA Vs 4 g/day EPA	Placebo	Completion rates of 88% and 78% in EPA and control groups, respectively In ITT analyses, 1 g/day group had significant improvements in $HAMD_{17}$*, $MADRS$**, and BDI** in 1 g/day group compared to baseline and controls, and 53% of subjects (compared to 29% in placebo) had 50% reduction in $HAMD_{17}$ No significant differences in 2 g/day and 4 g/day groups compared to baseline and placebo
Nemets et al. [63]	RCT Adjunct (SSRI, MAOI, mirtazapine) 4 weeks	20 recurrent unipolar depression subjects on maintenance therapy	$HAMD_{24} \geq 18$ despite antidepressant medications at for at least 3 weeks	2 g/day EPA	Placebo	Significant*** reduction in HAMD score compared to placebo. Six patients in the active treatment group (compared to 1 in placebo) achieved 50% reduction in HAMD score
Su et al. [96]	RCT Adjunct (SSRI, MAOI) for all except for one subject 8 weeks	28 subjects with MDD	MDD despite treatment with medications for at least 4 weeks before enrolment	Omega-3 PUFA (9.6 g/day) capsules (EPA 2.2 g and DHA 1.1 g)	Placebo	Completion rates of 86% and 71% in omega-3 and control groups, respectively Significant reduction in $HAMD_{21}$ compared to placebo group
McNamara et al. [56]	Open label Adjunct (SSRI) 10 weeks	14 SSRI-resistant MDD adolescents	Baseline CDRS-R score of >28 and <40 despite standard therapeutic dose of SSRI for minimum 6 weeks	Low-dose fish oil at 2.4 g/day (EPA 1.6 g and DHA 0.8 g) vs High-dose fish oil at 16.2 g/day (EPA 10.8 g and DHA 5.4 g)	None	Completion rates of 86% and 71% in omega-3 and control groups, respectively In ITT analysis, significant reduction in CDRS-R***. Symptom remission in 40% and 100% in low- and high-dose groups, respectively

CDRS-R Children's Depression Rating Scale-Revised, *DHA* docosahexaenoic acid, *EPA* ethyl eicosapentanoate, *HAMD* Hamilton Depression Rating Scale, *ITT* intention-to-treat, *MAOI* Monoamine oxidase inhibitor, *PUFA* polyunsaturated fatty acids, *RCT* randomized controlled trial, *SSRI* selective serotonin reuptake inhibitor, *TCA* tricyclic antidepressant

*$p < 0.05$, **$p < 0.01$, ***$p < 0.001$

apy, and it is inferred that treatment for a minimum of 4 weeks is required for benefits to manifest, although dose requirements remain unclear due to the wide range of evaluated doses (1 g/day in Peet & Horrobin [72] vs 10.8 g/day in McNamara et al. [56]). There is general agreement that EPA content is more relevant than DHA. Completion rates were high, ranging from 70 to 98%. Commonly reported adverse effects included GI symptoms and headaches [56, 72, 96], and none of the studies reported serious AEs, suggesting good safety and adherence under the treatment parameters evaluated in the studies discussed herein.

12.3.2.2 SAM-e

S-adenosylmethionine (SAMe) is a natural physiological compound found throughout the body. It plays a role in several metabolic pathways, and it is uniformly distributed in the brain, where it serves as a major source of methyl groups required for the synthesis of catecholamines and neuronal membranes [4, 71]. Given the dominant role of catecholamines in the neuropathology of depression, SAMe is speculated to have a therapeutic role in the regulation of mood disorders, including depression. Proposed mechanisms mediating its antidepressant effects include increased monoamine synthesis and serotonin turnover, inhibition of norepinephrine reuptake, and augmentation of dopaminergic activity, as well as regulation of neurotrophic activity, inflammatory cytokines, and bioenergetics [71, 84].

Several clinical trials and meta-analyses support a therapeutic role of SAMe in the treatment of depression, with response rates reported to be comparable to that of tricyclic antidepressants when used as monotherapy [8, 12, 22, 70]. There is also some evidence to support SAMe as adjunct to antidepressant medications [22, 87]. Currently, guidelines recommend SAMe as a second-line adjunctive treatment for use in mild to moderate MDD [80].

Preliminary evidence for efficacy in TRD has come from several open trials. In the study by Rosenbaum et al. [84], open-label oral SAMe was administered as monotherapy for 6 weeks to patients with MDD, of whom some had a history of nonresponse to antidepressants, and significant improvements were observed by week 3. In a more recent open-label study, 6-week treatment with SAMe tosylate as add-on to ongoing antidepressant medication was found to be associated with significant improvements and 43% remission rates [1]. Finally, in the RCT by Papakostas et al. [71], adjunct SAMe for 6 weeks was associated with significantly higher remission rates than adjunct placebo, and a post hoc analysis revealed significantly greater improvements in the ability to recall information in the SAMe group [48].

The results of these studies suggest therapeutic potential of adjunct SAMe for TRD and that SAMe at 800–1600 mg/day for 6 weeks appears to confer augmentation benefits in TRD. It was well tolerated, with no serious adverse events. Common adverse effects were similar to those reported in MDD and were generally mild and transient. They included headaches, fatigue, nervousness, sleep disturbances, and gastrointestinal issues, such as nausea, diarrhea, constipations, and lack of appetite [1, 71, 84].

12.4 Conclusion

Partial or nonresponse to conventional pharmacotherapy is common in patients with MDD and often persists in a substantial proportion in spite of switch and augmentation strategies. Poor adherence frequently contributes to lack of response and chronicity. Many patients discontinue antidepressants due to troublesome adverse effects, such as weight gain and sexual dysfunction. These observations underscore the need for alternative and integrative therapeutic approaches that do not rely solely on pharmacotherapy. Because many CAM modalities act via mechanisms different than antidepressant medications, they can be viable options for patients that are resistant to standard pharmacotherapy and augmentation strategies, and for those who develop intolerable adverse effects to medications. Moreover, patients who have no access to standard care and/or cannot afford the cost of medications may also benefit from CAMs, as these tend to be more affordable and available without a prescription. Finally, the majority of CAM therapies are either self-directed physical and/or mind-based practices or derived from natural products. As such, they often appeal to patients who are not comfortable with the use of psychotropic medications and those who wish to adopt CAMs as part of an integrative approach to maximize therapeutic benefits (Table 12.9).

The evidence to support the use of CAM therapies in TRD is promising but currently limited.

Based on efficacy, safety, and practicality, the most robust evidence is for exercise, MBCT, and ω-3 FA supplements as adjunctive to ongoing pharmacotherapy. There is less evidence on efficacy of yoga, light therapy, and SAMe in TRD, but given their reported good safety profiles and relative ease of use, these treatment modalities may be useful. There are several other CAM therapies not reviewed here which may be beneficial on an individual basis, but for which there is currently insufficient evidence to support widespread use.

Table 12.9 S-adenosyl-L-methionine in TRD

Author	Study design	Sample size	Definition of resistance	Intervention	Control	Key findings
Rosenbaum et al. [84]	Open label Monotherapy 6 weeks	20 MDD subjects (9 with and 11 without history of nonresponse)	1 or more failed trials of at least 4 weeks each	Up to 1600 mg/day SAMe	None	Overall significant*** reduction in $HAMD_{21}$ score compared to baseline 6/11 non-treatment-resistant and 1/9 treatment-resistant subjects met criteria for full response
Alpert et al. [1]	Open-label Adjunct (SSRI, SNRI) 6 weeks	30 subjects with treatment resistance	Partial or nonresponse to SSRIs or venlafaxine trials of at least 4 weeks	SAMe tosylate at 800–1600 mg/day	None	77% completion rate In ITT analyses, significant*** reductions in $HAMD_{17}$, MADRS, BDI, and CGI-S compared to baseline 50% responders and 43% remitters in ITT analysis at end point
Papakostas et al. [71]	RCT Adjunct (SSRI) 6 weeks	73 subject with TRD	Trial of SSRI for at least 4 weeks	SAMe at 800 mg/day	Placebo	Completion rates of 70% and 79% in SAMe and placebo, respectively Although improvements in HAMD and CGI-S observed in both treatment arms, significantly higher response** (18 subjects in SAMe, 6 subjects in placebo) and remission* (14 subjects in SAMe and 4 subjects in placebo) rates in treatment group
Levkovitz et al. [48]	Post hoc analysis					Significantly greater improvement in ability to recall information* in SAMe than placebo group

BDI Beck Depression Inventory, *CGI–S* Clinical Global Impressions–Severity, *ITT* intention-to-treat, *HAMD*, Hamilton Depression Rating Scale, *MADRS* Montgomery-Åsberg Depression Rating Scale, *RCT* randomized controlled trial,, *SAMe* S-adenosylmethionine, *SSR* selective serotonin reuptake inhibitor
$*p < 0.05$, $**p < 0.01$, $***p < 0.001$

It is important to emphasize that pharmacological and/or psychological treatments remain the first-line recommendations for depressive disorders and, thus, should be considered ahead of CAM therapies. Moreover, clinical judgement should always be applied when evaluating suitability and safety of CAM modalities for individual patients. Although the CAMs discussed in this chapter have been reported to be safe and devoid of serious adverse effects, there is a dearth of information on long-term effects and on interactions between CAM therapies and conventional treatments or between different CAM therapies. This is complicated by the fact that CAMs such as herbal supplements and nutraceuticals are not as rigorously regulated as pharmaceuticals. Moreover, patients often do not disclose self-directed CAM use to clinicians, and clinicians may not ask [80], adding to the risk of dangerous interactions. Finally, due to limited research conducted in TRD, there are currently no standard guidelines for use in this population.

Despite these limitations, the growing body of evidence in support of specific CAMs indicates therapeutic potential in TRD. As such, CAM therapies as add-on to evidence-based first-line interventions may be considered as part of an integrative approach to the management of TRD. Given the paucity of long term and interaction safety data, and the absence of guidelines for use in TRD, it is recommended that clinicians discuss the risks and benefits of available CAM treatments with their patients and establish guidelines for use in an individually tailored manner.

References

1. Alpert JE, Papakostas G, Mischoulon D, et al. S-adenosyl-L-methionine (SAMe) as an adjunct for resistant major depressive disorder: an open trial following partial or nonresponse to selective serotonin reuptake inhibitors or venlafaxine. J Clin Psychopharmacol. 2004;24:661–4.
2. Appleton KM, Hayward RC, Gunnell D, et al. Effects of n-3 long-chain polyunsaturated fatty acids on depressed mood: systematic review of published trials. Am J Clin Nutr. 2006;84:1308–16.
3. Appleton KM, Sallis HM, Perry R, et al. Omega-3 fatty acids for depression in adults. Cochrane Database Syst Rev. 2015;11:CD004692.
4. Baldessarini RJ. The neuropharmacology of S-adenosyl-L-methionine. Am J Med. 1987;83:95–103.
5. Bauer M, Forsthoff A, Baethge C, et al. Lithium augmentation therapy in refractory depression-update 2002. Eur Arch Psychiatry Clin Neurosci. 2003;253:132–9.
6. Benedetti F, Colombo C. Sleep deprivation in mood disorders. Neuropsychobiology. 2011;64:141–51.
7. Bloch MH, Hannestad J. Omega-3 fatty acids for the treatment of depression: systematic review and meta-analysis. Mol Psychiatry. 2012;17:1272–82.
8. Bressa GM. S-adenosyl-L-methionine (SAMe) as antidepressant: meta-analysis of clinical studies. Acta Neurol Scand Suppl. 1994;154:7–14.
9. Brook OH, van Hout HP, Stalman WA, de Haan M. Nontricyclic antidepressants: predictors of nonadherence. J Clin Psychopharmacol. 2006;26:643–7.
10. Butler LD, Waelde LC, Hastings TA, et al. Meditation with yoga, group therapy with hypnosis, and psychoeducation for long-term depressed mood: a randomized pilot trial. J Clin Psychol. 2008;64:806–20.
11. Cano M, Cardoner N, Urretavizcaya M, et al. Modulation of limbic and prefrontal connectivity by electroconvulsive therapy in treatment-resistant depression: a preliminary study. Brain Stimul. 2016;9:65–71.
12. Carpenter DJ. St John's wort and S-adenosyl methionine as "natural" alternatives to conventional antidepressants in the era of suicidality boxed warning: what is the evidence for clinically relevant benefit? Altern Med Rev. 2011;16:17–39.
13. Chiesa A, Serretti A. Mindfulness based cognitive therapy for psychiatric disorders: a systematic review and meta-analysis. Psychiatry Res. 2011;187:441–53.
14. Chiesa A, Castagner V, Adrisano C, et al. Mindfulness-based cognitive therapy vs. psychoeducation for patients with major depression who did not achieve remission following antidepressant treatment. Psychiatry Res. 2015;226:474–83.
15. Chojnacka M, Antosik-Wójcińska AZ, Dominiak M, et al. A sham-controlled randomized trial of adjunctive light therapy for non-seasonal depression. J Affect Disord. 2016;203:1–8.
16. Cladder-Micus MB, Vrijsen JN, Becker ES, et al. A randomized controlled trial of mindfulness-based cognitive therapy (MBCT) versus treatment-as-usual (TAU) for chronic, treatment-resistant depression: study protocol. BMC Psychiatry. 2015;15:275.
17. Cooney GM, Dwan K, Greig CA, et al. Exercise for depression. Cochrane Database Syst Rev. 2013;12:CD004366.
18. Cramer H, Lauche R, Langhorst J, Dobos G. Yoga for depression: a systematic review and meta-analysis. Depress Anxiety. 2013;30:1068–83.
19. Cramer H, Anheyer D, Lauche R, Dobos G. A systematic review of yoga for major depressive disorder. J Affect Disord. 2017;213:70–7.

20. Dallaspezia S, Benedetti F. Chronobiological therapy for mood disorders. Expert Rev Neurother. 2011;11:961–70.
21. Dawson R, Lavori PW, Coryell WH, et al. Course of treatment received by depressed patients. J Psychiatr Res. 1999;33:233–42.
22. De Berardis D, Orsolini L, Serroni N, et al. A comprehensive review on the efficacy of S-adenosyl-L-methionine in major depressive disorder. CNS Neurol Disord Drug Targets. 2016;15:35–44.
23. Delion S, Chalon S, Herault J, et al. Chronic dietary alpha-linolenic acid deficiency alters dopaminergic and seronotonergic neurotransmission in rats. J Nutr. 1994;124:2466–75.
24. Delion S, Chalon S, Guilloteau D, et al. Alpha-linolenic acid deficiency alters age-related changes of dopaminergic and serotonergic neurotransmission in the rat frontal cortex. J Neurochem. 1996;66:1582–91.
25. Desai R, Tailor A, Bhatt T. Effects of yoga on brain waves and structural activation: a review. Complement Ther Clin Pract. 2015;21:112–8.
26. Echizenya M, Suda H, Takeshima M, et al. Total sleep deprivation followed by sleep phase advance and bright light therapy in drug-resistant mood disorders. J Affect Disord. 2013;144:28–33.
27. Eisenberg DM, Davis RB, Ettner SL, et al. Trends in alternative medicine use in the United States, 1990–1997: results of a follow-up national survey. JAMA. 1998;280:1569–75.
28. Eisendrath SJ, Delucchi K, Bitner R, et al. Mindfulness-based cognitive therapy for treatment-resistant depression: a pilot study. Psychother Psychosom. 2008;77:319–20.
29. Eisendrath SJ, Gillung E, Delucchi KL, et al. A randomized controlled trial of mindfulness-based cognitive therapy for treatment-resistant depression. Psychother Psychosom. 2016;85:99–110.
30. Fava M, Rush AJ, Wisniewski SR, et al. A comparison of mirtazapine and nortriptyline following two consecutive failed medication treatments for depressed outpatients: a STAR*D report. Am J Psychiatry. 2006;163:1161–72.
31. Freeman MP, Hibbeln JR, Wisner KL, et al. Omega-3 fatty acids: evidence basis for treatment and future research in psychiatry. J Clin Psychiatry. 2006;67:1954–67.
32. Galper DI, Trivedi MH, Barlow CE, et al. Inverse association between physical inactivity and mental health in men and women. Med Sci Sports Exerc. 2006;38:173–8.
33. Gaynes BN, Dusetzina SB, Ellis AR, et al. Treating depression after initial treatment failure: directly comparing switch and augmenting strategies in STAR*D. J Clin Psychopharmacol. 2012;32:114–9.
34. Giedke H, Klingberg S, Schwarzler F, Schweinberg M. Direct comparison of total sleep deprivation and late partial sleep deprivation in the treatment of major depression. J Affect Disord. 2003;76:85–93.

35. Golden RN, Gaynes BN, Ekstrom RD, et al. The efficacy of light therapy in the treatment of mood disorders: a review and meta-analysis of the evidence. Am J Psychiatry. 2005;162:656–62.
36. Grosso G, Pajak A, Marventano S, et al. Role of omega-3 fatty acids in the treatment of depressive disorders: a comprehensive meta-analysis of randomized clinical trials. PLoS One. 2014;9:e96905.
37. Güzel Özdemir P, Boysan M, Smolensky MH, et al. Comparison of venlafaxine alone versus venlafaxine plus bright light therapy combination for severe major depressive disorder. J Clin Psychiatry. 2015;76Ñ:e645–54.
38. Josefsson M, Lindwall M, Archer T. Physical exercise intervention in depressive disorders: meta-analysis and systematic review. Scand J Med Sci Sports. 2014;24:259–72.
39. Hibbeln JR, Salem N Jr. Dietary polyunsaturated fatty acids and depression: when cholesterol does not satisfy. Am J Clin Nutr. 1995;62:1–9.
40. Ho SC, Jacob SA, Tangiisuran B. Barriers and facilitators of adherence to antidepressants among outpatients with major depressive disorder: a qualitative study. PLoS One. 2017;12:e0179290.
41. Höfer P, Schosser A, Calati R, et al. The impact of serotonin receptor 1A and 2A gene polymorphisms and interactions on suicide attempt and suicide risk in depressed patients with insufficient response to treatment—a European multicentre study. Int Clin Psychopharmacol. 2016;31:1–7.
42. Kautto M, Kampman O, Mononon N, et al. Serotonin transporter (5-HTTLPR) and norepinephrine transporter (NET) gene polymorphisms: susceptibility and treatment response of electroconvulsive therapy in treatment resistant depression. Neurosci Lett. 2015;590:116–20.
43. Kennedy SH, Lam RW, McIntyre RS, et al. Canadian Network for Mood and Anxiety Treatments (CANMAT) 2016 clinical guidelines for the management of adults with major depressive disorder: section 3. Pharmacological treatments. Can J Psychiatr. 2016;61:540–60.
44. Kenny MA, Williams JMG. Treatment-resistant depressed patients show a good response to mindfulness-based cognitive therapy. Behav Res Ther. 2007;45:617–25.
45. Khoury B, Lecomte T, Fortin G, et al. Mindfulness-based therapy: a comprehensive meta-analysis. Clin Psychol Rev. 2013;33:763–71.
46. Knubben K, Reischies FM, Adli M, et al. A randomized, controlled study on the effects of short-term endurance training programme in patients with major depression. Br J Sports Med. 2007;41:29–33.
47. Lam RW, Levitt AJ, Levitan RD, et al. The CanSAD study: a randomized controlled trial of the effectiveness of light therapy and fluoxetine in patients with winter seasonal affective disorder. Am J Psychiatry. 2006;163:805–12.

48. Levkovitz Y, Alpert JE, Brintz CE, et al. Effects of S-adenosylmethionine augmentation of serotonin-reuptake inhibitor antidepressants on cognitive symptoms of major depressive disorder. J Affect Disord. 2012;136:1174–8.

49. Lin PY, Su KP. A meta-analytic review of double-blind, placebo-controlled trials of antidepressant efficacy of omega-3 fatty acids. J Clin Psychiatry. 2007;68:1056–61.

50. Lam RW, Levitt AJ, Levitan RD, et al. Efficacy of bright light treatment, fluoxetine, and the combination in patients with nonseasonal major depressive disorder – a randomized clinical trial. JAMA Psychiat. 2016;73:56–63.

51. Malhi GS, Byrow Y. Is treatment-resistant depression a useful concept? Evid Based Ment Health. 2016;19:1–3.

52. Mårtensson B, Pettersson A, Berglund L, et al. Bright white light therapy in depression: a critical review of the evidence. J Affect Disord. 2015;182:1–7.

53. Martiny K, Refsgaard E, Lund V, et al. A 9-week randomized trial comparing a chronotherapeutic intervention (wake and light therapy) to exercise in major depressive disorder patients treated with duloxetine. J Clin Psychiatry. 2012;73:1234–42.

54. Mather AS, Rodriguez C, Guthrie MF, et al. Effects of exercise on depressive symptoms in older adults with poorly responsive depressive disorder: randomized controlled trial. Br J Psychiatry. 2002;180:411–5.

55. McIntyre RS, Filteau MJ, Martin L, et al. Treatment-resistant depression: definitions, review of the evidence, and algorithmic approach. J Affect Disord. 2014;156:1–7.

56. McNamara RK, Strimpfel J, Jandacek R, et al. Detection and treatment of long-chain omega-3 fatty acid deficiency in adolescents with SSRI-resistant major depressive disorder. Pharma Nutrition. 2014;2:38–46.

57. Miller IW, Keitner GI, Whisman MA, et al. Depressed patients with dysfunctional families: description and course of illness. J Abnorm Psychol. 1992;101:637–46.

58. Mota-Pereira J, Silverio J, Carvalho S, et al. Moderate exercise improves depression parameters in treatment-resistant patients with major depressive disorder. J Psychiatr Res. 2011a;45:1005–11.

59. Mota-Pereira J, Carvalho S, Silverio J, et al. Moderate physical exercise and quality of life in patients with treatment-resistant major depressive disorder. J Psychiatr Res. 2011b;45:1657–9.

60. Mrazek DA, Hornberger JC, Altar CA, Degtiar I. A review of the clinical, economic, and societal burden of treatment-resistant depression: 1996-2003. Psychiatr Serv. 2014;65:977–87.

61. National Center for Complementary and Alternative Medicine. 2002. What is complementary and alternative medicine? National Institutes of Health. Available at [http:nncam.nih.gov/health/whatiscam/#su1].

62. Nemeroff CB. Prevalence and management of treatment-resistant depression. J Clin Psychiatry. 2007;68:17–25.

63. Nemets B, Stahl Z, Belmaker RH. Addition of omega-3 fatty acid to maintenance medication treatment for recurrent unipolar depressive disorder. Am J Psychiatry. 2002;159:477–9.

64. Niederhofer, Klitzing V. Bright light treatment as add-on therapy for depression in 28 adolescents: a randomized trial. Prim Care Companion CNS Disord. 2011;13:PCC.11m01194.

65. Noaghiul S, Hibbeln JR. Cross-national comparisons od seafood consumption and rates of bipolar disorders. Am J Psychiatry. 2003;160:2222–7.

66. Nyström MB, Neely G, Hassmén P, et al. Treating major depression with physical activity: a systematic overview with recommendations. Cogn Behav Ther. 2015;44:341–52.

67. Oldham MA, Ciraulo DA. Bright light therapy for depression: a review of its effects on chronobiology and the autonomic nervous system. Chronobiol Int. 2014;31:305–19.

68. Papakostas GI, Petersen TJ, Farabaugh AH, et al. Psychiatric comorbidity as a predictor of clinical response to nortriptyline in treatment-resistant major depressive disorder. J Clin Psychiatry. 2003;64:1357–61.

69. Papakostas GI. Managing partial response or non-response: switching, augmentation, and combination strategies for major depressive disorder. J Clin Psychiatry. 2009a;70:16–25.

70. Papakostas GI. The role of S-adenosyl methionine in the treatment of depression. J Clin Psychiatry. 2009b;70:18–22.

71. Papakostas GI, Mischoulon D, Shyu I, et al. S-adenosyl methionine (SAMe) augmentation of serotonin reuptake inhibitors for antidepressant non-responders with major depressive disorder: a double-blind, randomized clinical trial. Am J Psychiatry. 2010;167:942–8.

72. Peet M, Horrobin DF. A dose-ranging study of the effects of ethyl-eicosapentaenoate in patients with ongoing depression despite apparently adequate treatment with standard drugs. Arch Gen Psychiatry. 2002;59:913–9.

73. Peng HJ, Zheng HR, Ning YP, et al. Abnormalities of cortical-limbic-cerebellar white matter networks may contribute to treatment-resistant depression: a diffusion tensor imaging study. BMC Psychiatry. 2013;13:72.

74. Perera S, Eisen R, Bhatt M, et al. Light therapy for non-seasonal depression: systematic review and meta-analysis. B J Psych Open. 2016;2:116–26.

75. Piet J, Hougaard E. The effect of mindfulness-based cognitive therapy for prevention of relapse in recurrent major depressive disorder: a systematic

review and meta-analysis. Clin Psychol Rev. 2011;31:1032–40.
76. Pilu A, Sorba M, Hardoy MC, et al. Efficacy of physical activity in the adjunctive treatment of major depressive disorders: preliminary results. Clin Pract Epidemiol Ment Health. 2007;3:8.
77. Prasko J, Brunovsky M, Latalova K, et al. Augmentation of antidepressants with bright light therapy in patients with comorbid depression and borderline personality disorder. Biomed Pap Med Fac Univ Palacky Olomouc Czech Repub. 2010;154:355–61.
78. Prien R, Kupfer D. Continuation drug therapy for major depressive episodes: how long should it be maintained? Am J Psychiatry. 1986;143:18–23.
79. Qureshi NA, Al-Bedah AM. Mood disorders and complementary and alternative medicine: a literature review. Neuropsychiatr Dis Treat. 2013;9:639–58.
80. Ravindran AV, Balneaves LG, Faulkner G, et al. Canadian network for mood and anxiety treatments (CANMAT) 2016 clinical guidelines for the management of adults with major depressive disorder: section 5. Complementary and alternative medicine treatments. Can J Psychiatr. 2016;61(9):576–87.
81. Reynolds CF, Smith GS, Dew MA, et al. Accelerating symptom-reduction in late-life depression: a double-blind, randomized, placebo-controlled trial of sleep deprivation. Am J Geriatr Psychiatry. 2005;13:353–8.
82. Rao NP, Varambally S, Gangadhar BN. Yoga school of thought and psychiatry: therapeutic potential. Indian J Psychiatry. 2013;55:S145–9.
83. Rohan KJ, Mahon JN, Evans M, et al. Randomized trial of cognitive-behavioral versus light therapy for seasonal affective disorder: acute outcomes. Am J Psychiatry. 2015;172:862–9.
84. Rosenbaum JF, Fava M, Falk WE, et al. The antidepressant potential of oral S-adenosyl-l-methionine. Acta Psychiatr Scand. 1990;81:432–6.
85. Rosenbaum S, Tiedermann A, Sherrington C. Physical activity interventions for people with mental illness: a systematic review and meta-analysis. J Clin Psychiatry. 2014;75:964–74.
86. Rush AJ, Trivedi MH, Wisniewski SR, et al. Acute and longer-term outcomes in depressed outpatients requiring one or several treatment steps: a STAR*D report. Am J Psychiatry. 2006;163:1905–17.
87. Sarris J, Kavanagh DJ, Byrne G. Adjuvant use of nutritional and herbal medicines with antidepressants, mood stabilizers and benzodiazepines. J Psychiatr Res. 2010;44:32–41.
88. Segal Z, Williams JM, Teasdale J. Mindfulness-based cognitive therapy for depression. New York: The Guilford press; 2002.
89. Shapiro D, Cook IA, Davydov DM, et al. Yoga as a complementary treatment for depression: effects of traits and moods on treatment outcome. Evid Based Complement Alternat Med. 2007;4:493–502.
90. Sharma A, Barrett MS, Cucchiara AJ, et al. A breathing-based meditation intervention for patients with major depressive disorder following inadequate response to antidepressants: a randomized pilot study. J Clin Psychiatry. 2017;78:e59–63.
91. Silveira H, Moraes H, Oliveira N. Physical exercise and clinically depressed patients: a systematic review and meta-analysis. Neuropsychobiology. 2013;67:61–8.
92. Souery D, Oswald P, Massat I, et al. Clinical factors associated with treatment resistance in major depressive disorder: results from a European multicenter study. J Clin Psychiatry. 2007;68:1062–70.
93. Stephens I. Medical yoga therapy. Child Aust. 2017;4:12.
94. Strauss C, Cavanagh K, Oliver A, Pettman D. Mindfulness-based interventions for people diagnosed with a current episode of an anxiety or depressive disorder: a meta-analysis of randomized controlled trials. PLoS One. 2014;9:e96110.
95. Streeter CC, Gerbarg PL, Saper RB, et al. Effects of yoga on autonomic nervous system, gamma-aminobutyric-acid, and allostasis in epilepsy, depression, and post-traumatic stress disorder. Med Hypotheses. 2012;78:571–9.
96. Su KP, Huang SY, Chiu CC, Shen WW. Omega-3 fatty acids in major depressive disorder. A preliminary double-blind, placebo-controlled trial. Eur Neuropsychopharmacol. 2003;13:267–71.
97. Sublette ME, Ellis SP, Geant AL, et al. Meta-analysis of the effects of eicosapentaenoic acid (EPA) in clinical trials in depression. J Clin Psychiatry. 2011;72:1577–84.
98. Sundborn LT, Bingefors K. The influence of symptoms of anxiety and depression on medication non-adherence and its causes: a population based survey of prescription drug users in Sweden. Patient Prefer Adherence. 2013;7:805–11.
99. Thase ME, Kupfer DJ. Characteristics of treatment-resistant depression. In: Zohar J, Belmaker R, editors. Treating resistant depression. New York: PMA Publishing; 1987. p. 23–45.
100. Tindle HA, Davis RB, Phillips RS, et al. Trends in use of complementary and alternative medicine by US adults: 1997-2002. Altern Ther Health Med. 2005;11:42–9.
101. Trivedi MH, Rush AJ, Wisniewski SR, et al. Evaluation of outcomes with citalopram for depression using measurement-based care in STAR*D: implications for clinical practice. Am J Psychiatry. 2006a;163:28–40.
102. Trivedi MH, Greer TL, Grannemann BD, et al. Exercise as an augmentation strategy for treatment of major depression. J Psychiatr Pract. 2006b;12:205–13.
103. Tuunainen A, Kripke DF, Endo T. Light therapy for non-seasonal depression. Cochrane Database Syst Rev. 2004;2:CD004050.

104. Wirz-Justice A, Bader A, Frisch U, et al. A randomized, double-blind, placebo-controlled study of light therapy for antepartum depression. J Clin Psychiatry. 2011;72:986–93.

105. World Health Organization. The World Health Report – 2001: mental health: new understanding, New Hope. Geneva: World Health Organization; 2011.

106. Yamamura T, Okamoto Y, Okada G, et al. Association of thalamic hyperactivity with treatment-resistant depression and poor response in early treatment for major depression: a resting-state fMRI study using fractional amplitude of low-frequency fluctuations. Transl Psychiatry. 2016;6:e754.

Complex Cases of Comorbid Depression and Personality Disorder (PD)

13

Ramamohan Veluri and Vicky P.K.H. Nguyen

13.1 Introduction

We present cases of two patients with depressive illness complicated by comorbid personality disorders (PDs). "Barbara" and "Janet" each have more than one type of comorbid PDs. "Barbara" had depression and both avoidant and obsessive personality traits, which interfered with her recovery and return to work. "Janet" had depression and both dependent and borderline personality traits, which produced vulnerability to the sick role preventing her from returning to work and prolonging her depressive illness. Both patients were initially stabilized on psychopharmacology before cognitive behavioural therapy (CBT) was commenced. The CBT formulation of each patient was informed by case conceptualization methodology outlined in "Case Formulation in Cognitive Behavioural Therapy: The Treatment of Challenging and Complex Cases" edited by Tarrier [24]. What is the psychotherapeutic approach to these patients? How should the psychotherapist address personality traits that are interfering with recovery from primary depressive illness?

R. Veluri, MD, DPM, MRCPsych, FRCPC (✉)
Northern Ontario School of Medicine,
Sudbury, ON, Canada

Vicky P.K.H. Nguyen, MD, PhD
Psychiatry Resident, Northern Ontario School of Medicine, Sudbury, ON, Canada

13.2 Case 1 Presentation

Barbara is a 58-year-old former executive of an accounting firm that recently closed its doors. She is married and is a mother of two grown-up children. Her son is single, in his early 20s, and lives in another city. Her daughter, in her late 20s, lives with her husband and three children in another country. As the executive of the accounting firm, Barbara was responsible for the decision to sell the company and to let go of over 50 employees instead of taking drastic measures to save the company and the employee's jobs.

After the company closed its doors, she had her first major depressive episode with atypical features and had thoughts of suicide. She was successfully treated during a month-long stay in the hospital with a combination of sertraline, bupropion, and supportive psychotherapy and was discharged to outpatient psychiatric care. CBT was initiated following discharge. She continued to receive IPT after CBT was terminated. (Table 13.1, Fig. 13.1).

13.3 Clinical Questions

How would psychotherapy benefit Janet in addressing dependent tendencies and borderline traits, which contribute to maintaining her depression?

What approach should the psychotherapist take?

What psychotherapeutic modality would most benefit the patient?

© Springer International Publishing AG, part of Springer Nature 2018
K. Shivakumar, S. Amanullah (eds.), *Complex Clinical Conundrums in Psychiatry*,
https://doi.org/10.1007/978-3-319-70311-4_13

Table 13.1 Barbara's personal details and problem list

Family of origin	Eldest child of four and only daughter; took care of her brothers growing up; both parents worked low-pay jobs and had frequent arguments about finances; parents have depression and anxiety; worked part-time in retail since 16 to help her family
Current family	Married for 12 years to her second husband; she raised her children from a previous relationship as a single mother; her brothers live far away with their families and there is little contact; her parents are deceased
Social supports	No close friends of her own; she socializes with her husbands' family and friends; she frequently visits her son, with whom she shares a friendship as well as a mother-son relationship
Educational history	She dropped out of high school to take a full-time job to help her family when her mother lost her job; she completed adult education later on and completed college; credits from college were used towards a university education; she completed the degree of master of business administration part-time while working as a secretary at the accounting firm
Career history	She rose through the ranks over 15 years at the accounting firm to become a director
Activities of interest	Reading; long-distance running; tennis; golf; charity work
Developmental history	She had normal birth and development; as a child, school was challenging due to inattention and difficulty with perfectionistic tendencies; later on in life, she received coaching to manage these tendencies and excelled in her education; growing up she was her parents' helper/babysitter for her younger siblings; her value to her parents and family was the help she provided to them in child-rearing
Premorbid personality	Obsessive-compulsive personality disorder (OCPD), Avoidant personality traits
Past medical history	Generally healthy, her family physician followed her for mild elevation of liver enzymes
Substance use history	Started drinking alcohol on and off socially during her teen years; gradually through her 20s and 30s, she became a regular drinker; she struggled with alcohol use disorder in her 40s and required in-patient rehabilitation treatment; now in her 50s, she drinks 1 to 2 glasses of wine daily
Medications	Sertraline 150MG daily Bupropion 300MG daily
Baseline scales	BDI = 20 (moderately depressive symptoms) HAM-A = 17 (mild anxiety symptoms) Y-BOCS = 14 (mild obsessive-compulsive symptoms)
Problem list	1. Depression 2. Anxiety 3. Obsessive rumination 4. Overestimation of responsibility 5. Views herself as unattractive 6. Feels unloved/unwanted if her husband fails to initiate sex 7. Inhibited, lacks confidence in social situations 8. Blames herself for her son's substance use problems 9. Avoids talking to her husband about her feelings 10. Poor self-care during low moods 11. Perfectionistic about diet and exercise during better moods 12. Inconsistent in maintenance of healthy self-esteem/image 13. Problematic alcohol use and elevated liver enzymes

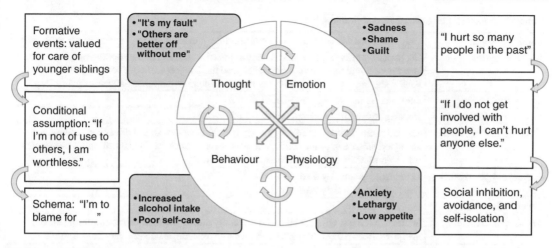

Fig. 13.1 CBT formulation for Barbara

13.4   Case 2 Presentation

Janet is a 24-year-old nursing student on disability for work stress and depression. She lives with her partner of 10 years and has no children. She experienced severe burnout during her final year of nursing school and took an extended sick leave. She found it difficult to balance between maintaining boundaries with her fellow nursing students. She would become overly involved in helping classmates with their work neglecting her own. Without healthy boundaries, she frequently got into conflicts with the same classmates. Without appropriate boundaries, she tended to become overly involved in patient care and emotionally affected by her patients' suffering. There is no self-harm behaviour. She had been in CBT group therapy for a few months before she was assessed by a psychiatrist and started on medication. Individual CBT was initiated in combination with specific techniques of dialectical behaviour therapy (DBT) [18] in order to adapt to the patient's presentation. (Table 13.2, Fig. 13.2).

13.5   Clinical Questions

How would psychotherapy benefit Janet in addressing dependent tendencies and borderline traits, which contribute to maintaining her depression?

What approach should the psychotherapist take?

What psychotherapeutic modality would most benefit the patient?

13.6   Literature Review

Personality disorder (PD) can be defined as a recurring pattern of maladaptive habits of thinking, behaving, and responding emotionally to the environment. Based on estimates by Samuels [21], 6–10% of the general population have one or more PD. Beckwith et al. [6] reviewed studies of estimates of prevalence of PD in clients of mental health services in the community and found that rates vary from low 42% to high 92%. Having a PD is a predictor of more severe mental health problems and resistance to psychological therapies and psychotherapy dropout [26]. Kuyken and colleagues [16] found PD sufferers had more severe mental illness at baseline prior to psychological treatment and more residual symptoms following termination of treatment. The authors also noted that it was not the PD, per se, that interfered with psychological intervention, rather, cognitive distortions such as avoidant and paranoid beliefs that determined therapy outcome. This observation by Kuyken and colleagues [16] would suggest PDs are perhaps ame-

Table 13.2 Janet's personal details and problem list

Family of origin	Only child; parents are financially comfortable; parents deny any mental health problems
Social supports	Her partner works full-time and is very supportive; she has many supportive friends; her grandmother and mother visit often; she also has support from her partner's extended family; she has a friendship with her mother instead of a mother-daughter relationship
Educational history	She excelled in nursing school until illness
Activities of interest	Drawing; gardening; sewing; crafts; scrapbooking
Developmental history	She had normal birth and development; as a child, school was challenging because she attempted suicide in grade school and was socially ostracized for the attempt; classmates were told by their parents not to associate with her
Premorbid personality	Borderline personality disorder Dependent personality disorder
Past medical history	Generally healthy
Substance use history	Started smoking marijuana on and off socially during her teen years; currently smokes marijuana once a day and drinks 2–3 alcoholic beverages one to three times a week
Medications	Bupropion 300MG daily Lisdexamfetamine dimesylate 60MG daily
Baseline scales	BDI = 15 (mild depressive symptoms) HAM-A = 10 (very little anxiety symptoms) ADHD adult self-rating scale = inattention
Problem list	1. Depression 2. Marijuana use 3. Work avoidance 4. Entrenched sick role disproportionate to measured symptom severity 5. Low self-esteem 6. Low distress tolerance 7. Sensitivity to rejection 8. Low skill in healthy boundaries 9. Low perceived self-efficacy 10. Poor emotional self-management

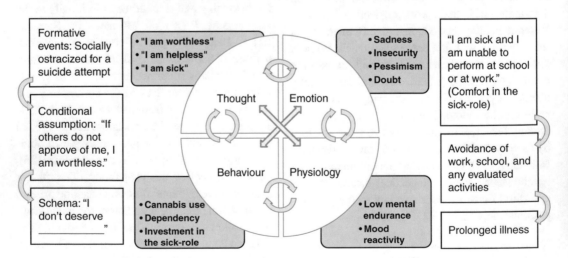

Fig. 13.2 CBT formulation for Janet

nable to cognitive and behavioural psychological interventions aimed at changing maladaptive patterns in thinking, feeling, behaving, and relating to others.

Generally, having a PD means living many years of significant distress and dysfunction in important social and personal domains without treatment. People with PD often fail to live up to their potential in achievement and happiness. They are at higher risk of developing mental illness, suicide, and dying prematurely than people without PDs [26]. Dixon-Gordon and colleagues [9] systematically reviewed studies of health outcomes associated with PDs and found evidence of correlations with obesity, propensity to develop an eating disorder (including binge eating), chronic pain, chronic illness including liver disease, cardiovascular disease, gastrointestinal disease, arthritis, venereal disease, hypertension, and atherosclerosis. Correspondingly, sufferers of PDs tended to have high rates of health service utilization. Having a diagnosed PD carries almost a life sentence of stigma and vulnerabilities that is yet to be adequately addressed by clinical psychiatry. However, tremendous effort by some researchers and clinicians has led to the beginnings of effective treatment strategies combining both pharmacotherapy and psychotherapy [2, 20].

Unfortunately, treatment recommendations for PD are tentative at best and not yet based on sufficient evidence for confident implementation [2]. Development of treatment of PD is challenged by absence of diagnostic and assessment tools sensitive and specific to the wide range of personality pathology, disorder severity, safety implications, and prognosis. To further complicate matters, developers of the International Classification of Diseases (ICD) and of the Diagnostic and Statistical Manual of Mental Disorders (DSM) have radically different approaches to PD characterization [25]. How PD is characterized will determine how we collectively design our approach to psychological and psychosocial therapies for sufferers of PD and for mental health issues in people with PD.

Contrary to popular belief that any PD is a permanent, long-term, and unchangeable condition, Seivewright et al. [22] found high variability in prognosis of various PDs defined by the DSM-III in their 12-year study. The authors found "Cluster B" personality traits (antisocial, histrionic) tended to wane over the years. Contrastingly, "Cluster A" (schizoid, schizotypal, and paranoid) and "Cluster C" (obsessive, avoidant) personality traits tended to worsen over time without

treatment directly targeting the PD. Significant for clinical psychiatry is evidence that the presence of comorbid PD in primary psychiatric disorder predicts treatment outcome for depression. Hardy and colleagues [12] found symptoms of depression tended to be more severe at baseline in patients with "Cluster C" PD, who also showed significantly less improvement following treatment compared to those without PD. Thus, having a PD means an added vulnerability for high burden of mental illness and poorer quality of life.

Not only are sufferers of PDs tend not to respond as well to psychotherapy, they also tend to drop out of therapy at higher rates than other therapy recipients. According to a recent meta-analysis of randomized clinical trials for individual psychotherapy for depression by Cooper and Conklin [7], comorbid PD was a predictor of therapy dropout. Not surprising, given that hypothesized impaired capacity for attachment is likely responsible for intrapsychic dysfunction and impoverished interpersonal relationships common to all PDs [17]. Supporting this hypothesis are findings by Joyce and colleagues [13], in their randomized clinical trial that personality traits negatively affected treatment response to interpersonal psychotherapy (IPT) but not to cognitive behavioural therapy (CBT) for depression. The severity of the PD was associated with poorer outcome from IPT, which requires the capacity to trust others and take risks in the interpersonal domain for clinical gains.

Attachment theory as it pertains to PD is still a relatively new area of research. Evidence is still insufficient for a precise description of types of attachment problems associated with each PD. It is a still promising area of inquiry given the implications for approaches to psychotherapeutic treatment for PDs. For example [8], proposed that clinicians treating PD with psychotherapy need to be aware of individual maladaptive interpersonal schemas in order to create lasting or meaningful change. Generally, the author characterized PD sufferers as having highly pessimistic expectations of others in fulfilment of their attachment needs; PD sufferers operate under the assumption that others would not "nurture" them but will "reject, control, or abuse" them [8]. This means treating sufferers of PD requires competent and sensitive clinicians willing to go the extra mile to adapt to and address their individual patient's interpersonal challenges.

Given favourable therapeutic alliance between well-matched psychotherapist and patient, evidence so far suggests that PD can be treated with limited success [8]. In resource-limited settings, the treatment of PD is often impractical unless the PD is severe and causing significant distress. Realistically, when patients with PD or "Axis II" present to clinical psychiatry, psychiatric diagnoses historically labelled as "Axis I" are the foci of therapy. PDs are subject to clinical attention only when they have implications for treatment of primary psychiatric disorders such as depression. In retrospect, this approach may have led to positive outcomes for those with PD according to evidence gathered and reviewed by Shea et al. [23]. The authors found evidence that patients with depression and borderline PD receiving treatment for issues related to the PD had better outcomes in residual symptoms and in the domains of social, occupational, and global functioning than patients with PD but without depression. As another example, depressed men, with comorbid opioid use disorder and antisocial personality disorder treated with CBT and addiction counselling, showed significant improvement in psychiatric symptoms, employment, drug use, and illegal activities, compared to men who did not have depression [23]. Depression was a positive prognostic factor for these patients with antisocial and borderline PD. Despite significant challenges of treating patients with comorbid PD, these pieces of data would suggest to us reason for cautious optimism.

Indeed, some studies have suggested that when patients with an "Axis II" diagnosis of a PD are properly engaged in treatment, there may be unexpected concomitant reduction in symptoms of PD during the course of treatment for the presenting/primary "Axis I" psychiatric illness. Indeed, Keefe et al. [14] compared CBT treatment outcome for 33 patients with major depression without PD and 26 patients with major depression and comorbid PD. The authors found

that early psychotherapeutic work on maladaptive core beliefs resulted in significant reductions in both symptoms of depression and symptoms of comorbid PD. Patients in this study had "Cluster B" and "Cluster C" personality issues. These are descriptions of a handful of studies of treatment for patients with anxiety or depression and a comorbid PD. The results somewhat lend support to a cognitive approach to PDs.

Data on the psychological treatment of mental illness in people with PDs is limited for good reason. The majority of randomized controlled trials up to date address the psychotherapeutic treatment of only approximately 50% of the population of mental health patients: those *without* a comorbid PD. Most clinical trials also measure outcomes of rigorously applied manual-based or "manualized" psychotherapy. It is a well-known fact that the psychotherapy performed on research subjects do not mirror well the psychotherapy that is actually done in practice [11]. Furthermore, clinical trials exclude participation of countless patients who refuse manual-based therapy or are unable to participate in manual-based therapy due to cognitive limitations (e.g. learning disabilities). Keeping in mind these caveats, recent meta-analyses evaluating the efficacy of psychological therapies for depression have consistently shown robust effect sizes for manualized or manual-based CBT and IPT.

In a meta-analysis of 198 randomized controlled trials involving 15,118 adults with major depressive disorder, Barth and colleagues [3] found each of seven psychotherapeutic modalities (IPT, behaviour activation, CBT, problem-solving therapy, social skills training, psychodynamic therapy, supportive counselling) superior to control (usual care or waitlist) with moderate to large effect sizes. Not surprisingly because other studies echo similar findings, CBT, behavioural activation, and IPT emerged as the modalities with the most robust response. There was no heterogeneity in pooled measured reductions in depressive symptoms as a result of psychotherapy [3]. In general, CBT has accumulated the most evidential support in the literature for the treatment of "Axis I" disorders.

The literature on CBT as a treatment modality for PDs lacks strong meta-analyses like the one by Barth and colleagues. Matusiewicz and colleagues [19] performed a less systematized review of studies on cognitive psychotherapies for PD published between 1980 and 2009. The authors found a generally favourable outlook for the usefulness of cognitive approaches to PDs. The absence of quality randomized controlled trials on psychological treatment of mental illness in people with comorbid PDs means an absence of rigorously validated psychological treatment protocols designed specifically for sufferers of PDs. No CBT manual exists to guide the psychotherapeutic treatment of depression or anxiety in patients with comorbid PD. Currently, the most clinically instructive and comprehensive guide to the psychological treatment PDs is the book by the inventor of CBT, Dr. Aaron T. Beck, and his colleagues, Dr. Denise D. Davis and Arthur Freeman, entitled "Cognitive Therapy of Personality Disorders" [5].

13.7 Treatment Course and Response

Barbara received 4 months of weekly CBT for a total of 16 sessions. CBT goals were collaboratively decided upon with patient input. CBT was conducted with heavy emphasis on cognitive changes. Goals included more realistic estimation of her personal responsibility for the consequences of her company's closure, for her son's substance use, and generally for others' actions, behaviours, and circumstances beyond her control. She developed more balanced views of her influence on her children, particularly her son. Gradually she improved in mood and anxiety. Barbara returned to work as a manager at a social enterprise and enjoyed her job. However, she had problems with attention and concentration despite a euthymic mood. Lisdexamfetamine dimesylate 40MG was added to her medication regime to good effect.

Despite improved mood and cognition, Barbara was still socially anxious and inhibited, which interfered with her abilities to network for her work. With the patient's consent, she was transitioned from CBT to IPT with a focus on interpersonal deficits/sensitivity over the next 3 months. CBT booster sessions were integrated with IPT sessions. IPT was provided using guidelines and instructions from the "Clinician's Quick Guide to Interpersonal Psychotherapy" by Weissman et al. [27]. Deficits in her relationship with her husband were also addressed using IPT techniques. When asked to compare her experiences of the two psychotherapeutic techniques, she indicated that she felt more comfortable with IPT because her habits of thinking and perceiving were not targeted for change, but IPT seemed to help her achieve similar level of improvement in mood.

Janet received 3 months of weekly CBT for a total of 12 sessions. CBT was provided with heavy emphasis on behavioural activation to encourage stepping out of the sick role . CBT goals collaboratively decided upon with patient input included goal setting, improving decisiveness, problem-solving skills, return to school or to work, reducing cannabis and alcohol use, and improving self-efficacy. DBT skills from the "Skills Training Manual for Treating Borderline Personality Disorder" [18] were taught concurrently as CBT proceeded to address various interpersonal difficulties. For example, the skill of mindfulness was used to address inattention; interpersonal effectiveness skills were used to address problems with boundaries. Janet gradually improved but made the decision not to return to nursing school. She decided not to be involved in any kind of work requiring prolonged and deep involvement with people. She started a part-time position at a friend's local business. She was eventually discharged from outpatient psychiatric care.

13.8 Summary

We described two patient cases illustrating challenges in the treatment of depression with psychotherapy. In the first case (Barbara), CBT helped the patient to resume full-time employment. However, after CBT termination, the patient had significant interpersonal deficits, which were better addressed using techniques of IPT. In the second case (Janet), the patient was heavily invested in the sick role. IPT would have been inappropriate for Janet given that IPT relies on the temporary sick role in order to help the patient accept psychotherapeutic help and increase help-seeking behaviour from his or her trusted social network.

Barber and Muenz [1] previously hypothesized that cognitive therapy (CT) was more effective than IPT in depressed patients who were also avoidant, whereas IPT was more effective for depressed patient who had obsessive tendencies. Joyce and colleagues [13] did not replicate this finding. They tended to find both avoidant and obsessive-compulsive PDs to interfere with IPT. In Barbara's case, avoidant traits likely would have interfered with her homework exercises for IPT. CBT was required to change the self-belief that she was worthless unless others relied upon her and to reduce her skewed sense of responsibility for other's health and welfare. Barbara had reduced avoidant tendencies when she returned to work. By then, she was prepared to do assignments between therapy sessions aimed at reducing social isolation and interpersonal sensitivity or deficits with IPT.

Joyce and colleagues [13] reported from their randomized trial comparing IPT with CBT in depressed patients that personality traits were more likely to interfere with IPT than with CBT treatment further supporting the chosen sequence of CBT followed by IPT. In their discussion, Joyce and colleagues articulated the hypothesis that perhaps outcomes of other "dynamic" psychotherapies may also be adversely affected by patient neuroticism, thereby putting into question the traditional clinical belief that dynamic psychotherapies are indicated for patients with personality disorders.

The answer to this question came partially this year, when Kikkert and colleagues [15] replicated the study by Barber and Muenz [1] for CBT versus psychodynamic supportive psychotherapy. The authors found that the severity of avoidant or obsessive-compulsive personality did not influence the outcome of therapy in the treatment of depression. Therefore, for Barbara and for similar patients, clinician experience and judgement combined with collaboration with the patient remain the best method of deciding which psychotherapy modality and when to apply in the treatment of depression.

Like Barbara, Janet also had significant interpersonal stressors, but they were better addressed using interpersonal skills of DBT, which augmented the main psychotherapeutic modality used: CBT. For Barbara, emphasis was on cognitive therapy during her CBT sessions. For Janet, emphasis was on behaviour activation to mobilize her out of the sick role during her CBT sessions. Both patients were not provided manual-based CBT but modified CBT adapted to suit their individual clinical presentation. Adaptations were made in collaboration with the patient themselves. We illustrate here the reality of psychotherapeutic treatment in clinical psychiatric practice not describable in clinical trials.

It is known for a decade and a half that specific maladaptive core beliefs are associated with various personality disorders [4]. More recently, Keefe et al. [14] observed that in depressed patients with comorbid personality disorders, early cognitive work aimed at dysfunctional core beliefs predicted better outcomes for both depressive and personality disorder symptoms. In the case of Janet, she had traits of borderline and dependent personality disorders comorbid with her depressive symptoms. The personality pathology in Janet was addressed insofar as it contributed to her recovery from her mood disorder. Often in the case in many clinical settings, there is neither available resource nor psychotherapist hour to target the personality pathology itself. If the goal is functional recovery, targeting the personality pathology may not be necessary or advised. We have already seen evidence that personality pathology may not interfere with outcome of therapy for depression [14].

According to Fournier et al. [10], personality pathology is marked by dysfunctional cognitions that can be identified and targeted. In case 1, Barbara was identified to have an overestimation of responsibility for others that contributed to her mood symptoms. In case 2, Janet was identified to have an underestimation of her capacity to cope and excessive need for approval and care from others. Janet was entrenched in the sick role because it helped her escape from disapproval and fulfilled the need for attentive care from others. In both cases, personality pathology was addressed insofar as it improved the patient's chances of functional recovery.

Currently, systematic bedside assessment tools validated for use in clinical psychiatry to objectively determine type and measure severity of personality pathology, are only in the developmental stage. The clinical value of such tool is uncertain. Until our state of knowledge improves, we advocate for attention to personality pathology only so far as it helps to conceptualize cognitive distortions and beliefs contributing to the patient's presenting complaints. CBT-based conceptualization of the patient combined with a CBT-based psychotherapeutic course adapted to the patient remain the most well-studied and practical approach to any mental health patient with comorbid personality disorders. Typically, patients with maladaptive avoidant and paranoid beliefs have more severe depressive symptomatology at baseline intake and are more likely to have residual symptoms upon psychotherapy termination [16]. Generally, we recommend that goal and focus of therapy be directed at the presenting psychiatric complaint, and the physician needs to work collaboratively with the patient towards the goal of functional recovery.

Disclosure Statement No grants received for this work. There was no conflict of interest with any person or organization.

References

1. Barber JP, Muenz LR. The role of avoidance and obsessiveness in matching patients to cognitive and interpersonal psychotherapy: empirical findings from the treatment for depression collaborative research program. J Consult Clin Psychol. 1996;64(5):951–8.
2. Bateman AW, Gunderson J, Mulder R. Treatment of personality disorder. Lancet. 2015;385(9969):735–43.
3. Barth J, Munder T, Gerger H, Nüesch E, Trelle S, Znoj H, Jüni P, Cuijpers P. Comparative efficacy of seven psychotherapeutic interventions for patients with depression: a network meta-analysis. PLoS Med. 2013;10(5):e1001454.
4. Beck AT, Butler AC, Brown GK, Dahlsgaard KK, Newman CF, Beck JS. Dysfunctional beliefs discriminate personality disorders. Behav Res Ther. 2001;39(10):1213–25.
5. Beck AT, Davis DD, Freeman A. Cognitive therapy of personality disorders. 3rd ed. New York: The Guilford Press; 2015.
6. Beckwith H, Moran PF, Reilly J. Personality disorder prevalence in psychiatric outpatients: a systematic literature review. Personal Ment Health. 2014;8(2):91–101.
7. Cooper AA, Conklin LR. Dropout from individual psychotherapy for major depression: a meta-analysis of randomized clinical trials. Clin Psychol Rev. 2015;40:57–65.
8. Dimaggio G. Integrated treatment for personality disorders: an introduction. J Psychother Integr. 2015;25(1):1–2. https://doi.org/10.1037/a0038765.
9. Dixon-Gordon KL, Whalen DJ, Layden BK, Chapman ALA. Systematic review of personality disorders and health outcomes. Can Psychol. 2015;56(2):168–90.
10. Fournier JC, Derubeis RJ, Beck AT. Dysfunctional cognitions in personality pathology: the structure and validity of the personality belief questionnaire. Psychol Med. 2012;42(4):795–805.
11. Havik OE, VandenBos GR. Limitations of manualized psychotherapy for everyday clinical practice. Clin Psychol Sci Prac. 1996;3:264–7.
12. Hardy GE, Barkham M, Shapiro DA, Stiles WB, Rees A, Reynolds S. Impact of Cluster C personality disorders on outcomes of contrasting brief psychotherapies for depression. J Consult Clin Psychol. 1995;63(6):997–1004.
13. Joyce PR, McKenzie JM, Carter JD, Rae AM, Luty SE, Frampton CM, Mulder RT. Temperament, character and personality disorders as predictors of response to interpersonal psychotherapy and cognitive-behavioural therapy for depression. Br J Psychiatry. 2007;190:503–8.
14. Keefe JR, Webb CA, DeRubeis RJ. In cognitive therapy for depression, early focus on maladaptive beliefs may be especially efficacious for patients with personality disorders. J Consult Clin Psychol. 2016;84(4):353–64.
15. Kikkert MJ, Driessen E, Peen J, Barber JP, Bockting C, Schalkwijk F, Dekker J, Dekker JJM. The role of avoidant and obsessive-compulsive personality disorder traits in matching patients with major depression to cognitive behavioral and psychodynamic therapy: a replication study. J Affect Disord. 2016;205:400–5.
16. Kuyken W, Kurzer N, DeRubeis RJ, Beck AT, Brown GK. Response to cognitive therapy in depression: the role of maladaptive beliefs and personality disorders. J Consult Clin Psychol. 2001;69(3):560–6.
17. Levy KN, Johnson BN, Clouthier TL, Scala JW, Temes CM. An attachment theoretical framework for personality disorders. Can Psychol. 2015;56(2):197–207.
18. Linehan MM. Skills training manual for treating borderline personality disorder. New York: Guilford Press; 1993.
19. Matusiewicz AK, Hopwood CJ, Banducci AN, Lejuez CW. The effectiveness of cognitive behavioral therapy for personality disorders. Psychiatr Clin North Am. 2010;33(3):657–85.

20. Nathan PE, Corman JM. A guide to treatments that work. New York: Oxford University Press; 2015. Chapters 27 and 28. p. 851–94.

21. Samuels J. Personality disorders: epidemiology and public health issues. Int Rev Psychiatry. 2011;23(3):223–33.

22. Seivewright H, Tyrer P, Johnson T. Change in personality status in neurotic disorders. Lancet. 2002; 359(9325):f2253–4.

23. Shea MT, Widiger TA, Klein MH. Comorbidity of personality disorders and depression: implications for treatment. J Consult Clin Psychol. 1992;60(6):857–68.

24. Tarrier N, editor. Case formulation in cognitive behaviour therapy: the treatment of challenging and complex cases. London/New York: Routledge, Taylor & Francis Group; 2006.

25. Tyrer P, Crawford M, Mulder R. ICD-11 working group for the revision of classification of personality disorders. Reclassifying personality disorders. Lancet. 2011;377(9780):1814–5.

26. Tyrer P, Reed GM, Crawford MJ. Classification, assessment, prevalence, and effect of personality disorder. Lancet. 2015;385(9969):717–26.

27. Weissman MM, Markowitz JC, Klerman GL. Clinician's quick guide to interpersonal psychotherapy. Oxford/New York: Oxford University Press; 2007.

A Complex Case of a Personality Disorder

14

Brad D. Booth and Michelle D. Mathias

14.1 Introduction

As noted in the *Diagnostic and Statistical Manual of Mental Disorders*, 5th edition (DSM-5 [4]), a personality disorder is "an enduring pattern of inner experience and behavior that deviates markedly from the expectations of the individual's culture." This pattern can affect cognition, affect, interpersonal function, and impulse control. The pattern is inflexible, pervasive in multiple settings, and fairly stable throughout the person's life.

Significant revisions to the diagnostic criteria and approach for this group of disorders were proposed to be included in the DSM-5 [5]. However, these were ultimately rejected, and the traditional diagnostic approach was maintained. A hybrid dimensional-categorical model was placed in a separate section, as an option for clinicians to consider. Despite generally maintaining the *status quo*, one very significant change was made – removing the "arbitrary boundaries between personality disorders and other mental disorders." This served to recognize that personality disorders are true primary psychiatric entities.

Regardless of the different perspectives regarding diagnostic criteria, individuals with primary or secondary personality disorders or the associated dysfunctional personality traits can pose clinical conundrums for even the most experienced of clinicians. Individuals with personality disorders compose up to 14% of the general population [13, 35]. In addition, such diagnoses are often associated with psychiatric comorbidity, including psychosis, affective disorders, anxiety disorders, and alcohol/substance problems. They are also associated with high use of psychiatric services [13]. Those without full-blown personality disorders may present in a crisis situation wherein their dysfunctional personality traits emerge.

With this background, we present a case and discussion of one of the more challenging personality disorders, namely, antisocial personality disorder (ASPD).

B.D. Booth, MD, FRCPC (✉)
Integrated Forensic Program, Royal Ottawa Mental Health Centre, Ottawa, ON, Canada
e-mail: brad.booth@theroyal.ca

M.D. Mathias, MD, FRCPC
Division of Forensic Psychiatry,
Department of Psychiatry,
University of Ottawa, Ottawa, ON, Canada
e-mail: michelle.mathias@theroyal.ca

14.2 Case Example: Antisocial Personality Disorder (ASPD)

Mr. Randy Smith is a 45-year-old man who presents to the psychiatric emergency in significant distress, demanding admission. He is experiencing auditory hallucinations and fears for his

© Springer International Publishing AG, part of Springer Nature 2018
K. Shivakumar, S. Amanullah (eds.), *Complex Clinical Conundrums in Psychiatry*,
https://doi.org/10.1007/978-3-319-70311-4_14

safety. He believes government agents are trying to poison him and remove his brain. He is worried he is going to hurt someone or himself. He is agitated and has an intimidating and threatening demeanor. A urine toxicology screen is negative. His file reveals a history of ASPD, substances, schizoaffective disorder (depressive type), social anxiety disorder, generalized anxiety disorder, attention deficit disorder (ADHD), and possible post-traumatic stress disorder (PTSD).

Randy had a disrupted childhood, suffering significant physical abuse at the hands of his biological father until age 10, when his father left the picture. Injuries from the abuse would include frequent abrasions and bruising from open hand slaps, punches, and hits with a belt or hanger. He also had a fractured wrist on one occasion and had a cigarette put on his back on three occasions as punishment. He was then raised by his mother who had a string of unstable, abusive male partners. Randy was diagnosed with ADHD in grade 2, but was never really treated for the disorder given his mother was opposed to this. He had severe behavioral problems throughout school. He had early oppositional defiant disorder symptoms, such as talking back to teachers and swearing when upset. As he grew older, he lashed out physically to other students who teased him. By age 13, he was initiating these fights. He gravitated to the "partying crowd" in middle school, starting to use alcohol and cannabis regularly by age 13. He also started to run into legal problems, including break and enters, thefts, and mischief charges around the same age. He continued to show impulsive aggression and anger.

By age 15, Randy's drug use escalated, experimenting with "magic mushrooms," opiates, and amphetamines and snorting cocaine. By 18, he was addicted to crack cocaine, which would remain his drug of choice throughout life, though he was able to maintain prolonged periods of abstinence from all substances, both in and out of jail.

At age 16, Randy dropped out of school and continued having non-violent legal problems primarily to support his drug habit. However, at age 19, he was convicted of his first violent crime – an assault causing bodily harm on a drug-using friend while high on cocaine. He served 11 months for this offense. He had a number of other non-violent offenses, including fraud, thefts, stolen property, and breaches. His second serious violent offense was an attempt murder charge, at 24 years old. It has been a drug deal "gone wrong." The charge was pleaded down to aggravated assault, and he served 7 years in a federal penitentiary. At the time of his current presentation to the emergency, he did not have any other violent charges in his legal history. His last conviction was around 5 years ago for possession and distribution of cocaine. In total, he had 25 previous sentencing dates and had served about 12 years of his adult life in jails.

Despite his substance use and other problems, Randy maintains close ties with his mother, who worked as a nurse and is now retired. He was also skilled in carpentry, learning this from a close uncle. He has worked intermittently in construction, noting he did not want anyone supporting him and would refuse to apply for social assistance when out of work. He is currently in between jobs and sleeping at friends' places.

From a relationship perspective, Randy had a number of short-term heterosexual relationships early in life. He had one common-law girlfriend of 3 years, prior to his 7-year federal sentence, at the age of 24. The relationship had been very stormy and was characterized by mutual physical and emotional abuse. She was also addicted to crack cocaine and likely had some borderline personality traits. Since then, however, he has been single. He noted that he always "picks unstable women," and it's better to be alone. Despite his tumultuous common-law relationship, he has no domestic violence history and elaborated, "Real men don't hurt women." He does not believe he has any children and explained that he would never want to put a child through what he did growing up.

Physically, Randy has osteoarthritis in numerous joints, in addition to severe low-back pain. He has hepatitis C, though his liver enzymes are stable. He is otherwise healthy.

Randy's family psychiatric history was relevant for bipolar type 1 in his maternal uncle, depression in his mother, and schizophrenia in his paternal grandfather and a paternal cousin. His father and several relatives on both sides of the family had alcohol problems.

As a child, Randy was very shy and easily embarrassed. He hated being the center of attention, which was difficult given his ADHD. Starting in adolescence, he drank to cope with his anxiety in social situations. Similarly, he has always tended to worry over small issues, which worsened his sleep and ability to focus. In early adulthood, Randy started to develop chronic and worsening depressive episodes that appeared separate from, though worsened by, substance use. He would also use substances to cope with "bad childhood memories" and anxiety.

While incarcerated for his attempt murder charge, Randy maintained complete abstinence. However, about 2 years into the sentence, at the age of 26, he had a psychotic episode. At the time, he had been held "in the hole" (i.e., 24-h seclusion) for 3 months for talking back to guards and "causing problems." He had started to think the guards were reading his mind and trying to poison him. He also started hearing auditory hallucinations. Initially, he was selective about the foods he was eating and then stopped eating completely. He was not forthcoming about symptoms. After his weight dropped to a dangerously low level, however, he eventually saw the prison's general practitioner. He was diagnosed with schizoaffective disorder and treated with oral antipsychotic medications. He agreed to take medications in jail to "sleep his time away," but he did not believe he was ill. On completion of his sentence, he stopped his medications, which resulted in a relapse of his psychosis. Since then, he has been hospitalized on three occasions for psychosis and suicidal thoughts. He continues to have a pattern of medication non-compliance, intermittent substance use, and recurrence of his psychosis. Obtaining follow-up has been difficult, and he has been refused from most mental health facilities given his criminal history.

14.3   Discussion

Randy's case may appear atypical to those who do not work regularly with those with criminal histories, particularly given that Randy is not "just another personality disorder." In fact, equally complex presentations are frequent in many individuals with primary or comorbid personality disorders. While patients with mental health issues can face stigma, those with personality disorders are particularly at risk of stigma, even within the psychiatric field [12, 34]. This is likely in part due to misperceptions about and lack of experience with these populations, therapeutic nihilism, and countertransference.

The reality, however, is that personality disorders are mental disorders that have significant overlap with other mental disorders. Further, many of the sequelae and symptoms of personality disorders have effective interventions.

14.3.1 Diagnosis and Epidemiology

ASPD is one of the ten personality disorders outlined in the DSM-5 [4]. As one of the few diagnoses that can only be given to those who are 18 and older, individuals must show evidence of antisociality, in the form of conduct-disordered behavior, before the age of 15. This might include rule violations, lies, theft, aggression, and destruction of property.

Approximately 40–70% of adolescents with conduct disorder go on to meet criteria for ASPD [3]. The latter diagnosis of ASPD is characterized by a pervasive pattern of disregard for, and violation of, the rights of others that begins in childhood or early adolescence and continues into adulthood. As with all personality disorders, these traits must be inflexible, pervasive, and persisting.

Diagnosing any personality is difficult in a single interview without collateral information, given one must establish that the traits go back to adolescence, are inflexible, and are not due to other causes. In fact, full-blow antisocial personality is relatively rare in the general population, with a prevalence of approximately 3% of adults. Conversely, adult antisocial behavior is seen in approximately 12% of individuals [14, 30]. Higher rates of 40–60% are seen in prison populations [30].

While ASPD is not common, antisocial behavior is more common and can have numerous causes. Such behavior, however, is often mistakenly equated with an antisocial personality disorder. The DSM-5 takes efforts to differentiate such behavior as either stemming from mental disorders or from other causes. For example, one can give a V-code diagnosis of "Adult antisocial behavior (V71.01)" for someone showing criminal, aggressive, or other antisocial behavior that comes to clinical attention but "is not due to a mental disorder." Examples include professional thieves, drug dealers, or racketeers. Thus, an ill individual with schizophrenia, who assaults under the influence of psychosis, would not be given this label. Similarly, a diagnosis of ASPD would not be given if the antisocial behavior is seen exclusively in the course of bipolar disorder or schizophrenia. Some clinicians may overlook psychosis or mania in those presenting with aggression and anger. Alternatively, they may mislabel similar aggression and anger from a stress state as antisocial, when the cause may simply be anxiety, depression, or another temporary state of distress.

For all personality diagnoses, clinicians should apply the DSM-5 criteria longitudinally, to the lifespan of the patient. Many individuals with ASPD have similar childhood experiences [30]. They often have childhood adversity with exposure to physical violence. They demonstrate early difficulties with attention and impulsivity, and many gravitate to use of alcohol or illicit substances.

Of note, many individuals will erroneously use ASPD and psychopathy interchangeably. This confusion unfortunately clouds the literature, making evidence-based conclusions difficult. Noteworthy distinctions are that psychopathy is often characterized by a lack of empathy, lack of emotions, and callousness, which are not seen in ASPD. Individuals must score high on the Psychopathy Checklist (PCL-R). Only approximately 15% of individuals with ASPD have psychopathy [25]. It is unlikely that Randy, as described above, would qualify for a diagnosis of psychopathy.

14.3.2 Transinstitutionalization

Much of the psychiatric literature shows that there is an inverse relationship between the number of long-term psychiatric beds and the numbers of people in prison. Given the current lack of long-term beds, there has been an exponential growth of individuals with mental illness/intellectual disabilities in prisons [24, 36].

Unfortunately, prisons were not developed to care for mentally ill individuals. As such, these individuals may be placed in long-term seclusion for illness-motivated behaviors. They may have difficulties getting appropriate medications. They also have problems getting appropriate supports upon release from jail, given mental health providers may feel uncomfortable about treating a "criminal."

14.3.3 Comorbidity

While many clinicians may think that those with ASPD are cold, callous, and without emotions, in fact, many ASPDs have significant dysregulation in mood and anxiety. Large-scale studies indicate these individuals are at increased risk of mood and anxiety disorders [1, 23]. More than 50% of individuals with ASPD have an anxiety disorder, about twice the rate of non-ASPD individuals. Most common is social phobia (31%), followed by PTSD (21%). GAD, panic disorder, and agoraphobia are also prevalent. Rates of depression are around 20%, escalating to 40% if an anxiety disorder is present. Alcohol use disorder affects 54% of ASPDs, escalating to 70% if comorbid anxiety is present. Substance use disorders affect 40%. Thus, a fair summary is that anxiety, depression, and substances are the norm. It could be hypothesized that these individuals, who often have early trauma, develop anxiety disorders with subsequent anxiety. They then turn to substances to self-medicate these disorders.

Suicidal ideation and suicide attempts are also common in ASDPs. Nearly 50% of individuals have suicidal ideation, if suffering depression and anxiety.

14.3.4 Etiology

As with all personality disorders, the cause of ASPD is multifactorial. There appears to be heavy genetic influences, as supported by large-scale twin, adoption, and family studies [26, 29, 32]. Specific genes have been purported to be most important, including those related to monoamine oxidase (MAO). It is likely that this genetic loading only makes an individual more vulnerable to the effects of an adverse environment. Caspi [11] showed variable number tandem repeats (VNTR) creating a functional polymorphism in the promoter region of the MAO-A gene located on the X-chromosome. This polymorphism results in decreased activity of MAO. Individuals with severe abuse and maltreatment were much more likely to have antisocial behaviors if they had this MAO-A polymorphism.

In addition to genetic influences, sympathetic hypoarousal has been noted in individuals with ASPD and aggression, which is apparent in very young children [31, 37]. Frontal lobe dysfunction has also been seen in those with ASPD [9, 38]. This may contribute to impaired executive function, with ensuing cognitive rigidity, impaired problem-solving ability, and abnormal attention. The potential result is an impaired ability to recognize contextual cues in the environment. Further, this may lead to difficulties formulating plans, the reduced ability to reason or recognize consequences, limited ability to maintain concentration and focus on long-term goals, difficulties with behavioral regulation, lack of guilt, and unstable moods.

Further to neurotransmitter and sympathetic nervous system differences, it is hypothesized that individuals with ASPD also have differences in brain structures. In particular, impaired amygdala and hippocampal function may interfere with emotional regulation, aversive conditioning, and social learning [21]. Abnormalities in pre-

frontal gray matter have also been highlighted [10, 21].

Social factors and the resulting psychological sequelae also likely play a role in development of ASPD. In particular, dysfunctional family and peer influences have been hypothesized to be important. This includes psychopathology in parents, coercive parenting styles, physical abuse, and family conflict [32]. These factors likely have impact, particularly on those with genetic and physical vulnerabilities to developing ASPD.

14.3.5 Natural Course and Prognosis

Unfortunately, there are limited studies on ASPD. However, the natural course of ASPD appears to be similar to other personality disorders, with gradual but important improvements and a portion "burning out" [7]. Many struggle with addiction, mental health issues, and the related sequelae. Individuals have elevated rates of early natural death and unnatural death (suicide, homicide, and accidents). In 1966, Robins published data pertaining to 523 child guidance clinic patients who were seen between 1922 and 1932 [33]. In the mid-1950s, nearly 90% of these patients were located, and, of them, 94 individuals met lifetime criteria for ASPD. Of these individuals, 12% remitted, 27% improved but had not remitted, and 61% had not improved. While more than one-third had improved, many had ongoing interpersonal difficulties, irritability, or marital discord.

Similarly, the Gluecks [22] followed 500 boys deemed to be delinquent. Follow-up interviews were conducted at ages 25, 32, and 45 years. Childhood antisocial behavior predicted worse educational, economic, employment, and family status in adulthood. Job stability and marital attachment, however, were associated with improvement.

One study examined 39 individuals with ASPD, aged 41–67 [6]. Criminality was noted to decrease from 27 years of age and onward. In another study of 68 men with ASPD [8], with an average follow-up of 29 years, approximately 24% had died, 27% had remitted, 31% had improved but not remitted, and 42% had not improved.

14.4 Approach and Treatment of ASPD

When faced with individuals suffering from ASPD, it important to have an organized, multidimensional approach. As noted above, many individuals with ASPD present with psychiatric comorbidity, substance use problems, and potential violence.

14.4.1 Clarification of Issues

A thorough biopsychosocial assessment should be completed. The interview should initially focus on primary psychiatric disorders, including mood disorders, psychosis, anxiety disorders, substance, and ADHD. These can mimic or worsen antisocial symptoms. The history should confirm childhood adversity and conduct disorder. Collateral information can also be helpful. Comorbid medical issues should be clarified, as many individuals with ASPD may have hepatitis, HIV, or other illnesses related to a high-risk lifestyle. Intoxication and recent substance use should be ruled out with urine alcohol and drug screens. Further, it is vital to do formal evaluations for risk of violence and risk of suicide.

In the complex case above, it would helpful to make a problem list, which would include:

- Acute and chronic risk of violence and self-harm
- Substance use issues
- Medication non-compliance
- Schizoaffective disorder
- Anxiety disorders (social anxiety disorder, generalized anxiety disorder, PTSD)
- ADHD
- Lack of stability/housing/supports

The next step would be to develop a treatment plan prioritizing the above needs.

14.4.2 Risk Assessment and Risk Management

As with any psychiatric patient, it is important to evaluate the risk individuals pose to themselves and others. Individuals with ASPD have increased rates of suicide and of violence. As such, a formal risk assessment should include evaluating the risk of violence and risk of suicide. Semi-structured violence risk assessment tools may assist, such as the HCR-20 [15]. This is not, however, required. Some individuals can present in crisis in the context of dysfunctional interpersonal relationships and may be at risk for partner violence. Once risk factors for self-harm and violence are identified, the clinician should develop a safety management plan addressing the most important risk factors.

When an inexperienced clinician faces someone showing anger and aggression, they may incorrectly assume the person simply has ASPD. While those with ASPD can become aggressive, if it is motivated strictly by personality, then this aggression is often predictable. Many will respond well and settle with de-escalation techniques such as support, empathy, and reassurance. Anger is usually only directed at care providers when an adversarial approach is taken or when denying them something they are seeking (e.g., substances).

While many individuals with ASPD will not be violent in the healthcare setting, some may act out, if intoxicated with alcohol or substances. Alternatively, this may occur, should they have altered thinking due to psychosis, mania, or other illnesses affecting rational thought. In severe cases, individuals may require firm limits, sedating medications, or seclusion/restraint. Police or security may also be required, when de-escalation techniques are not working.

Risk management plans may include hospitalization, though it is recommended to clarify expectations of behavior prior to doing so, though safety of staff and other patients should trump treatment needs of the patient. At times, some individuals with ASPD may have legal issues at hand. However, it cannot be assumed that police will hold the individual or get the person appropriate psychiatric care if taken into custody. There may also be needs to warn potential targets of a real risk, such as an intimate partner.

14.4.3 Pharmacologic Treatment

As with all personality disorders, there are currently no validated treatments, specifically aimed at treating ASPD. There is, however, evidence that treatment of comorbid conditions, and related symptoms, may provide improvements in those targeted areas.

With this, the authors recommend the following principles:

- Treat comorbidities, including depression, anxiety, ADHD, psychosis, and substance abuse with evidence-based interventions.
- Avoid potentially abused medications or those with a high street value, such as narcotics, benzodiazepines, and short-acting stimulants.
- Choose agents that:
  - Have limited interaction with street drugs if it is an ongoing issue for the patient
  - Account for specific patient difficulties including impulsivity, suicidality, and lack of reliability – this may mean using longer-acting agents and those with less risk of withdrawal if missed or intoxicated if taken in overdose
  - Also assist other symptoms (e.g., choosing an antidepressant that helps with anxiety, sleep, and mood stability)
- Be aware of common comorbid physical diagnoses, such as HIV, hepatitis, and COPD to optimize medication selection.
- Many individuals with ASPD have very high tolerance to medications and may require high doses.
- Be clear on what you are treating, with ongoing evaluation of the specific treatment target.
- Avoid giving agents to appease the patient's request. Many will have "heard from friends" that a medication is good or may have tried specific medications on the street. That said, the patient may, at times, be right and may have actually found useful agents through their own trial and error.
- Continue to balance risks and benefits of any agent.
- Keep treatment goals realistic.

In addition to addressing primary psychiatric disorders that are comorbid, there is some limited evidence suggesting that medications may be helpful for specific target symptoms or behaviors. For example, when evaluating criminality, one very large study [27] noted that while on appropriate treatment for ADHD, men with ADHD had a 32% decrease in the criminality rate and women had a 41% decrease. Of course, the clinician would want to prescribe medications with less abuse potential.

Addressing aggression as a specific target has some variable evidence but could be tried in many patients, all the while weighing the risks and benefits. As noted above, if the individual has another psychiatric disorder, it is appropriate to choose an agent for that disorder and have reduced aggression as a secondary target.

Specific agents that have evidence for off-label use include valproic acid/divalproex sodium, carbamazepine, SSRIs, lithium, atypical antipsychotics, typical antipsychotics, and β-blockers [18–20]. Use these selectively, however, following the above principles and monitoring their effect on target symptoms.

14.4.4 Psychotherapeutic Options

The authors further recommend that psychotherapeutic treatment should follow many of the same principles as with pharmacologic treatment:

- Treat comorbidities, including depression, anxiety, ADHD, psychosis, and substance.
- Be clear on what you are treating, with ongoing evaluation of the specific treatment target.
- Continue to balance risks and benefits of therapy.
- Keep treatment goals realistic.

Gabbard [16] noted that patients with ASPD often "just go through the motions of treatment without being touched by it." However, a small portion may require or benefit from hospitalization, and thus the following principles are recommended:

- Have very clear treatment rules and regulations.
- Focus on the patient's faulty thought process, holding them accountable for their behavior and showing them that each behavior is a

learning experience. Many patients will repeatedly fail to anticipate negative outcome of their behavior.

- Help the patient insert thoughts between their impulses and action. If appearing impulsive, review with them what possible outcomes may occur.
- Keep a "here-and-now" focus.

While evidence is lacking, due to a paucity of quality studies, it is recommended to use psychological interventions, with the caveats noted by Gabbard above. While patients with ASPD may need hospitalization in crises or for comorbid conditions, the therapist must be cognizant that they may be more likely to exploit vulnerable copatients. They may also have lower frustration tolerance. Similarly, they will, at times, induce dysfunctional countertransference within the clinical team. It can be helpful to use motivational techniques focused on changing behavior to avoid the negative results that have occurred. In fact, use of cognitive-behavioral interventions, augmented with motivational techniques, may have the best success.

There has been some evidence that dialectical behavior therapy (DBT) approaches may also provide some benefits [28]. Modifications were made to traditional DBT, including agreements at the beginning, treatment targets, skills training groups, and dialectical dilemmas. For example, they included an additional skills module entitled "Crime Review."

A Cochrane review of psychological interventions for ASPD noted that there was a paucity of high-quality studies focused on expected targets of ASPD treatment [17]. Three interventions (contingency management with standard maintenance, CBT with standard maintenance, and an anti-drunk driving program with incarceration) had evidence for improving outcomes, particularly around substance use. Similar results were found by the NICE guidelines [3].

While psychotherapy techniques have a lack of evidence in ASPD, there is significant evidence in the correctional literature focused on reducing criminality. One of the best-supported

interventions is the risk, need, and responsivity (RNR) model. In this model, treatment is matched to the risk posed by individual offenders (*risk*), specifically targets criminogenic needs (*needs*), and is adapted to the individual learning styles and abilities of offenders (*responsivity*) [2].

The theory describes eight risk factors, known as "The Big 8," which are tied to recidivism and are as follows:

- Criminal history
- Procriminal companions
- Procriminal attitudes
- Antisocial personality pattern
- Education/employment
- Family/marital
- Substance abuse
- Leisure/recreation

One of the "responsivity factors" includes issues such as mental illness, which would interfere from an individual benefiting from any intervention. Thus, a clinician may need to treat depression, psychosis, or ADHD to allow the individual to improve in therapy.

14.4.5 Other Interventions

In addition to risk assessment/management, pharmacological treatments, and psychological treatments, clinicians may need to consider alternate interventions. For example, individuals who present with aggression, violence, and/or ASPD often invoke negative countertransference reactions. These may interfere with accurate diagnosis and inappropriate treatment and interventions. Furthermore, while the behavior of an individual with ASPD may not be purely motivated by mental illness, any negative outcomes like assaults or death would put high scrutiny on the clinician. As such, clinicians would likely benefit from consulting colleagues around the case. Further, consultation to a forensic psychiatrist or forensic psychologist may also be helpful as many have significant experience with complex cases involving those with ASPD. These professionals may also provide assistance with risk assessment and management, as needed.

In the case of individuals with extreme ASPD and associated violence, the criminal justice system may become involved. There are provisions in many jurisdictions to incarcerate or civilly commit individuals who show extreme and recurrent violence. At times, individuals with ASPD and comorbid severe mental illness will commit offenses under the influence of their illness. For example, in our case example, Randy may assault someone motivated primarily by delusional beliefs. In such a case, he may qualify as not criminally responsible due to mental illness. The courts or his legal counsel would potentially pursue this. Generally, the forensic psychiatry system, which focuses primarily on managing risk of ill individuals, has greater resources to manage such difficult individuals.

14.5 Recommendations

In working with individuals who have ASPD or any other personality disorder, clinicians face numerous challenges as outlined. With this, it is recommended that the clinician:

- Be aware of their own skills and knowledge, including limitations which may prevent them working with this complex population.
- Be aware of the diagnostic criteria for personality disorders, including literature regarding the relationship to offending and risk.
- Be comfortable recognizing and treating comorbid diagnoses, which commonly occur in those with personality disorder.
- Ensure complete risk assessments and risk management for suicide and violence, which are essential when dealing with individuals with ASPD.
- Use pharmacological and psychotherapeutic interventions, in addition to any possible consultations, when needed.

Disclosure Statement "The authors have nothing to disclose."

References

1. Alegria AA, Petry NM, Liu S-M, Blanco C, Skodol AE, Grant B. Sex differences in antisocial personality disorder: results from the national epidemiological survey on alcohol and related conditions. Personality Disorders: Theory, research and treatment. 2013; 4(3):214–22.
2. Andrews DA, Bonta J. The psychology of criminal conduct. 5th ed. New Providence: Matthew Bender & Company Inc.; 2010.
3. Antisocial Personality Disorder: Treatment, Management and Prevention. Leicester/London: The British Psychological Society and the Royal College of Psychiatrists; 2009.
4. APA. Diagnostic and statistical manual of mental disorders. 5th ed. Arlington: American Psychiatric Publishing; 2013a.
5. APA. 2013b. Personality disorders. Retrieved from http://www.dsm5.org/Documents/Personality%20 Disorders%20Fact%20Sheet.pdf.
6. Arboleda-Florez J, Holley HL. Antisocial burnout: an exploratory study. Bull Am Acad Psychiatry Law. 1991;19(2):173–83.
7. Black DW. The Natural History of Antisocial Personality Disorder. Can J Psychiatr. Revue Canadienne de Psychiatrie. 2015;60(7):309–14.
8. Black DW, Baumgard CH, Bell SE. A 16- to 45-year follow-up of 71 men with antisocial personality disorder. Compr Psychiatry. 1995;36(2):130–40.
9. Blair RJ. Neurocognitive models of aggression, the antisocial personality disorders, and psychopathy. J Neurol Neurosurg Psychiatry. 2001;71(6):727–31.
10. Blair RJ, Peschardt KS, Budhani S, Mitchell DG, Pine DS. The development of psychopathy. J Child Psychology and Psychiatry and Allied Disciplines. 2006;47(3–4):262–76. https://doi.org/ 10.1111/j.1469-7610.2006.01596.x.
11. Caspi A, McClay J, Moffitt TE, Mill J, Martin J, Craig IW, Taylor A, Poulton R. Role of genotype in the cycle of violence in maltreated children. Science. 2002;297(5582):851–4. https://doi.org/10.1126/ science.1072290.
12. Catthoor K, Feenstra DJ, Hutsebaut J, Schrijvers D, Sabbe B. Adolescents with personality disorders suffer from severe psychiatric stigma: evidence from a sample of 131 patients. Adolesc Health Med Ther. 2015;6:81–9. https://doi.org/10.2147/AHMT.S76916.
13. Coid J, Yang M, Tyrer P, Roberts A, Ullrich S. Prevalence and correlates of personality disorder in Great Britain. Br J Psychiatry. 2006;188(5):423–31. https://doi.org/10.1192/bjp.188.5.423.
14. Compton WM, Conway KP, Stinson FS, Colliver JD, Grant BF. Prevalence, correlates, and comorbidity of DSM-IV antisocial personality syndromes and alcohol and specific drug use disorders in the United States: results from the national epidemiologic survey on alcohol and related conditions. J Clin Psychiatry. 2005;66(6):677–85.

15. Douglas KS, Hart SD, Webster CD, Belfrage H. HCR-20 (Version 3): Assessing risk for violence. Burnaby: Mental Health, Law, and Policy Institute, Simon Fraser University; 2013.

16. Gabbard GO. Psychodynamic psychiatry in clinical practice. 4th ed. Arlington: APA Press; 2005.

17. Gibbon S, Duggan C, Stoffers J, Huband N, Völlm B, Ferriter M, Lieb K. Psychological interventions for antisocial personality disorder. Cochrane Libr. 2010;16(6):1–110.

18. Glancy GD, Knott TF. Part I: The psychopharmacology of long-term aggression - toward an evidence-based algorithm. Can Psychiatr Assoc Bull. 2002;34(6):13–8.

19. Glancy GD, Knott TF. Part II: The psychopharmacology of long-term aggression - toward an evidence-based algorithm. Can Psychiatr Assoc Bull. 2002;34(6):19–24.

20. Glancy GD, Knott TF. Part III: The psychopharmacology of long-term aggression - toward an evidence-based algorithm. Can Psychiatr Assoc Bull. 2003;35(1):13–8.

21. Glenn AL, Raine A. The neurobiology of psychopathy. Psychiatr Clin North Am. 2008;31(3):463–75. https://doi.org/10.1016/j.psc.2008.03.004

22. Glueck S, Glueck E. Unraveling juvenile delinquency. Cambridge, MA: Harvard University Press; 1950.

23. Goodwin RD, Hamilton SP. Lifetime comorbidity of antisocial personality disorder and anxiety disorders among adults in the community. Psychiatry Res. 2003; 117(2):159–66.

24. Harcourt BE. From the asylum to the prison: rethinking the incarceration revolution. Texas Law Review. 2006;84(7):1751–86.

25. Hare R. Hare Psychopathy Checklist Revised (PCL-R). 2nd ed. Toronto: Multi-Health Systems; 2003.

26. Jacobson KC, Prescott CA, Kendler KS. Genetic and environmental influences on juvenile antisocial behaviour assessed on two occasions. Psychol Med. 2000;30(6):1315–25.

27. Lichtenstein P, Halldner L, Zetterqvist J, Sjölander A, Serlachius E, Fazel S, Långström N, Larsson H. Medication for attention deficit–hyperactivity disorder and criminality. N Engl J Med. 2012;367(21):2006–14. https://doi.org/10.1056/NEJMoa1203241.

28. McCann RA, Ball EM. DBT with an inpatient forensic population: the CMHIP forensic model. Cogn Behav Pract. 2000;7:447–56.

29. Mednick SA, Gabrielli WF Jr, Hutchings B. Genetic influences in criminal convictions: evidence from an adoption cohort. Science. 1984;224(4651):891–4.

30. Moran P. The epidemiology of antisocial personality disorder. Soc Psychiatry Psychiatr Epidemiol. 1999;34(5):231–42.

31. Oosterlan J, Geurts HM, Knol DL, Sergeant JA. Low basal salivary cortisol is associated with teacher-reported symptoms of conduct disorder. Psychiatry Res. 2005;134:1–10.

32. Rhee SH, Waldman ID. Genetic and environmental influences on antisocial behavior: a meta-analysis of twin and adoption studies. Psychol Bull. 2002;128(3):490–529.

33. Robins LN. Deviant children grown up: a sociological and psychiatric study of sociopathic personality. Baltimore: Williams & Wilkins; 1966.

34. Sheehan L, Nieweglowski K, Corrigan P. The stigma of personality disorders. Curr Psychiatry Rep. 2016;18(1):11. https://doi.org/10.1007/s11920-015-0654-1.

35. Torgersen S, Kringlen E, Cramer V. The prevalence of personality disorders in a community sample. Arch Gen Psychiatr. 2001;58(6):590–6. https://doi.org/10.1001/archpsyc.58.6.590.

36. Torrey EF, Kennard AD, Eslinger D, Lamb R, Pavle J. More mentally ill persons are in jails and prisons than hospitals: a survey of the states Alexandria. Virginia: National Sheriffs Association; 2010.

37. van Goozen SH, Fairchild G. Neuroendocrine and neurotransmitter correlates in children with antisocial behavior. Horm Behav. 2006;50(4):647–54. https://doi.org/10.1016/j.yhbeh.2006.06.021.

38. Yang Y, Raine A, Lencz T, Bihrle S, LaCasse L, Colletti P. Volume reduction in prefrontal gray matter in unsuccessful criminal psychopaths. Biol Psychiatr. 2005;57(10):1103–8. https://doi.org/10.1016/j.biopsych.2005.01.021.

A Complex Case of Attention Deficit Hyperactivity Disorder in an Adult

15

Kuppuswami Shivakumar, Shabbir Amanullah, and Adnan Rajeh

15.1 Case Example of Adult Attention Deficit Hyperactivity Disorder (ADHD)

DJ is a 44-year-old divorcee and father of five from three different relationships. He was recently fired from his job where he was discovered to have been under the influence of alcohol. He is currently on welfare and has to pay a fine for a speeding ticket that he was recently issued. When seen by the family physician, he was diagnosed with generalized anxiety disorder (GAD) and depression whereupon he was referred to your services for further assessment and management.

He was seen in your outpatient clinic. On assessment, he was complaining of having generalized anxiety disorder (GAD) symptoms includ-

K. Shivakumar, MD, MPH, MRCPsych(UK), FRCPC (✉)
Department of Psychiatry, Northern Ontario School of Medicine Psychiatry Department, Sudbury, ON, Canada
e-mail: kshivakumar@hsnsudbury.ca

S. Amanullah, MD, DPM, FRCPsych(UK), CCT,FRCPC
University of Western Ontario, Woodstock General Hospital University of Western Ontario, Woodstock, ON, Canada
e-mail: samanullah@wgh.on.ca

A. Rajeh, MD
Victoria Hospital and Children's Hospital of Western Ontario, London, ON, Canada

ing excessive worry, fatigue, muscle tension, sleep problems (e.g., difficulty falling asleep, shutting his mind off), restlessness, and having difficulty concentrating. He also reports feeling tense except when he drinks. He complains of low mood, easy boredom, and irritability. These symptoms were prominent when he was at work where he was unable to focus on tasks at hand. His appetite is erratic, and he tends to indulge in fast food and claims that when he gets around to cooking a meal, he can eat it well. He denies any significant weight loss and strongly denies any sustained periods of elation, euphoria, or excessive spending.

His daily routine consists of waking up at around 11:00 AM, typically starting his day by heading out for coffee and bagel. He showers on occasion and tends to connect with friends over the phone, primarily to discuss whose house they will have a drink at in the evening. The patient does little else at home, and despite many reminders to update his resume or pay bills, he never gets around to doing it. His kitchen sink is filled with unwashed dishes, and he hasn't done his laundry in many weeks. Newspapers and magazines litter his living space, and his friends have often said his house is "like a pig stye." Contact with children was reduced out of concern from the child protection services about the patient's erratic behavior and difficulty sticking to the times that he said he would pick up the children. His children have grown distant, and this worries the patient quite a lot as he says he's "a good father." He denies any significant preoccupation with suicide or wanting to be dead and claims that when he is with friends, he feels happy and can enjoy their company.

The patient reports that his relationships never seem to last more than a few years as he doesn't like to be told what to do. The last relationship he had was among the most stable ones but ended after a series of arguments about his procrastination. His inability to complete tasks and quick temper were issues both at work and at home. He denies any features in keeping with obsessive-compulsive disorder (OCD).

At work, where he was often late and was frequently told that tasks needed to be completed within a limited time frame, he received many warnings, but these were to no avail. His workplace was disorganized with sheets of paper strewn across the table with no notes or bookmarks to help guide with task completion. He also reported that his disorganization was because the other workers talked loudly on the phone or were otherwise distracting.

Given the above presentation, it is felt that further clarification is needed to look for specific features of ADHD. This includes a collateral history from family members, especially his parents (developmental perspective), in addition to information from his school if available. A comprehensive assessment also includes the use of rating scales like Adult ADHD Self-Report Scale (ASRS) or Conners Adult ADHD Rating Scales.

As he did not show any acute withdrawals from alcohol, nor did he express any suicidal or homicidal ideas, he was asked to come back after completing the above tasks with his mother (with his consent).

On follow-up, he presented with his mother who gave a history of being disruptive (e.g., often disrupting the class, disturbing and distracting the other children) at home and at school. In fact, he was recommended by his teachers for a psychiatric consultation, but unfortunately, this was not completed. The mother also stated that when her son was growing up, he was always on the go and restless, had difficulties paying attention, and was frustrated when asked to do chores which required concentration such as homework. He was also suspended from his school on a number of occasions for challenging authority and being the class clown. His mother reports that he had few close friends as he found it hard to wait his turn when playing games.

15.1.1 Key Findings from the History

Although the predominant complaints are of anxiety and feeling tense, the underlying presentation strongly suggests adult ADHD. The history obtained from his mother strongly supports this diagnosis.

15.2 Discussion

15.2.1 Diagnosis and Epidemiology

The condition, which has assumed many labels over the past century (Fig. 15.1), has a prevalence rate in school age children ranging between 3% and 10% with a worldwide mean of 5.3% [1–5]. ADHD key features, distinguishing features, and the associated comorbid conditions are described in Table 15.1.

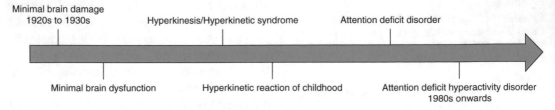

Fig. 15.1 Evolution of terms used to describe adult ADHD over the years

15.3 ADHD: Key Features

Table 15.1 Major key features of ADHD, distinguishing features and the associated comorbid conditions

Inattention
  Failure to give attention to details/makes careless mistakes
  Difficulty with organization/easily sidetracked and distractible
  Reluctance to engage in activities that require sustained attention
  Forgetful in daily activities/careless mistakes at work/failure to complete household chores or tasks at the workplace
  Does not seem to listen when spoken to/forgets to return calls/pay bills
  Failure to follow through instructions/inefficiency
  Procrastination which can be paralyzing
  Difficulty with fine print/difficulty in reviewing lengthy papers/meeting deadlines

Hyperactivity
  Feeling restless/rash driving
  Likes hands-on jobs or those that are "active"
  Being uncomfortable in meetings, restaurants that involve sitting for an extended period of time
  Low frustration tolerance
  Difficulty waiting one's turn
  Intrusive in conversations
  Inefficiency at work

DSM-IV TR	DSM 5
Classified as disruptive behavior disorders seen in childhood and adolescence	Classified as neurodevelopmental disorder
Two subtypes, predominantly attention deficit and impulsivity/hyperactivity	Subtypes have moved to specifiers
Age criteria: before 7	Age criteria: Before 12

*Symptoms must be present in at least two distinct settings (e.g., home, work). Symptoms interfere with academic, occupational, or social functioning. More than five symptoms from each category as in DSM-5 (Diagnostic and Statistical Manual of Mental Disorders, Fifth Edition, APA).

Distinguishing features and prevalence rates of comorbid conditions

Anxiety disorders and OCD

Generalized anxiety disorder (53%)	Obsessive-compulsive disorder (13%)	Social anxiety disorder	Panic disorder (15%)
Lack of energy	Ego dystonic thoughts, images, impulses, fears	Fear centered around social situations	Palpitations
Feeling tense	Repetitive or intrusive thoughts	Fear symptoms will be evaluated negatively	Tremors
Somatic symptoms of anxiety		Tendency to avoid social situations	Shortness of breath
Excessive worry		Social situations promote intense anxiety	Feelings of impending doom
Sleep problems			Depersonalization/derealization
6-month period of the above			Fear of loss of control
			Abdominal discomfort
			Crescendo/decrescendo pattern
			Feelings of light-headedness/dizziness

Mood disorders		

Major depressive disorder (15–75%)
  Sustained low mood
  Feelings of worthlessness and
  hopelessness
  Weight loss or gain
  Suicidal thoughts/thought of death
  Anhedonia
  These are episodic
	Dysthymia
	(15–75%)
	  Overeating
	  Depressed mood
	  Feelings of
	  hopelessness
	  Low self-esteem
	  Duration of 2
	  years
	  Low energy
	  Fatigue
		Bipolar disorder (20–30%)
		  Episodic but sustained mood changes
		  from baseline
		  Elation or euphoria
		  Decreased need for sleep
		  Expansive ideas or grandiose delusions
		  Pressure of speech/flight of ideas different
		  from baseline
		  Excessive involvement in activities that
		  could lead to painful consequences

Personality disorders

Borderline personality disorder
  Over idealization/devaluation
  Fears of abandonment
  Suicidal threats
  Chronic feelings of emptiness
  Quick mood fluctuations
  Self-harm
  Poor identity/poor sense of self

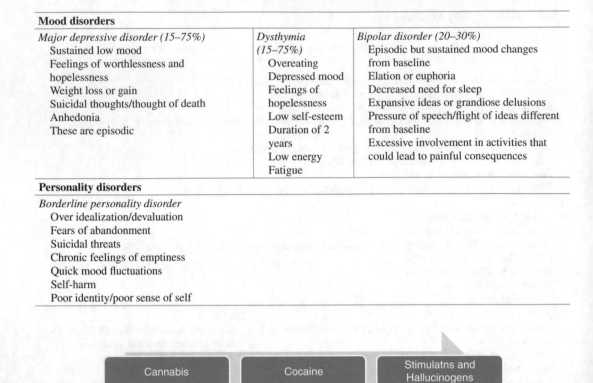

Fig. 15.2 Directional preference for other non-alcohol substances in adults with ADHD

15.3.1 Substance Use Disorders in Among Adults with ADHD

Given the similarities in the neurophysiological basis of ADHD and SUD, the causation is likely multifactorial. One can hypothesize there is a significant genetic component that includes synaptosomal-associated protein 25 (SNAP-25) and D2 and D4 receptor signaling pathway. Animal studies have shown that deletion of the SNAP-25 gene may have been implicated in the susceptibility to ADHD. The risk of SUD in ADHD is attributed by some authors to impulsivity. While prevalence rates are the same in those without ADHD, those with ADHD drink alcohol excessively. There are certain unique characteristics in adults with ADHD and those without ADHD. The cohort with ADHD began

using at an earlier age, used more often, and continued for a longer period. The diagram below depicts in descending order the preferences for other non-alcohol substances in adult ADHD (Fig. 15.2).

Studies have examined the symptoms subtypes of ADHD and shown that hyperactive-impulsive symptoms were more consistently associated with substance use and SUD compared to inattentive symptoms.

15.4 Approach and Treatment of ADHD

Given that ADHD in itself is not an acute condition but rather a chronic one emphasis should be laid on collecting and corroborating information about the individual before initiating a treatment plan. The following integrative management principles can be used in someone with complex ADHD [6–8].

1. Clearly define objectives that include current symptoms, differential diagnosis, comorbidity, psychosocial problems, and any other associated legal issues.
2. Patient psychoeducation: This is of paramount importance for the patient to improve self-awareness, to reduce stigma, and also to improve compliance. Giving brochures and connecting them with self-help groups may improve the long-term commitment to the treatment.
3. Family education plays a key part in reducing stigma and increasing the long-term treatment success.

The approach to the treatment of adult ADHD depends strongly on the severity of comorbid conditions, any forensic issues, and if acute admission is needed. Individuals with substance abuse comorbidity, especially alcohol dependence with a history of delirium tremens/seizures, will need to be admitted and managed accordingly so to those with psychosis secondary to substance abuse. Many individuals with substance abuse comorbidity may have sustained head injuries, and this will need to be addressed as part of acute management. Suicidal ideas or individuals with active suicidal plans need to be admitted and managed accordingly.

15.5   Management Options

15.5.1 Pharmacologic Treatment

Before initiating pharmacotherapy, one has to rule out potential cardiac risk factors given the side-effect profile of these medications. The history would include fainting spells, seizures, palpitations with exercise, a family history of unexplained death, and QTc prolongation. It will also be good to get corroborative information from the family physician for any other cardiovascular morbidity. A note of involuntary movements and tic disorders should be made.

15.5.2 Initiating Treatment

Discussing treatment options with the patient constitutes good practice. The discussion of side effects, duration of treatment, and expectations helps with not just compliance but also for the patient to be an active part of the treatment process. The FDA has approved certain drugs that include the following (Table 15.2):

Third-line strategies include use of medications like tricyclic antidepressants (e.g., nortriptyline, desipramine); however, the data currently supports the use of stimulants with over 90% response during the acute phase of treatment. One of the drawbacks is the wearing off of the effects of the stimulants. Common side effects include a loss of appetite which, consequently, can result in weight loss, and some patients may

Table 15.2 Drugs which are approved or used off-label to treat ADHD

FDA		
Approved		Not approved/off-label
Stimulants	Non-stimulants	Buproprion
Methylphenidates, including OROS (osmotic-controlled release of oral delivery system)	Atomoxetine	Alpha-2 agonists-immediate release
Lisdexamfetamine	Alpha-2 agonists-slow release	Second generation antipsychotics/atypicals
D-Amphetamine	Clonidine	Modafinil
D-Methylphenidate	Guanfacine	

find this very troubling. Dry mouth and headaches are also well-known, hence the importance of discussing this with patients. One of the mechanisms by which a more sustained benefit can be achieved without fear of effects wearing off is to use long-acting preparations. Of the more commonly used medications is Concerta or extended-release methylphenidate, and the dose starts at 18 mg/day up to a maximum of 72 mg/day.

The use of medications like lisdexamfetamine is associated with a lower risk of abuse as stimulants can be inhaled or injected. One would usually start at a lower dose of about 20 mg/day and gradually increasing based on tolerability and response up to a maximum of 70 mg/day.

The non-stimulants have a low response rate and are considered second line. One of the main advantages with this group of medications is the very low abuse potential and should be given serious consideration with those in whom there is a high risk for stimulant misuse or due to side effects emerging from stimulants. Atomoxetine dosing is based on body weight of the individual with ranges between 1.2 and 1.4 mg/kg body weight. Maximum daily dosing is 100 mg/day. It is recommended that one starts at lower doses to minimize side effects. Caution should be exercised given its breakdown by cytochrome 2D6 and the potential for drug interactions, for example, fluoxetine.

The use of alpha-2 agonists (e.g., clonidine and guanfacine), although approved for use in children and adolescents, has occasionally been used in adults and been found to have a positive therapeutic role in individuals with inattention, and there are suggestions for combining it with stimulants. However, one should err on the side of monotherapy before looking into combining.

Sedation is a side effect along with fatigue, abdominal pain, and dizziness among others and hence the need to monitor blood pressure. Starting at the lowest possible dose is very important, for example, in clonidine, 0.1 mg/day with a target range of 0.1–0.2 mg, twice per day.

There will be individuals who require a combination of extended release and immediate release, and this could be due to the need for "coverage" at specific times including work, school, or all day coverage. An inadequate response may warrant a discussion on compliance, side effects, and to rule out any comorbid psychiatric conditions. Dosing may be increased or switching may be an option. Compliance has been found to be an issue, and evidence shows noncompliance within 2–3 months in a majority of patients. Long-acting medications have better compliance. At times, adjunctive agents may be required which include neuroleptics, SSRIs, mood stabilizers, and regiments involving combination treatments.

15.5.2.1 Psychological Interventions

Coaching can offer supportive therapy in a structured manner either individually or in groups, and CBT is capable of treating many comorbidities associated with ADHD (Fig. 15.3). However, psychotherapy alone cannot treat the wide spectrum of ADHD symptoms and problems. It has many more beneficial effects in comparison with pharmacotherapy in the long-term treatment plan of ADHD. Many recent articles state the increased benefit of combined therapy, especially CBT plus stimulants in the treatment of ADHD. Psychotherapy, generally, leads to the improvement of behavioral, social, cognitive, and executive impairments.

Fig. 15.3 A visual representation of non-pharmacological interventions

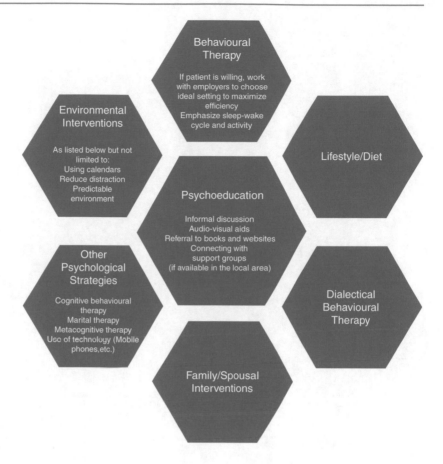

References

1. Faraone SV. Report from the third international meeting of the attention-deficit hyperactivity disorder molecular genetics network. Am J Med Genet A. 2002;114(3):272–6.
2. Faraone SV, Sergeant J, Gillberg C, Biederman J. The worldwide prevalence of ADHD: is it an American condition? World Psychiatry. 2003;2(2):104.
3. Kooij SJ, Bejerot S, Blackwell A, Caci H, Casas-Brugué M, Carpentier PJ, Edvinsson D, Fayyad J, Foeken K, Fitzgerald M, Ginsberg Y, Henry C, Krause J, Lensing MB, Manor I, Niederhofer H, Nunes-Filipe C, Ohlmeier MD, Oswald P, Pallanti S, Pehlivanidis A, Ramos-Quiroga JA, Rastam M, Ryffel-Rawak D, Stes S, Asherson P, Gaillac V. European consensus statement on diagnosis and treatment of adult ADHD: The European Network Adult ADHD. BMC Psychiatry. 2010;10(1):67.
4. Levin FR, Evans SM, Kleber HD. Prevalence of adult attention-deficit hyperactivity disorder among cocaine abusers seeking treatment. Drug Alcohol Depend. 1998;52(1):15–25.
5. Polanczyk G, de Lima MS, Horta BL, Biederman J, Rohde LA. The worldwide prevalence of ADHD: a systematic review and metaregression analysis. Am J Psychiatr. 2007;164(6):942–8.
6. Searight HR, Burke JM, Rottnek FRED. Adult ADHD: evaluation and treatment in family medicine. Am Fam Physician. 2000;62(9):2077–86.
7. Solanto MV, Marks DJ, Mitchell KJ, Wasserstein J, Kofman MD. Development of a new psychosocial treatment for adult ADHD. J Atten Disord. 2008;11(6):728–36.
8. Willcutt EG. The prevalence of DSM-IV attention-deficit/hyperactivity disorder: a meta-analytic review. Neurotherapeutics. 2012;9(3):490–9.

Complex Cases of PTSD: Importance of Sociocultural Factors in the Sri Lankan Context

16

Daya Somasundaram and T. Umaharan

16.1 Introduction

What are the consequences of disasters?
What are the factors influencing the experience of trauma?
Why is it important to understand social and cultural factors in the management of trauma?

On average 700 natural and man-made disasters kill 100,000 and affect 255,000,000 people each year (International Federation of Red Cross and Red Crescent Societies, 2010). Although impacts and mental health consequences of disasters have many similarities, nature, type, and severity of trauma can cause differences. Manmade disaster also known as war produces countless deaths and injuries of civilians as well as combatants and displacement of large numbers of populations. Disaster-stricken communities often experience disruption of family and community life, work, normal networks, institutions, and structures [1]. Members of the community exposed to disasters can develop loss of motivation, dependence on relief, hostility, and despair.

It has been understood that disasters disproportionately strike the socioeconomically deprived, minorities, and marginalized and that their consequences may be more serious and chronic in these groups.

Disasters cause a variety of psychological and psychiatric sequelae [2].These range from a number of maladaptive behavioral patterns to diagnosable psychiatric disorders as well as adaptive and resilient coping responses in the face of catastrophic events to understandable non-pathological distress. Conditions like acute stress reaction (ASR, the old disaster syndrome), post-traumatic stress disorder (PTSD), depression, anxiety, somatoform disorders, and substance abuse (especially alcohol) can occur in a significant number of survivors, although most people recover remarkably well [2, 3]. Chronic trauma, particularly interpersonal where escape is not possible, can lead to complex PTSD [4], enduring personality changes [5] or Disorders of Extreme Stress Not Otherwise Specified (DESNOS) [6].

There even appears to be a neurobiological basis to PTSD that is reflected in changes in brain structures such as the amygdala, hippocampus, and prefrontal cortex and their functioning, memory networks, neurotransmitter systems such as noradrenalin and serotonin, and the endocrinal axis. Perception of trauma is influenced by many factors: age, sex, culture, past experience, preparedness, and dimensions of trauma such as

D. Somasundaram (✉)
Department of Psychiatry, Faculty of Medicine, University of Jaffna, Jaffna, Sri Lanka

School of Medicine, Faculty of Health Sciences, University of Adelaide, Adelaide, Australia

T. Umaharan
Post Graduate Institute of Medicine, University of Colombo, Colombo, Sri Lanka

duration, intensity/magnitude, continuity, and type.

It is becoming clear that social and cultural values, beliefs, and perceptions shape how traumatic events impact on an individual, family, and community and the way they respond [1, 7, 8]. There are social and cultural factors which make trauma; and hence PTSD is complex and difficult for straightforward interventions. On the other hand, the same factors, social, cultural, and personality, can exert favorable effects in expression, duration, and recovery process of PTSD and adherence to treatment. Therefore understanding social, cultural, and personality factors is of paramount importance in managing PTSD. This chapter tries to elaborate the values of these factors through the study of several complex cases.

16.2   Methodology

What are the adverse effects of the civil war in Sri Lanka?
What is meant by the term "collective trauma?"

Sri Lanka faced multiple devastating disasters, both man-made and natural, in the recent past. Individuals, families, and communities in Sri Lanka, particularly of the Northern and Eastern provinces and the border areas of Sri Lanka, have undergone 25 years of war trauma, multiple displacements, injury, detentions, torture, and loss of family, kin, friends, homes, employment, and other valued resources [9].

Sri Lankan ethnic conflict, at its extreme, manifested as war for about three decades and led to casualties of more than 100,000. The war also caused permanent disability (both physical and psychological), internal and external (overseas) displacement of civilians, and exceptional destruction of properties, social structure, and ecosystems [10–18]. The armed manifestation of the Sri Lankan ethnic conflict emerged in the mid-1970s and was brought to an end in May 2009 resulting in more than 40,000 deaths of civilians with indiscriminate shelling and bombing by the state as the rebels held the civilian population hostage, and many more injuries and unacknowledged war crimes [19–25].

In addition to widespread individual mental health consequences [26, 27] such as PTSD (13%), anxiety (49%), and depression (42%) among internally displaced persons (IDPs) from the war-affected zones [26] of Sri Lanka, families and communities have been uprooted from familiar and traditional ecological contexts such as ways of life, villages, relationships, connectedness, social capital, structures, and institutions [9] and have resulted in tearing of the social fabric, lack of social cohesion, disconnection, mistrust, hopelessness, dependency, lack of motivation, powerlessness, and despondency. Social pathologies like substance abuse, violence, gender-based abuse, and child abuse have been increased. The social disorganization led to unpredictability, low efficacy, low social control of antisocial behavior patterns, and high emigration, which in turn cause breakdown of social norms, anomie, learned helplessness, thwarted aspirations, low self-esteem, and insecurity. The long-lasting impact at the collective level or some have called it tearing in the social fabric would then result in the social transformation [28] of a sociopathic nature that can be called collective trauma that in turn, through breakdown in social support systems and social capital, would adversely impact on individual traumatization, prognosis, and recovery.

This chapter is based on qualitative analysis of individuals with PTSD and analysis of cases encountered in clinical practice (see the Annex) whose predisposing factor was traumatic exposures in the war. This chapter reports on familial and sociocultural factors influencing the manifestation and course of the PTSD. The findings discussed in this chapter are therefore clinical outcomes and observations obtained from the case series and qualitative interviews.

16.3   Sociocultural Factors Making Trauma (PTSD) Complicated

What are the sociocultural factors complicating trauma (PTSD)?
How do these factors make trauma (PTSD) complicated?

16.3.1 Ostracization

Ostracization maintains PTSD. It has many social, economical, familial, occupational, and interpersonal impacts. Trauma survivors find no one listening them, to provide necessary supports, and to incorporate them into family and community and refusal of employment and relationship problems. Labeling (as mad) and consequences of stigmatization further traumatize PTSD sufferers. Some families treat PTSD sufferers as a mental case. This is noted to happen predominantly to female survivors. Some even assault survivors to "control" them. Such survivors are again noted to be women mostly.

> Mrs. A. was viewed as incapacitated to look after her child. Her family including her daughter stopped talking and relating to her. Mrs. A. said "I used to wander while crying. This was a shame to my family. They misunderstood as I behaved deliberately (as mad). They even punished (assaulted) me for behaving madly. They think that their prestige was damaged by my illness, medicines I take for the illness and attendance to mental health services."

16.3.2 Social Isolation (Lack of Support Systems)

Social isolation has huge impacts on trauma and recovery. Survivors living alone or experiencing enforced isolation show symptoms of PTSD in greater intensity, chronicity of illness, and very slow recovery even with appropriate and vigorous interventions. The opposites are noted among survivors with no social isolation or loneliness. PTSD symptoms are less in number and intensity among sufferers not isolated or not experiencing loneliness. They also show com-

paratively faster and greater recovery. The survivors come out with the fact that when they are supported or surrounded by others they are less frequently and less intensely intruded with PTSD symptoms. They further state that such social opportunities provide them ways of occupying themselves.

Survivors with huge disease burden, chronicity of illness, or frequent hospitalization invariably claim that they do not share their trauma or sufferings because no one is available. This results from greater number of loss in survivors' families or networks or migration of family members or members in networks due to the disaster. Some survivors maintain a formal network with people in their environment. But they do not share because other people in network are also in a similar status, i.e., with traumatic exposures and/or losses, and they express no or minimum interest to listen. Failure to share maintains PTSD and trauma. For some survivors social isolation is enforced, because families of sufferers are reluctant to accept survivors due to stigmatization. Such survivors have to live alone, and loneliness or enforced isolation perpetuates and maintains trauma symptoms.

> Mrs. A. stated "the war wiped out all my family members from my world. I have been made to experience enforced isolation. Loneliness is extremely unbearable to me. This further aggravated my illness."

In some instances survivors are exposed to a different type of enforced isolation caused by initial trauma. Many survivors found all family members killed in war or displaced from the war area. Sometimes relatives keep survivors away from them because of accurate or misperception of involvement of survivors in war activities. In such instances relatives are highly anxious to support survivors as they believe that they would be punished for such actions.

> Mrs. A. further stated "I was followed by military intelligence for my involvement with campaigns against enforced disappearance and participation in protests for missing in the war. This produced greater amounts of anxiety to my family. My family were scared that they would fall into troubles with the military. This had been the main reason for my family's unwillingness to become involved in my activities and behaviors, refusal to relate and communicate with me and keeping themselves away from me."

Some patients are noted to perceive loneliness or isolation in absence of such thing. Absolute or perceived lack of emotional warmth is the usual cause for this. Lack of emotional warmth can be resulted from poor family dynamics, exhaustion of family following long-term interventions to a chronic sufferer, continuing circumstances which caused trauma such as chronic war in which people's primary concern is to save their lives, or complete investment of time to manage consequences of disaster or basic needs of life.

Enforced isolation or loneliness sometimes results from PTSD withdrawal symptoms causing weakness of support system. Irritability, aggression, and violent or destructive behavior expressed by survivors are noted to be the causes for this. Such survivors are noted to be chronic sufferers or possess post traumatic personality change. When patients express these maladaptive behaviors, members in their support system do not understand this as expression of disease and instead view as deliberate or with noxious intention. The result is exclusion of patients. Weakened support system exerts deleterious effects on patients' mental status and recovery from trauma.

Sometimes family members precipitate or perpetuate PTSD symptoms. They do this without their knowledge. But by doing this, they construct an environment maintaining and/or exacerbating disease. Many survivors who missed their children in disasters are repeatedly told by family members that their children have been killed and survivors' struggles to find the missing were meaningless. In such circumstances, survivors experience a sudden increase in their symptoms. In some instances survivors are forced to accept views of their family members and give up searching for the missing (Fig. 16.1).

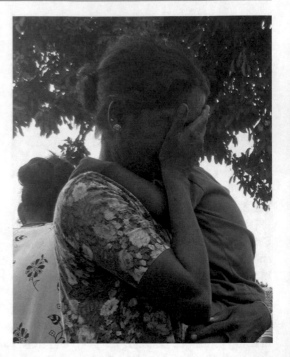

Fig. 16.1 Grieving mother

Enforced isolation or loneliness has another manifestation. In a war-affected zone, commonly female survivors and uncommonly male survivors are at risk to be sexually exploited by the military, or at least survivors perceive fear of sexual exploitation (commonly females). Sometimes fear of sexual exploitation emerges after an experience of sexual violence. In general, isolated or lonely survivors become prey to such violence. Recurrent sexual exploitation or fear of sexual exploitation carries the risk to perpetuate symptoms and signs of PTSD or make PTSD resistant to treatment. Also sufferers appear to be less interested into interventions in such situation.

> Mrs. A. said "my family and husband's family used to tell repeatedly that my daughter would not be alive and she would have been killed. They were very firm in their judgment. In their view, my efforts to find my daughter and crying for my children and husband were useless and meaningless. They even verbalized this straight forwardly to me as 'dead and disappeared never return by crying'. My family forced me to obey them and behave according to their commands/expectations."

> Mrs. A. stated "the military attempting to exploit me sexually was a persistent problem. Sometimes the attempts manifested as threats. These attempts and threats increased the tendency to be overwhelmed with the flashbacks and memories of the war. Reliving experiences were also due to the compulsion to see the military because I had to see them, for a considerable time in a day, walking around my dwelling. Sometimes this was caused by my imagination because I had been anxiously imagining the military and their presence around my house."

16.3.3 Environment

Most survivors with war trauma say changes made by war in their environment distress them. They see environment altered by disaster as not belonging to them. They feel uneasy with their altered environment. The surrounding appears unfamiliar, unfavorable, and unsuitable to them or not to the extent of their expectation. There are many reasons for such interpretation and perception; altered physical structure of environment by war; exodus or evacuation of people from the war environment; persistent exposure to people with physical consequences of war such as loss of vision or amputated limbs; alterations in behavior of people caused by collective trauma and which include submissive, unmotivated, and depressed population; and presence of the military in the environment and military vehicles and ammunitions. Survivors in such altered environment show less interest to adhere to interventions for PTSD. Survivors in an altered environment continue to perceive impending traumas. Also transitioned surrounding persistently provides triggers to sufferers to reexperience past traumas.

> Mrs. A. claimed "there is a huge change in my environment after the war. I see and experience a huge vacuum around me. This has greatly been caused by the absence of my husband and daughters; also by the absence of other people who were my relatives, friends and neighbors. They were killed in the war."
> Mrs. B. admitted "I do not want to be in my village… because being there triggers memories/flashbacks of my children and subsequently what happened to them in the war and what I did… when I am away from my village intensity and frequency of memories and flashbacks are comparatively less."
> Mrs. B. also said "there are few in my village. They voluntarily provide support to me. This helps me. Their words pacify my suffering. Before the war there were sufficient people with such quality in my neighborhood. But the war either killed or displaced those people in high quantity. I see a significant difference in between the numbers of such people before and after the war. If such people could have been in my surrounding I would have been better alleviated."

War destroys and alters structure of landscapes. It wipes out, either by killing or displacement, civilians from villages. Trauma survivors perceive that their environment and surroundings have been shrunken. They see their villages contain few families and are saturated with army soldiers, in contrast. Therefore villages are not the same as in the past to them. Hence sufferers feel villages are not their own; environment is less familiar; altered set up of the village does not provide what it yielded in the past, i.e., support, connectedness, and happiness. The results are impairment in support systems and refusal to be in an altered environment. When they do visits to their villages or stay there, they feel strange and lonely.

> Mr. C. said "I do not want to be in my village… because being there triggers memories/flashbacks of my daughter and subsequently what happened to her in the war. Seeing army soldiers… listening their language… watching military vehicles… produce tremendous agony to me… I imagine and feel the military and their vehicles walk and run over my daughter."

16.3.4 Economical Status

Importance of economical status varies according to the economical strength of survivors and magnitude of trauma. Survivors with greater number of losses and traumatic experiences are not alleviated with economical subsidiaries. Economical strength has little value for patients with complex PTSD. They are also noted to be poorly motivated to practice routine coping practices and collective measures of community mental health. Economical assistance does not prompt them to practice these measures. Some survivors were paid compensation for their losses in the war. They indicated that raised economical status does not alter their sufferings and trauma. Some patients with PTSD and traumatic loss hold an opinion that adequacy of economy and spending on name of dead pacify them. They attribute part of their suffering to poor economical strength and subsequent failure to do rituals, customs, and other traditional last rites to the dead. Those patients are found to be economically deprived even before their trauma. They believe that if their economical status could have been better, they could have done more customs, rituals, and other traditional measures, and by doing these activities, their sufferings and trauma would have been improved. However, survivors with same traumatic experiences, but economically better off, claim that their economical strength does not bring any impact on their suffering and trauma. They do not associate their economical status with their suffering and complexity of trauma.

Patients' economical status at time of trauma associates with trauma symptoms. Socioeconomically deprived patients believe that if their economy could have been better at time of trauma, they could have well managed trauma, and its consequences would have been less. Such interpretation makes the trauma experience more dynamic and prevents healing.

> Mr. C. said "until the moment my daughter died she did not experience a comfortable life. I agree that I did not let her to experience poverty, but on the other hand I could not provide her a life without deficiencies. The final war and its consequences further aggravated the socio-economical condition of my family. When my daughter was killed, economical status of my family was worse. My family's economy has now improved and we have been experiencing a fairly good socio-economical well being. I ruminate about the past (socio-economical situation) of my family and compare it with the present status. In such circumstances, I feel ashamed and depressed because my daughter's suffering the deprived status and now she is no more to have the current improved life strikes my mind. I would have been better if my daughter could have had a comfortable life when she was alive."

Patients who lost their family members in disasters feel relief when they do economical assistance to poorer. They claim this satisfies them. These survivors expect the merits of their acts will pass onto the dead. Some feel they are possessed with souls of the dead and acts are done by those souls.

16.3.5 Belief System

Multiple losses of family members alter the belief system of patients. Such patients start to think that there is no meaning to continue life in the absence of their family members and they are not entitled to have a life in the world where their family members are no more. The altered thinking pattern leads to committing or attempting suicide. These survivors are also found to be chronically and severely ill.

Family members are essential parts of the world of people of collectivistic cultures. Therefore when trauma is associated with sudden loss of family members, they feel that their life ends with death of intimates. The perception of the shrinking of world proportionately increases with increasing number of losses. Survivors perceiving their world is lost do not show interest to replenish their world with other measures. They continue suffering and do not attend to mental health services and adhere to treatment. In such circumstances PTSD becomes chronic. These patients are simultaneously and persistently invaded with the thoughts "my family members are no more," "therefore I have no more life," and "I do not need happiness" in addition to intruding PTSD memories/flashbacks. These patients commonly say "I am not interested to involve with pleasurable activities" and "I do not need the happiness which was not possible to my family members killed in the war."

Evaluation of relationships plays an important role in the recovery process of PTSD. When patients believe that particular relationships are genuine and important to them, they struggle to acknowledge losses. In such circumstances losses appear unbearable and irrecoverable. These beliefs magnify symptoms and prolong duration of illness.

> Mrs. B. said "if my sons were unkind it would have been easier to me to calm myself. They had never had such characteristics."
>
> Mr. C. said "the relationship between my daughter and me was more than a daughter-father relationship. I know she was exceptionally different from other children. She was very concerned about me. She did not allow my other children to overrule, ill-treat or emotionally abuse me. She was very much emotionally supportive to me. She was the child who completely understood my problems, views, sufferings. She was consciously aware that I brought up them (children) with enormous hurdles after the death of my spouse. She knew how much I sacrificed my life for them. She used to point out these facts when she argued with others for me. She was never apart from me when she was alive. She did not sleep without my presence; she need me to sleep."

Evaluation of loss is another factor. Almost all patients with traumatic loss are very concerned about value of loss. If perceived value of loss is greater, then they are at risk to develop severe and chronic symptoms. Value is directly associated with survivors' life context (social, economical, familial), future plans, and social acceptance. When a member in a family is lost in a traumatic way and if the member's perceived value is greater, survivors' hope about life, future, and family are lost, and they perceive it irreplaceable and a chronic gap in their life which then maintains the PTSD.

> Mr. C. said "she was so clever... in study..., sports..., leadership qualities... She was an all-rounder. She loved the family. She was highly concerned about the family. She also acted as an advisor to me. I had lot of hopes about her. She had an aim to provide me a comfortable life and to care for me. She had many ambitions in her life... to study well... to enter university... to have a best employment... She wanted to give a meaning for the struggles I had overcame for the family. In times when I was not well, she used to become stressed. In those times, she cared for me very well. She used to order my other children to take care of me."

PTSD and associated grief symptoms continue when patients believe losses cannot be replenished. Patients who are ready to replace loss with appropriate substitutes recover earlier than others who are reluctant to do the same. Such measures expand the support system of sufferers or make survivors occupied.

> Mrs. B. claimed "I am not ready to replace anyone in my sons' positions. My elder sister killed in the war has another son. My brother-in-law requested me to treat him as my son. But I refused. I can never imagine others in my sons' positions. I do not think this will help to heal my trauma. I lost what I owned. I do not want to own others' assets."
> Mr. C. claimed "when I spend times at my house, my first daughter's daughter (first grand-daughter) joins to stay with me for accompaniment. She sleeps on my right arm, similar to my daughter. This is a surprise to me. I prefer this to happen again and again. When my granddaughter sleeps on my right arm she appears as my daughter to me."

Some patients show reluctance to practice coping mechanisms daily and for prolonged times at home. They believe this would be an annoyance to other family members; and this might hurt them.

They even imagine disagreement from family members for this and increase their suffering by disagreement. Such reluctance and imagination maintain trauma and delay recovery.

> Mrs. B. said "flashbacks and memories of my sons could only be managed with lamenting. When I fail to lament, the agony turns into severe head discomfort. Therefore I try to lament as much as possible. But this is not possible all the times. Therefore I do this mostly in washrooms."
> Mrs. B. further said "crying is not acceptable in ceremonies of happiness. Youngsters in such ceremonies remind me my children. This instantly causes me to weep. But I cannot cry because when I cry by looking at youngsters their parents might think that would bring misfortune to their children. I do not want to destroy others' happiness by crying."

Many patients do comparison of their life with pre- and posttrauma contexts. In disasters trauma is usually associated with destruction of wealth and relationships, and therefore patients are made socioeconomically, emotionally, and biologically deprived. Comparison unwraps their trauma and makes them to be chronic sufferers.

> Mr. C. said "I see girls, who were colleagues of my daughter but performed less well in the school compared to my daughter. When I see them I instantly think that if my daughter could have been alive she would have been shining more than them. Subsequently this thought brings abundance of sorrow. This is unmanageable to me."
> Mrs. A. said "when I become severely ill, my mind spontaneously recalls and thinks how I was served by my children and husband and how far I would have been served by them if they could have been alive."

16.3.6 Collective Bereavement

PTSD turns into complex and chronic when it is associated with loss of family members. This phenomenon is additionally complicated when survivors find lack or no space to grieve for killed. Sufferers show severe and intractable features when they cannot get space to grieve for their loved ones.

> Mrs. A. said "There was no time to grieve. I could not do what I was supposed to do for my husband and daughters. I should have grieved at the time for them. Their souls could have been pacified, if."

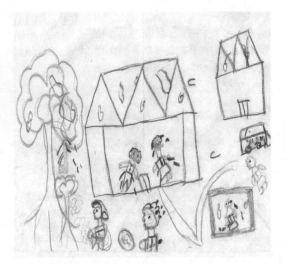

Fig. 16.2 Showing the girl's drawing of the scene of a shell blast (Note the child drew a cut leg hanging in the tree. Materials depicted in red are other body pieces)

When whole families are affected, when some are killed, while others are injured or some are separated, the consequences can be complicated by the lack of family support and interactions with uncertainty and helplessness. The following description and drawing by a child brings out the complex context (Fig. 16.2):

> "My mom was giving a shower to my elder brother's son. My elder sister was assisting her daughter to bath. She requested me to bring talcum powder for her daughter. While I was bringing it, I heard a blasting sound of a shell. When I regained consciousness, I found I was thrown on the ground. I noticed other members in my family also on the ground; my dad was on one side of me and my mom and elder sister were on the other side. I noted I had an injury. I rushed here and there in the house and found all of my family members who were injured. My dad's elder brother had severe injuries. Uncles (rebels) in the environment quickly took all of us into a lorry. I, my mom and younger brother were then taken in a boat."

16.4 Recovery from Trauma

What are the sociocultural factors helping in the recovery from trauma (PTSD)?

How can these factors be used to improve recovery from trauma (PTSD)?

Box 16.2 Sociocultural Factors Helping in Recovery

Social support system

Normalization

Practice of routine coping strategies

Practice of rituals, customs, and other traditional measures

Expression of grief

16.4.1 Social Support System

A good social support system helps survivors recover significantly and relatively quickly from PTSD. It provides emotional, intellectual, physical, and social supports and keeps survivors occupied with members of support system or some kind of activities or responsibilities. In such instances, survivors devote their attention and concentration to activities or responsibilities or interact with members of support system that appears to reduce experiencing traumatic flashbacks, memories, and reliving. Activities also increase survivors' motivation. Survivors feel protected and develop insights when support systems provide emotional and intellectual help. They understand that someone is available to care for them and find meaning to continue their life. They also feel obliged to repay what they receive and a sense of responsibility to survive for others who provided support to them.

> Mrs. A. feels considerably better with remarriage. She admitted "I needed support from at least some one. So when one gentleman who also lost his entire family in the war requested me to remarry I accepted. He is very supportive to me. After remarriage, intensity of my illness has been reduced. My remarriage has provided at least someone to interrupt my tendency of sinking into flood of memories and flashbacks of my children and husband persistently."
>
> Mrs. A. also said "my immediate family was not supportive (emotionally) to me. But few of my far relatives are. This helps me. I think trust on others is important for recovery process from trauma. Support from few of my relatives helps me in this aspect. If I could have received my family's support my recovery could have been better, I believe."
>
> Mrs. B. said "my second son maintained few aquariums. When I returned to my village from the

internment camp, the tanks were found undamaged, but without contents. Each time when I saw the tanks I developed head discomfort elicited by the traumatic memories. My family noted this and removed the tanks to prevent this."

A good support system assists to trauma sufferers in another way. Sufferers frequently say they are prompted to function when they observe others functioning well. Observation reminds them of responsibilities and necessity to function. Further it stimulates and nourishes motivation. When survivors are surrounded with a good support system and people functioning well, they start to function voluntarily and progress gradually. This has an energizing effect on functional and cognitive recovery of sufferers. The same effect is noted when survivors' environment is normalized. This effect is time dependent, i.e., progresses with time and early restoration have more favorable outcome.

> Mr. C. claimed "my children and relatives do not allow me to be preoccupied with the memories of my daughter and flashbacks of her death. My mother used to admonish me when she saw me crying or preoccupying with the thoughts of my daughter. She used to make sure that I was not alone or isolated. My father used to say that he might die anytime as he was in the latter half of elder hood and once he died, he would join my daughter and take care of her; and therefore, to not worry. My father died with the exodus from the Vanni region. My elder brother was so supportive to me, economically, physically and emotionally. He took additional care of me after the death of my daughter. He used to guide and counsel me. With deaths of these three people, my support system has shrunk."

A good support system helps patients to deal with suicidal thoughts. Patients emotionally resisted suicidal thoughts and subsequently they regain hope.

16.4.2 Normalization

Trauma survivors from war zones were immediately placed in internment camps. Internment camps did not have basic needs such as food, shelter, sanitary facilities, and water that are part of normal life. Moreover, survivors were prevented from moving freely (out of the camps), and most of them had to face continuous and severe security threats to their lives. Detention in

internment camps prevented trauma sufferers from practicing routine coping mechanisms and rituals, customs, religious ceremonies, and other traditions for those killed in the war. Survivors clearly recalled that when they were kept inside the camps, their symptoms were overwhelming. However, they found their symptoms improved markedly once they were freed from camps. Release from camps made them to be freely mobile, fulfill their needs, settle in their own way and have their own life, and importantly practice routine coping measures and collective traditional rites. Once they established a routine life, they found their recovery further increased.

A comparison between PTSD patients was made with the time periods they were kept inside internment camps. Those who spent more time in camps, which in turn reflected delay in normalization, presented with posttraumatic personality changes, more somatic symptoms, comorbid depression, and resistant type of illness. In contrast trauma sufferers with early normalization or those who spent less time in internment camps showed less disease burden and relatively quick response to treatment.

Some patients are slow to recover. They continuously encounter cues in their surrounding or environment and subsequent intrusion of traumatic flashbacks, memories, and reliving experience. These patients avoid public places, events, and to be freely mobile. They choose a place with minimum or no cues and fix their life into the particular environment. However, when these patients are encouraged to return to normal routine or placed so as to be flooded with clues eliciting their traumatic experiences, PTSD symptoms are noted to be improved with continuous exposures.

> Mr. C. said "in the first few months of my internment camp life I could not do monthly ritual ('Maalayam') for my daughter. This caused me lot of torment; I was anxious that my daughter would feel uneasy by the failure. However after about 4/5 months of entrance into the camp, a temporary temple was set up inside the camp. This relieved my frustration as I could continue doing rituals and customs."

Normalization is also important to caregivers. Normalized caregivers display more acceptance, empathy, and commitment to care for survivors.

Caregivers not normalized are reluctant to do the necessary as their primary concern is to be normalized. Therefore normalization indirectly shapes support system.

Normalization has another dimension. It is an essential component for therapeutic alliance. Normalized patients show more interest to access and communicate with healthcare workers than patients not normalized. Healthcare workers also find it easier to reach and treat normalized patients.

A Statement About Internment Camp Experience Written by a Survivor

No facilities are available to fulfill our basic needs in the camp where we are kept. There is a severe shortage for drinking water. We have to be in a queue for at least 2 h to get 1.5 liter water in a bottle. We are issued rice not properly boiled with either eggplant or pumpkin curry, daily. Sometimes we find worms, beetles, and flies in the curry. We have no access to get nutritious food. We

have been experiencing security threats continuously and in any form from the army. This has made us just as cadaveric creatures. The camp contains very minimum medical facilities. Sanitary condition of the camp is very poor. At least two people die daily in the camp. The cooking areas have been structured next to the temporary toilets. Drainages from the toilets leak and cause sewage to be flooded around the toilets and cooking areas. This has been persistently producing and keeping a very bad, foul odor in the camp. We have been living by enduring these struggles and sufferings. There are no closed facilities for women. In summary this (camp) is an open prison. Some army soldiers try to seduce and abuse identified female ex-combatants and mentally ill. They attempt to fulfill their intention by giving valuable gifts to them. Labeled ex-combatants are taken by force or threatening in nights and this is explained as inquiry.

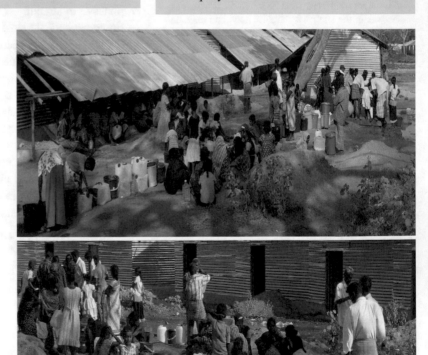

Figs. 16.3, 16.4, 16.5 and 16.6 Internment camps after the end of the war in Sri Lanka

Figs. 16.3, 16.4, 16.5 and 16.6 (continued)

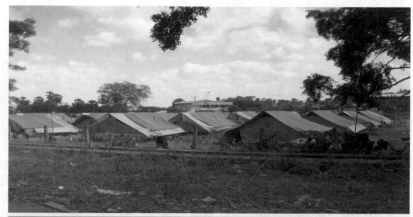

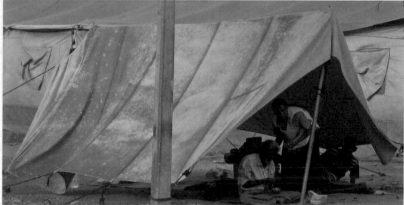

16.4.3 Practice of Routine Coping Strategies

Return to routine practices of coping can produce significant improvement in the mental status of trauma sufferers. While these practices reduce severity and frequency of symptoms and signs, they also empower survivors and recreate or strengthen their motivation. Many patients, especially patients who lost their intimates in traumatic ways, lose faith on god or religion after trauma. This is a feature of phase one reaction of grief, and it is a defense mechanism (displacement). This occurs as they believe that their god failed to save or rescue their loved ones. Religion and faith on god are well-known coping mechanisms, and they also act as a matrix to produce other coping mechanisms in Eastern communities. Therefore when a victim loses faith on god or religion, he/she also loses trust on other coping practices. It is noted that survivors who lose interest or are unmotivated to

practice routine coping strategies are to be chronic and intense sufferers of PTSD. They seek repeated hospitalization and function poorly. These patients concomitantly express loss of faith on practicing rituals, customs, and other traditional activities. Loss of faith appears to be a manifestation of loss of drive or motivation resulted from PTSD itself or comorbid depression or traumatic grief reaction.

However when these patients are enrolled into an organized coping activity, improvement is noted in disease burden and functional capacity. In the beginning of such enrollment, patients will be passive, and once they start to feel improvement, they convert into active. Therefore entry into routine coping practices is one of the channels for recovery.

The following is the experience of Mr. C. "I heard that souls died without water wander and will not reach the god. This must not happen to my daughter's soul. So in nights I keep water in containers beside flowering plants and in places where she used to occupy or spend times. I do not sleep in nights and look at the plants and places to make sure my daughter's arrival to drink water. I want my daughter's spirit to be peaceful. I keep photographs of my daughter all the times with me. When I am urged to see her I see her photographs. This pacifies me and gives some satisfaction."

Mr. C. further said "I feel relief by attending temples, praying gods and doing 'Pooja'. These measures lift up my mind. I feel I do something for my daughter. I keep a routine to give meal for at least 200 people on each annual remembrance day of my daughter. I do economical assistance to poorer. I feel my daughter will be happy by these acts, because she used to help to poorer and be supportive to marginalized people. When I do these I pray the gods to deserve the outcomes or merits ('Punniyam') to my daughter. I trust these measures will help to heal my daughter's sufferings. I beg at the gods to fulfill her needs and desires and keep comfortable and happy. When I perform these acts I feel they are done by my daughter; I feel I am possessed by my daughter."

Mrs. A. admitted "I attend to temples daily, morning and evening. I devote flowers and sing devotional poems ('Thaevaaram') with absolute love to gods. I paint and keep holy ass in my forehead all the times. I put currencies or coins into tiller boxes in temples. I do all these measures to soothe my children. I supplicate at god to take my children into heaven. By doing them I feel comfortable."

16.4.4 Practice of Rituals, Customs, and Other Traditional Measures

Patients put in places like internment camps or asylums where no facilities found to practice traditional measures or routine coping practices show relatively severe and lengthy illness than patients who obtain such opportunities. From this observation it becomes evident that practicing routines and traditions prevents deep routing of trauma.

Many patients with history of traumatic deaths of their intimates admit that disease burden becomes less, and they recovered motivation and functioning with institution of customs, rituals, and other traditional measures. When practicing these measures, survivors believe and are convinced that they devote something to dead; intimates (dead) will receive outcomes of the measures, and souls of dead would be soothed. They further believe souls of killed will forgive them for not taking rescue measures (perceived guilty). Some sufferers feel themselves as equipped or possessed by the dead, and these activities are carried out by the dead. Survivors are pacified by practicing these measures regardless of such interpretations. For survivors who lost their intimates in trauma, practicing these measures is partly an undoing action of defense mechanism and partly a continuing service to intimates lost in trauma. However survivors with trauma of missing their intimates in disasters are not in a position to practice these activities for the missed. Traditional compulsion to commit these measures, but insufficient evidences to confirm assassination of missed, and absolute unwillingness to do traditional practices resulting from denial of probable catastrophe to missed make survivors indecisive and distressed and keep alive trauma.

Mr. C. said "there were 4 students including my daughter from my neighborhood killed in the war. They studied in the same school. They were buried beside each other in the seashore of my village. Villagers and relatives of the dead planted flowering plants, herbs and trees in the land of burial. The place was maintained as a sacred place. I used to visit the place daily when I was in my village until I was displaced. I used to devote flowers, aroma and incense sticks to my daughter and do lament ('Oppaari'). I used to do lament until my sufferings subsided. I used to sleep beside my daughter (sepulture). I used to pour water to the plants. Each time when I poured water I felt my daughter was cooled. These measures helped to me a lot. I practiced this as a routine. But the war and displacement stopped me from practicing them. It was a huge drawback to me in dealing my trauma. When I returned to my hometown with the resettlement program, I was shocked. There was a military camp in the land where we buried our children. We explained to the military the importance of the place and pleaded them to return the land to us. But the army refused to leave the place. This reenacted my sufferings. I could not accept military feet over my daughter. It meant to me that my daughter was disgraced. I am frustrated. I feel I am stopped from caring my daughter; I am prevented to devote meal ('Padaiyal') to my daughter; I am blocked from interacting with my daughter; I am held away from expressing my grief; and I am halted from practicing annual remembrance day in the place where she was seeded. When I see or imagine that army soldiers walk above my daughter (sepulture), I immediately and increasingly become melancholic. This had been the main reason for my leaving the village. When I had visits to my village I avoided visiting to the land where I seeded my daughter. I also have to resist the thoughts that my daughter is trampled by the military."

Mrs. B. said "once I was resettled in my village I did almsgiving ceremony ('Anthiyeddy' and 'Veeddukirithikam') and for next one year practiced monthly remembrance day ('Maalayam') for my children. A year after completion of last monthly remembrance day I started to practice annual remembrance day ('Thivasam') and I continue practicing this on annual basis. These practices calm my mind. I started to visit temples last year onward to pray and do rituals for my children. I did special 'Pooja' ('Moadcha-archanai') for my children to be united with the god. I granted 2 traditional lambs to a temple for the names of my children. I gave meal ('Annathaanam' and 'Moathaka-poosai') to poor people. This year I visited to Car ('Thaer') festival of a popular temple. I am satisfied that I do something for my kids. I will definitely continue these measures until I die."

Mr. C. told "I lost faith on gods and traditions after the death of my daughter. But after doing them I felt there was a reduction in the turbulence in my mind. The Mental Health Unit, General Hospital, Vavuniya conducted annual, traditional fasting ('Aadi-Amaavaasai Viratham') ceremony inside the camp for the people who lost their intimates in the war. I participated and felt some relief."

16.4.5 Expression of Grief

Survivors hold different opinions about visiting places where their loved ones were disposed or just left to be following their death (killing). Some prefer to visit frequently. These patients are found to lament instantly once they entered such places. They feel better following abundant and free lamentation. But some patients are reluctant to visit such places because it becomes unbearable and agonizing. These patients are found to be victims with multiple losses and chronic sufferers. Nevertheless, these patients also admit that expression of their grief pacifies them. They are ready to lament in appropriate places. Here the term appropriate is used because patients struggle to find appropriate places. There is a misunderstanding about lamenting. Family members, caregivers, and even therapists misunderstand that lamenting triggers severe illness. But the fact is opposite. It has an alleviation effect.

> Mrs. B. stated "I want to do frequent visits to the place where I put my second son and the place where my first son was buried. But my family and psychiatrist do not allow. They are afraid that I would develop another episode of severe illness. When I visit the place I am readily prompted to lament for my children by striking my head and chest with palms and it continues for long time ('Oppari'). I continue this without my awareness. This is why I am not allowed by my family and psychiatrist to do visits. But at the end I feel pacified. When I am flooded with the memories and flashbacks of my sons, I am tormented by them. The torment could only be managed by lamenting intensely and for long time. Suppressing the torment causes severe suffering (severe head discomfort). My family stops me from visiting to prevent falling into illness (severe head discomfort). But they do not know the value of lamenting. Flashbacks and memories of my sons and trauma could only be managed with lamenting. When I fail to lament, the agony turns into severe head discomfort. Therefore I try to lament as much as possible."

Lamenting is an important measure to patients to cope with PTSD and grief. Especially this measure significantly alleviates grief and reduces heaviness of mind of female survivors with traumatic loss. Sufferers find place of burial is the best place to lament. But some patients find places where they buried their family members are occupied by the military and therefore have fewer opportunities to lament. These patients are noted to develop more grief. They reason out that their loved ones are disgraced by military presence. Patients lamenting freely show greater coping than patients with less opportunities to lament.

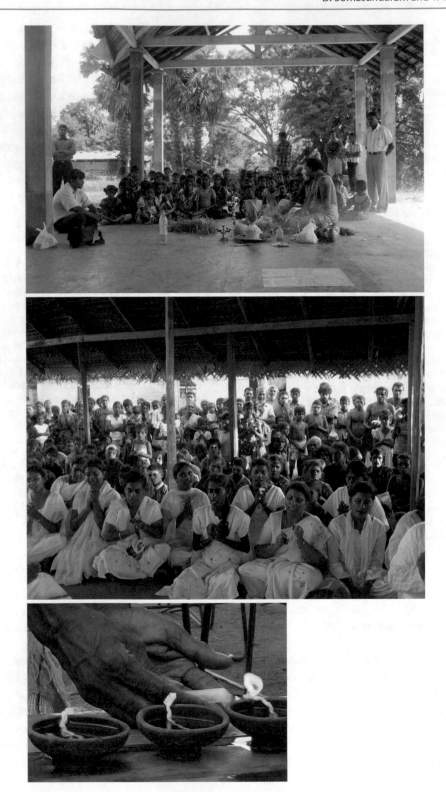

Figs. 16.7, 16.8, 16.9, 16.10, 16.11 and 16.12 Practice of routine coping strategies, rituals, customs, and other traditional measures in the internment camps in Sri Lanka

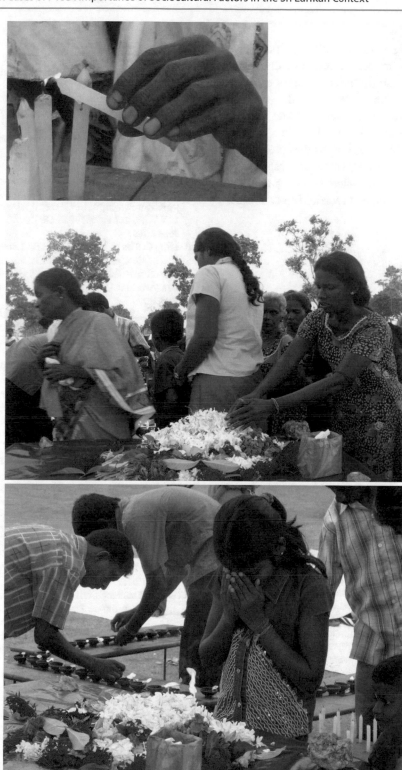

Figs. 16.7, 16.8, 16.9, 16.10, 16.11 and 16.12 (continued)

Conclusion

Some insight and holistic understanding of trauma, its impact not only on individuals but also on the family and community, grew out of extensive experience with the man-made disaster, the chronic civil war, and the natural disaster, the Asian tsunami of 2004. Psychosocial interventions designed to alleviate these systemic, ecological repercussions would have to be tailored to work at the family, community, and societal levels in order to be effective.

References

1. Richard AB, Gallagher GC, Lisa G, et al. Mental health and social networks after disaster. Am J Psychiatry. 2017;174:277–85. https://doi.org/10.1176/appi.ajp. 2016.15111403. Accessed 25 Nov 2016.
2. Green B, Friedman M, editors. Trauma, interventions in war and peace: prevention, practice, and policy. New York: Kluwer/Plenum Press; 2003.
3. Green B. Psychosocial research in traumatic stress: an update. J Trauma Stress. 1994;7:341–62.
4. Herman H. Trauma and recovery: the aftermath of violence from doemstic abuse to poltical terror. New York: Basic Books; 1992.
5. World Health Organization. Mental disorders: glossary and guide to their classification in accordance with the tenth revision of the international classification of diseases (ICD-10). Geneva: WHO; 1992.
6. De Jong J, Komproe I, et al. DESNOS in four post conflict settings: cross-cultural construct equivalence. J Traum Stress. 2005;18:13–23.
7. Wilson J. In: Tang CS, editor. Cross cultural assessment of psycholgoical trauma and PTSD, International and cultural psychology series. New York: Springer; 2007.
8. Wong P, Wong L. Handbook of multicultural perspectives on stress and coping, International and cultural psychology series. New York: Springer; 2006.
9. Somasundaram D. Collective trauma in northern Sri Lanka: a qualitative psychosocial-ecological study. Int J Mental Health Systems. 2007;1(Suppl 1):5.
10. Byman D. Keeping the peace: lasting solutions to ethnic conflicts. Baltimore (MD): John Hopkins University Press; 2002.
11. Cordell K, Wolff S. Ethnic conflict. Cambridge, UK: Polity; 2010.
12. Council NP. MARGA: cost of the war. Colombo: National Peace Council; 2001.
13. Eller JD. From culture to ethnicity to conflict: an anthropological perspective on international ethnic conflict. Ann Arbor: University of Michigan Press; 1999.
14. Esman M. An introduction to ethnic conflict. Cambridge, UK: Polity; 2004.
15. Horowitz D. Ethnic groups in conflict. 2nd ed. Berkeley: University of California; 2000.
16. Jesse N, Williams K. Ethnic conflict: a systematic approach to cases of conflict. Washington, DC: CQ Press; 2011.
17. Ross MH. Cultural contestation in ethnic conflict. Cambridge, UK: Cambridge University Press; 2007.
18. Smith A. Nationalism and modernism: a critical survey of recent theories of nations and nationalism. London: Routledge; 1998.
19. Commission of Inquiry. Report of the commission of inquiry on lessons learnt and reconciliation. Colombo: Government of Sri Lanka; 2011. http://www.priu.gov.lk/news_update/Current_Affairs/ca201112/FINAL%20LLRC%20REPORT.pdf. Accessed 22 June 2013
20. Philp C. The hidden massacre: Sri Lanka's final offensive against Tamil Tigers. In: Times online. London: The Times; 2009. http://www.timesonline.co.uk/tol/news/world/asia/article6383449.ece. Accessed 29 May 2009.
21. Stein G. War stories. In: Segus G, editor. Dateline. Crows Nest, New South Wales: SBS; 2010. http://www.sbs.com.au/dateline/story/watch/id/600331/n/War-Stories. Accessed 22 June 2013.
22. University Teachers for Human Rights- Jaffna (UTHR-J). Let them speak: truth about Sri Lanka's survivors of war. In: University Teachers for Human Rights-Jaffna (UTHR-J), editor. Special report. Colombo (Sri Lanka): UTHR-J; 2009. http://www.uthr.org/SpecialReports/Special%20rep34/Uthr-sp.rp34.htm. Accessed 22 June 2013.
23. United Nations Secretary General's Panel of Experts. Accountability in Sri Lanka. New York: United Nations; 2011. http://www.un.org/News/dh/infocus/Sri_Lanka/POE_Report_Full.pdf. Accessed 22 June 2013.
24. United Nations. Report of the secretary General's internal review panel of the United Nations action in Sri Lanka. New York: UNO; 2012. http://www.un.org/News/dh/infocus/Sri_Lanka/The_Internal_Review_Panel_report_on_Sri_Lanka. pdf. Accessed 22 June 2013
25. Wax E. Fresh reports, imagery contradict Sri Lanka on civilian no-fire zone. In: Washington Post. Washington, DC: Washington Post; 2009. http://www.washingtonpost.com/wp-dyn/content/article/2009/05/29/AR2009052903409.html?nav5emailpage. Retrieved May 30, 2009.
26. Husain F, Anderson M, Cardozo BL, et al. Prevalence of war related mental health conditions and association with displacement status in postwar Jaffna District, Sri Lanka. J Am Med Assoc. 2011;306:522–31.
27. Somasundaram D, Sivayokan S. War trauma in a civilian population. Br J Psychiatry. 1994;165:524–7.
28. Bloom SL. By the crowd they have been broken, by the crowd they shall be healed: the social transformation of trauma. In: Tedeschi RG, Park CL, Calhoun LG, editors. Posttraumatic growth: positive changes in the aftermath of crisis. Mahwah: Lawrence Erlbaum Associates, Inc; 1998. p. 179–213.

Psychiatric Emergencies: A Complex Case of Overdose and Assessment in the Emergency Department

17

Bruce Fage and Jodi Lofchy

Abbreviations

BPD   Borderline personality disorder
DBT   Dialectical Behaviour Therapy
ED   Emergency department
Project BETA   Best Practices in Evaluation and Treatment of Agitation

17.1 Chapter Objectives

- Review risk assessments for patients with chronic or recurrent suicidal ideation.
- Present therapeutic techniques for managing personal reactions.
- Explore the interface between medical and psychiatric issues in the emergency setting.
- Discuss a trauma-informed approach to managing agitation and distress.

B. Fage, MD
Department of Psychiatry, University of Toronto, Toronto, ON, Canada

J. Lofchy, MD, FRCPC (✉)
Psychiatry Emergency Services, Department of Psychiatry, University Health Network, University of Toronto, Toronto, ON, Canada
e-mail: Jodi.Lofchy@uhn.ca

17.2 A Complex Case History

Jennifer is a 33-year-old female living in a rented apartment in downtown Toronto, Canada. She supports herself by working as a server. She has a partner, but is vague about the details of her current romantic relationship, which has been strained as of late. She has no children, but her partner has one child from a previous relationship.

Jennifer was advised to go to the emergency department (ED) by a physician at a walk-in clinic after she expressed suicidal ideation. The physician had not seen her before and was concerned about her vague suicidal plan, but was not concerned enough to certify her under the mental health act. In the ED, she refused to engage with nursing staff, stating "I suggest you read my record" and preferring to wait and tell her story to "the doctor". There were a number of urgent trauma and resuscitation cases in the ED and she waited 4 h before being assessed. Jennifer lamented the wait and was rude and condescending to the nurses, demanding to be seen immediately. Her tone shifted when the emergency physician assessed her, and she intimated in a quiet, childlike manner that she was feeling unsafe, her medications were not working, and her partner was not returning her calls after an

© Springer International Publishing AG, part of Springer Nature 2018
K. Shivakumar, S. Amanullah (eds.), *Complex Clinical Conundrums in Psychiatry*,
https://doi.org/10.1007/978-3-319-70311-4_17

intense argument earlier this morning. She admitted to drinking two glasses of wine but did not appear clinical intoxicated. She was terrified that she would be at risk of harming herself if left alone in her apartment, and she had not been having regular appointments as her psychiatrist had been away on vacation for the past 3 weeks. Fortunately, he was returning next week, and an appointment had been scheduled at that time. She did not endorse any specific plan or intent to harm herself. The emergency physician agreed to review the clinical record.

Jennifer had gone to the ED with similar concerns a week ago and discharged by the emergency physician with a plan to follow up with the Psychiatric Urgent Care Clinic. When the clinic staff phoned 2 days later to book a time for an assessment, it became evident that she did not meet criteria for the referral as she was already connected with an outpatient psychiatrist at another city hospital. Thus, the referral was cancelled, and Jennifer felt frustrated with the lack of support.

As she denied suicidal intent, the initial disposition plan was to discharge her home. The emergency physician encouraged her to follow up with her psychiatrist next week and mobilize available friends to help her cope over the weekend. Jennifer became distraught, angrily declaring that she had purchased a large bottle of extra strength acetaminophen and would swallow a lethal amount if not admitted to hospital. Frustrated and unsure, the emergency physician decided to refer for psychiatric consultation. She provided brief handover of the known facts with the emergency psychiatry day team, who were wrapping up their shift. Thus, Jennifer waited a further 3 h before being assessed by the junior psychiatry resident on call.

The wait, and some dinner, had served to soften Jennifer's tough exterior. When assessed, she was engaged and felt validated to be speaking with "the psychiatrist". Despite attending weekly psychiatric appointments and a monthly women's support group, Jennifer was upset about her lack of support and stated that her mood had been

"up and down" over the past few months. She reported that she had recently been accepted into a Dialectical Behaviour Therapy treatment program (DBT). While this provided some hope, the 1 year wait list was incredibly disheartening, and she admitted that she needed assistance dealing with her history of trauma. She identified an ongoing conflict with her partner as a significant trigger and was unsure of his whereabouts at the moment. She became tearful when asked about what happened, and reported that, a week ago, she had found out that her partner had been having an affair with his ex-partner, who is the mother of his child. She had initially demanded that he leave the apartment, which she pays for, but felt devastated when he actually did. He returned to collect his belongings 2 days ago, and the couple briefly reconciled. He stayed the night but left this morning after another fight. When she was unable to connect with a close friend, Georgia, she went to a walk in-clinic to find some help.

A review of psychiatric symptoms indicated that she had been experiencing low mood and poor sleep for the past week, though her energy and appetite were normal. Suicide had been on her mind for many years, but over the last week, her thoughts had intensified. Her suicidal plan included acetaminophen overdose, but she said she would never go through with it. She denied significant symptoms of anxiety and no symptoms of mania or psychosis.

She had long struggled with mood swings, particularly in the context of interpersonal stressors. Seven months ago, she had quickly fallen in love with her current partner after they met on a dating app. She described him as "her saviour", attentive and emotionally supportive. She was happy to have met him at a very vulnerable time, almost immediately after the dissolution of her previous relationship. Though she had not self-harmed for many months, she disclosed that she had superficially cut after finding out about the affair, but as she had promised herself, she would never cut again; she felt deeply ashamed. Cutting had been a coping mechanism for a number of years, but a significant part of her work with her outpatient psychiatrist had been developing alternative strategies, including yoga, mindfulness, and calling friends. Alcohol use had been an off and on concern, but she had recently cut down to 4–6 drinks per week. At one point she had been drinking closer to 10–15 drinks per week, but she has no history of withdrawal seizures. She reported a remote history of marijuana use, but no other illicit drugs.

Jennifer had, at one point or another, been diagnosed with persistent depressive disorder, post-traumatic stress disorder, alcohol use disorder, and borderline personality disorder. The most recent discharge summary from 8 months ago indicated "complex post-traumatic stress disorder" with a referral to DBT services. She had had three previous psychiatric admissions, two of which had been in her mid- to late-20s, the longest having been 3 months. She had been doing relatively well for a number of years after being connected with her outpatient psychiatrist, until an impulsive suicide attempt 14 months ago following the death of her mother. She ingested a large number of acetaminophen and alprazolam tablets and was brought to hospital after calling 911 immediately post-ingestion. She spent 3 days in the intensive care unit, followed by 2 days on the general medical unit before a 5-day psychiatric admission.

Her current psychiatric medications include escitalopram 20 mg by mouth daily, clonazepam 1 mg by mouth at night, and quetiapine 300 mg by mouth at night as well as 25 mg by mouth, three times daily, as needed for anxiety. Typically, she does not use the extra medication but has lately started taking all three tablets at night for sleep. She is also taking dienogest 2 mg by mouth daily for chronic pelvic pain from suspected endometriosis. Otherwise, her past medical history is noncontributory.

She is the youngest of three siblings, born in Kingston, Ontario. She met her developmental milestones on time. She was a lively child and an average student, who started dating early with a string of sexual partners when she was 15. She had a therapeutic abortion at age 16 after an unplanned pregnancy. She graduated high school on time and attended university, studying 2 years of art history before leaving to work as a server. She reported being sexually abused by her father between the ages of 9 and 14. When it happened, she told her mother who did not believe her. When her older brother discovered what was happening and confronted her father, it caused a significant conflict within the family. She no longer has contact with her father, and her mother died 14 months ago in a motor vehicle accident. Her mother had been struggling with depression for a long time, and it is suspected that her death may have been a suicide, a fact Jennifer vehemently refutes.

On mental status, Jennifer is a 33-year-old female who appears younger than her stated age, wearing a fitted tank top and jeans. Her speech is soft and high pitched, and despite her initial reluctance, she is cooperative with the assessment. Her mood is "okay", her affect mildly dysphoric. Her thought form is linear and goal directed, focused on her interpersonal stressors. There is no psychotic content evident, and she does not appear to be responding to internal stimuli. She harbours suicidal ideation, a previously expressed plan, but denies intent. Insight and cognition are preserved, but a history of impulsivity is noted.

Jennifer and the resident worked together to develop a safety plan, and Jennifer called a friend to pick her up. She felt validated and heard after the assessment, stating "I don't want to kill myself, I just don't want to be alone". The resident was uncertain about the best course of action, but was loathed to admit a "frequent flying BPD" patient and felt pressured by the nursing team who stated she "didn't need to be here". Jennifer had grown weary of waiting in the hospital and wanted to leave. As she had an upcoming appointment next week with her psychiatrist, denied suicidal intent, and had managed to connect with her friend, the staff felt that she would be safe for discharge. She was asked to return to the ED if suicidal intent developed.

17.3 Assessing Suicide Risk in a Patient with BPD and Chronic or Recurrent Suicidality

As a core diagnostic feature of borderline personality disorder (BPD), recurrent suicidal behaviour, gestures, or threats present a challenging management experience [1]. With a 10% prevalence among psychiatric outpatients and between 15% and 25% in an inpatient population [2], patients suffering from this disorder are commonly encountered in the ED. In a study of patients admitted to a psychiatric hospital through the ED for suicidal behaviours, 56% met criteria for BPD [3]. As the portal of entry for a number of psychiatric services, clinicians in the emergency setting must provide a thorough and effective risk assessment. Though it may be easy to underestimate the acute risk of suicide in a patient with chronic suicidality, multiple studies have converged on an approximate 10% rate of completed suicide, or one in ten patients diagnosed with BPD [4].

At the core of any suicide risk assessment is an empathic understanding of the patient's current presentation from a biopsychosocial perspective. An acute and frantic ED may not be the ideal setting for developing rapport. Patients, such as Jennifer, typically explain their story to multiple staff members before receiving a thorough risk assessment. Finding a comfortable and private environment and clearly explaining your role and the purpose of the assessment are therapeutic first steps [5]. Validating the patient's distress, highlighting his or her strengths, and respecting the decision to come for help as an alternative to suicide can make the patient feel heard and understood. Developing this sense of respect is key to engaging and eliciting important information from a patient who may have difficulty trusting an unfamiliar process. If a patient is guarded or frightened, directly asking about suicidal ideation may not provide accurate or complete information [6]. Validation is critical; a 2006 study of consumer experiences in the ED following a suicide attempt indicated that fewer than 40% of patients felt listened to and taken seriously by providers [7].

Inquiry into the nature of the suicidality, with attention to intent and plan, is paramount. Intent is a reflection of the intensity of ideation and can be accompanied by a plan with varying degrees of specificity and lethality. Assess the practicality of the plan and what steps the patient has taken towards implementation. Plans with immediate and deadly consequences such as jumping from a height or shooting oneself are particularly concerning, though elucidating the patient's presumption of the lethality of their plan remains important. Patient intent cannot be discounted even if a suicide plan is unlikely to end in death. Patients with chronic suicidality may have a long history of multiple attempts with varying degrees of lethality and intent. Assessing and documenting past attempts, including features such as the situation, method, intent, and consequence of each attempt, provides essential backstory to place the current suicidality into context [6]. In Jennifer's case, her previous attempt occurred in the context of significant interpersonal loss following the death of her mother. Though she sought emergency assistance after the toxic ingestion, her ICU admission suggests that her attempt was of high lethality. The present context of interpersonal conflict places her at higher than baseline risk. Notably, the conflict is ongoing, and relationship status not yet determined. There is the potential that further distress is imminent pending interaction with her partner. While clinicians cannot predict the future, discussing the patient's hopes and fears about what may happen to him or her and how that will affect suicidality can clarify the level of risk.

Impulsivity is a recognized risk factor for suicidal behaviour [8, 9]. A predilection for acting on a whim, without forethought or careful consideration, is a frightening reality for many patients (and similarly, their caregivers and providers) [1]. Though detailed plans are generally associated with a greater risk of suicide, a history of impulsive behaviour is cause for concern and difficult to assess [6]. Jennifer's previous suicide attempt occurred impulsively, with limited premeditation and planning. In patients without a clear history of prior suicide attempts, screening for other potentially dangerous behaviours such as substance abuse, high-risk sexual behaviours, and deliberate self-injurious behaviours can paint a picture of impulsivity in various contexts [8]. This is not to suggest that all dangerous behaviours are indicative of suicidality, though presence of self-mutilation has been reported to double the risk of suicide [10]. Reported reasons for self-injurious behaviour vary and include interpersonal frustration, attention seeking, lessening internal distress, and numbing emotional pain [11]. A history of childhood physical and sexual abuse is associated with an increased risk of attempted suicide and self-destructive behaviour [12]. Jennifer reported a history of both impulsive and non-impulsive wrist cutting, and her prior suicide attempt was not extensively premeditated. Jennifer's ability to maintain her physical safety in the context of further interpersonal difficulty could be compromised by her impulsivity. Further increasing her suicide risk is the lingering question of substance abuse. Though she had worked hard to reduce her weekly alcohol intake, the presence of intoxication or a comorbid substance use disorder increases the risk of suicide attempts [12]. Though in sustained partial remission, her alcohol use had long been a coping mechanism, and reports of intoxication in the ED were concerning.

Helpful Things to Say

1. It sounds like you are incredibly frustrated right now. What is the worst part about this whole situation?
2. Is there anyone I could talk to who really understands what you've been experiencing?
3. You have had really difficult experiences in relationships. It makes sense that you are feeling this distressed.
4. What helps when things are this bad?

Clinicians in the emergency psychiatric setting will develop a level of familiarity with a number of frequently presenting patients. While this familiarity can be useful in developing longer-term rapport and comfort with engagement, a key component of the assessment must be a longitudinal view of the current pattern of behaviour and presentation. An "acute-on-chronic" model of

suicidality recognizes the baseline elevated risk but also acknowledges that current stressors may elevate the acute likelihood of a suicide attempt [13]. For patients with chronic ideation and recurrent utilization of healthcare services, assess what has changed and what is new. Consider the pattern: Jennifer had a past history of ED presentations but had been doing well in the community and had only been reappearing in the ED over the past week. In cities with multiple hospitals and crisis centres, finding out if there have been multiple emergency visits across the region can help establish the pattern. If available, contact friends and family for collateral information. The escalation of presentations, coupled with her substance use, interpersonal conflict, and impulsivity, increases Jennifer's acute risk of suicide.

Key Points to Consider

- BPD is commonly encountered in the ED and carries a significant lifetime risk of suicide.
- A therapeutic rapport helps to ensure a thorough risk assessment.
- Note previous suicide attempts and the context in which they occurred.

17.4 Documenting Risk in the Chronically Suicidal Patient

A key part of risk assessment is accurate documentation. The acronym CAIPS (*C*hronic and *A*cute factors, *I*mminent warning signs, *P*rotective factors, and *S*ummary statement) is a tool to construct a suicide risk assessment that is clinically sound and legally defensible [14]. The resident summarized Jennifer's risk as follows:

> Jennifer's previous suicide attempts, history of substance abuse, impulsivity, and diagnosis of BPD place her at a chronically elevated baseline risk of suicide. Acutely, she is in the midst of a difficult breakup that increases her level of risk. She has acted on a plan by purchasing a bottle of acetaminophen for use in overdose. However, she denies current intent or hopelessness, is not intoxicated, and wants to follow up with her outpatient supports. She has sought help in the ED as an alternative to self-harming and can present a coherent plan of

treatment as an outpatient, engaging friends and crisis supports, and returning to the ED if needed. In summary, Jennifer is at a chronically elevated risk of suicide that is currently increased due to interpersonal conflict. Despite this, she is denying intent and future oriented, with a clear treatment plan in place, and is at low risk of acute suicide.

17.5 Managing Their Personal Reactions to Patients in the Emergency Setting

Due to the volume of patients with BPD assessed in the ED, providers must be mindful of their own feelings and reactions to patients in this setting [15]. The fast-paced, loud, and chaotic nature of the ED can be frightening to patients who are unsure about what they are experiencing or what may happen to them. Psychiatric presentations to EDs are increasing [16], leading to longer wait times for patients who may not realize that emergency staff have been working hard to ensure patients are assessed in a safe and timely manner. Time and resource demands, coupled with unsociable hours, may not allow front-line staff the requisite time to build a therapeutic alliance and understand a patient's uncertainty and distress. Patients may be brought to the ED by coercive means, and collateral may not be readily available. Thus, factors associated with the emergency setting can worsen or exacerbate the crisis experience for patients with BPD. Debriefing any negative aspects of the ED experience, in a supportive and nondefensive manner, can build rapport and give insight into the patient's concerns.

There are a number of practical steps that emergency staff can take to understand a patient's distress and provide the excellent care each patient deserves and requires. If possible, finding a calm, quiet, and private space to speak can provide the patient a sense of control and safety. Attend early to concrete and physical needs like hygiene and hunger so that patients can readily engage in a fulsome discussion of their crisis needs. Dialectical Behaviour Therapy (DBT) is an empirically supported, structured therapeutic programme for the treatment of BPD [17]. As the core dialectic in DBT, the tension between accepting oneself and recognizing the need for change may be exacerbated in a crisis [18].

Techniques from DBT can be adapted for the emergency setting. Validation of the person's experience is a critical first step in crisis de-escalation [15]. It is essential to presume the distress the patient is feeling is real, and their inner experience is intolerable. It can be difficult to relate to patients who present with what appear to be relatively minor concerns; however, accepting that the crisis is having a significant impact is crucial. Validating the decision to come and seek help, as opposed to self-harming, can help the patient feel understood. Feeling understood could lead to better rapport, which is necessary for completing a thorough and accurate risk assessment.

When upset or distressed, patients with BPD can lash out at providers or attempt to "split" the team. Splitting is a common defence mechanism, whereby patients have difficulty holding opposing views of a person at the same time. In a healthcare setting, this can result in some team members being rejected and others adored. In Jennifer's case, she was angry and dismissive with the nursing staff and idealized the psychiatry resident. Recognizing these patterns can help interprofessional teams work together and handle personal reactions to these demanding scenarios. Patients with a diagnosis of BPD face significant stigma in healthcare settings, with staff in inpatient settings reporting less optimism and more negativity about their experience working with this population [19]. Attitudes of emergency staff are often mixed; despite expressing sympathy, front-line workers can feel that working with self-harming patients is not rewarding or a good use of ED resources [20].

Helpful Things to Say

1. This experience is unbearable, and it is really hard to cope right now.
2. I'm glad that you came for help instead of hurting yourself.
3. What lets you feel in control when you are this upset?
4. You are worried about your relationship. Let's think about what you need right now.

Emergency staff may feel that they do not have the necessary skills to assist patients with BPD who are experiencing a crisis, or worse, feel that managing these patients is impossible. It is important to recognize that the patient's distress is not about you. Jennifer is experiencing an interpersonal crisis and feeling angry, frustrated, and abandoned. In this moment of extreme distress, she is unable to use her coping skills to handle what she is experiencing. Address and contain the distress before trying to problem-solve. Taking breaks from discussing traumatic episodes allows for recovery time. Patients may have community teams, and linking with them is key, reinforcing the available supports [13]. It can be tough to feel empathic in the middle of the night when you are exhausted or burnt out. Providers who work in these settings need space and time to debrief about their experiences with colleagues and take opportunities to attend to self-care.

Healthcare workers may question the value of admission in patients with BPD, expressing frustration with "frequent flyers", or patients with recurrent ED presentations. Hospital volumes may also increase pressure to discharge patients due to a limited number of psychiatric beds. Limited resources can set up a power struggle between patient and clinician. Providers in training, as in Jennifer's case, feel pressure to avoid an admission that will be seen as unhelpful in the eyes of their senior colleagues. A more empathic approach is to listen to the patient and avoid making an a priori decision about admission. The role of admission in patients with BPD is controversial, and while there is a general clinical consensus that inpatient care should be minimized, the APA Practice Guidelines for the Treatment of BPD do suggest indications for admission [8, 9]. A clinical system that provides brief hospitalization or holding in a psychiatric ED can provide good clinical care during periods of acutely increased suicidal risk, avoiding the need for a long-term admission.

Key Points to Consider

- Be mindful of your feelings and reactions when working with this patient population.

- Validate the extreme vulnerability and level of distress that a patient is feeling.
- Take time for self-care and debrief with colleagues.

17.6   Case Part 2

The next evening, Jennifer returns to the ED. She is clearly intoxicated and admits to consuming a bottle of wine. Jennifer is irritable and sarcastic, swearing, with slurred speech. The same physician picks up her chart and asks Jennifer why she came back to the ED. Jennifer angrily states "I will only talk to a doctor who cares". She will not provide a history, but repeatedly states she needs to be in a safe place. Her vitals are within normal limits. The physician is frustrated by Jennifer's return and refers for psychiatric assessment.

Due to a high number of referrals, the psychiatry resident is not able to immediately assess Jennifer. Tired of waiting, Jennifer tells the emergency nurse she is leaving, gets up, and stumbles, knocking a tray of suturing instruments from the bay beside her onto the floor. The nearby emergency physician comes back to the bedside and tells her that because of her intoxication and safety concerns she is being detained under the mental health act and cannot leave until the morning. Jennifer becomes irate, screaming and attempting to push past the nurse on her way out, causing the nurse to fall back against the counter. A code white is called, with security guards rushing in, pinning Jennifer to the bed and placing her in restraints. She is struggling and spitting at staff. The emergency physician tells her she needs medication to "calm her down" and orders 25 mg of loxapine and 2 mg of lorazepam to be given intramuscularly. After receiving the injection, Jennifer starts crying and goes limp.

The psychiatry resident responds to the code, arriving after the medication is administered. The emergency physician angrily tells the resident that "this is not a good use of resources" and demands that he "go ahead and admit the patient". Jennifer is distraught and refuses to answer questions. The resident brings her some tissues and asks if she would be willing to stay if taken out of restraints. Tearfully, she agrees. The resident assists her out of restraints, and she is transferred to the psychiatric holding area in a quieter section of the ED.

Jennifer is not forthcoming with details but insists she does not feel safe at home. When pressed, she admits to suicidal ideation and intent but will not disclose a plan. She denies toxic or lethal ingestions. The history of her presenting illness is vague; based on the information from previous assessments, the resident feels comfortable with holding overnight for further assessment. She appears tired, and the resident ends the assessment and allows her to sleep.

Three hours later, the resident receives a stat page. During nursing rounds Jennifer is discovered unresponsive with vomitus beside her bed. A code blue is called. She is intubated and transferred to the intensive care unit.

17.7 Navigating the Medical and Psychiatric Interface in the Emergency Setting Using an Interprofessional Team

Patients suffering from psychiatric emergencies may present in a variety of settings, including general and psychiatric hospitals, crisis clinics, mobile teams, and to community practitioners [21]. As psychiatric patients have similar or greater risk for medical comorbidity when compared to the general population [22], the general hospital emergency physician provides the first-line screen for acute medical problems. Determining whether or not a patient's presentation is due to medical or psychiatric illness can be challenging, and evidence suggests that physicians may be prone to attributing symptoms to psychiatric illness and fail to screen for medical comorbidity [22, 23].

Providers struggle with determining whether or not a patient is medically stable for psychiatric assessment. Factors such as level of medical support on site and timing of referral will change the threshold at which a patient is deemed medically stable, and it is recommended that psychiatric consultants have an open discussion with the referring physician about how to best meet the patient's needs. This can be particularly problematic when the reason for referral is vague, or the lines between medical and psychiatric are unclear. While there is no universal standardized definition for medical stability [24], the American College of Emergency Physicians published comprehensive guidelines regarding medical clearance [25]. Medical assessment of patients presenting with psychiatric complaints should be guided by history and physical examination, and there are no recommended routine investigations. Routine urine toxicology screens on patients who are alert and cooperative do not affect emergency management and should not delay referral to psychiatry, as psychiatric teams are capable of ordering these investigations when clinically indicated. A common point of contention is when to refer an intoxicated patient for psychiatric assessment, as psychiatric complaints may resolve when the patient is no longer intoxicated. Ideally, referrals to psychiatry should be made when the patient is capable of participating in an interview so that an accurate risk assessment can be performed. This should be based on a patient's cognitive ability to participate in an interview and not a specific blood alcohol concentration [25]. Realistically, pressures on ED staff lead to referral prior to detoxification. Clinicians should be aware of the policies and culture of their institution [21]. Arguing over the appropriateness of a referral in the middle of the night is unhelpful, and strong, collaborative relationships between emergency and psychiatric services are essential to a well-functioning department.

In Jennifer's case, frustration with her multiple presentations may have led to inadequate screening for toxic ingestion. As a well-known "psychiatric patient", it would be easy to underestimate the acutely elevated level of risk. Based on her previous history of overdose, screening for alcohol, acetaminophen, salicylates, and other intoxicants may have provided useful information and changed management early. It may have been beneficial to request blood or urine screening to clarify. Collaboration between the psychiatric resident and emergency staff is key to ensure that she is in a monitored setting. It is unclear how long Jennifer was nonresponsive, and the added effect of chemical restraint complicates the clinical picture.

17.8 Proactively Reducing the Risk of Violence and Agitation

The ED is a stressful environment for people experiencing a psychiatric crisis. Long wait times, intoxicants, and uncertainty can combine to exacerbate a patient's stress level and increase the likelihood of violent behaviour. Despite the high prevalence of agitation and violence in the emergency setting, a lack of clear guidelines and best practices led many facilities to quickly employ physical and chemical restraint. The Best Practices in Evaluation and Treatment of Agitation project (BETA) was an attempt by expert working groups to synthesize the available literature into practical guidelines for clinicians [26]. Notably, agitation has a broad differential, and it is important to undertake a thorough medical and psychiatric evaluation and uncover the reasons for the distress. Aggressive behaviours, both physical and verbal, are a means of communicating that whatever is happening is not okay. Patients with BPD who present in crisis may be overwhelmed by their experience and have difficulty communicating their needs; enable containment of their distress and establish communication to prevent escalating behaviour. If possible, emergency psychiatric assessments should occur in a designated mental health space, away from the stressful, high-stimuli emergency setting [27]. Specialized equipment such as video monitoring, alarm buzzers, clear lines of sight to nursing stations, weighted furniture, and non-barricadeable doors are recommended design elements for a safe space for patients and providers [28]. Consider the potential of violence and work to mitigate risk factors. If available, review past charts and speak with the emergency team to determine if there is a history of aggressive behaviour. Observe the patient in the waiting area before assessment for signs of agitation, such as pacing or yelling. In Jennifer's case, the crowded emergency area, replete with IV poles and other potentially dangerous equipment, was a suboptimal environment for her assessment.

17.9 Trauma-Informed Approach to Help Patients Experiencing Agitation

With the growing recognition that many men and women receiving psychiatric care are survivors of physical and sexual trauma, providers in the emergency setting must recognize vulnerability and work to avoid re-victimizing patients who are presenting in crisis. Clinicians and patients struggle with the complicated dynamic of safety and autonomy. It is recognized that when some people are highly aroused and emotionally charged, they lose the ability to self-regulate and modulate their affect. One should be mindful of the patient experience and help promote an enhanced internal locus of control. Offer choices and opportunities for decision-making, as many trauma survivors experienced abuse at a time when everything seemed out of their control [29]. Providing time and space for verbal de-escalation may preclude the eventual use of physical and chemical restraints. As a clinical skill, verbal de-escalation requires training and practice with a number of technical domains [30].

Restraint practices can be harmful, unsafe, and traumatizing, even with the best of intentions [31]. Patients and families are faced with locked doors or detainment under mental health legislation in a system that can feel byzantine and unsupportive. At the same time, the safety of the distressed patient, other patients, and the clinical team is a top priority. Institutions may implement mandatory hospital gown policies, which provide an opportunity for searching and removal of belts, shoelaces, and any potential weapons but also represent a loss of autonomy. Physical and chemical restraints are an unfortunate, but sometimes necessary, last resort. Even in a restrictive ED environment, there are opportunities to facilitate patient autonomy. Explain what is happening, what medications are being administered, and what the potential side effects may be [32]. If clinically appropriate, seclusion rooms may avoid the need for mechanical restraints. Most institutions have policies regarding least restraint or minimum effective restraint to keep everyone safe. Restraints must be applied in a way that minimizes the

re-enactment of a prior sexual assault. Some organizations have instituted a policy about patient
debriefing following a restraint event, in which
a patient, at an appropriate time, is provided an
opportunity to discuss his or her experiences and
offered support. Though difficult during a first
meeting, co-creating a safety plan provides a
chance for patients to identify triggers and alternate methods of coping with distress. Clinicians
must be aware of this potentially coercive aspect
of psychiatric care and work to find solutions for
our vulnerable patients.

Helpful Things to Say
1. Would you like to have the interview
   here in the waiting room or in a more
   private interview room?
2. When you are yelling, it makes it difficult for me to hear you – I bet if we sit
   down, we could start to understand what
   is troubling you.
3. I can see you are very uncomfortable –
   can I offer you some medication to help
   you feel in control?
4. Jennifer, you are having a psychiatric
   emergency. Medication would be helpful right now. Would you like the medication by mouth or by needle?

17.10 Summary

Risk is a complex issue and a difficult part of
emergency psychiatric assessment. Our patients
who suffer from chronic suicidal ideation are
among the most difficult to help, both from a personal and systems perspective. One must recognize the level of risk and make a calculated
decision about discharge. It is of the utmost
importance to appreciate the challenges facing
this patient population in order to provide effective patient-centred care.

Disclosure Statement "The authors have nothing to
disclose."

References

1. American Psychiatric Association. DSM 5. American
   Psychiatric Association. Washington, DC: 27 May 2013.
2. Leichsenring F, Leibing E, Kruse J, New AS, Leweke
   F. Borderline personality disorder. Lancet. 2011;
   377(9759):74–84.
3. Hayashi N, Igarashi M, Imai A, Osawa Y, Utsumi
   K, Ishikawa Y, Tokunaga T, Ishimoto K, Harima H,
   Tatebayashi Y, Kumagai N. Psychiatric disorders
   and clinical correlates of suicidal patients admitted
   to a psychiatric hospital in Tokyo. BMC Psychiatry.
   2010;10(1):1.
4. Paris J. Chronic suicidality among patients with borderline personality disorder. Psychiatr Serv. 2002;53:
   738–42.
5. Perlman CM, Neufeld EA, Martin L, Goy M, Hirdes
   JP. Suicide risk assessment inventory: a resource
   guide for Canadian health care organizations.
   Toronto, ON: Ontario Hospital Association and
   Canadian Patient Safety Institute; 2011. https://www.
   oha.com/KnowledgeCentre/Documents/Final%20
   -%20Suicide%20Risk%20Assessment%20
   Guidebook.pdf. Accessed 25 Sep 2016.
6. Jacobs DG, Baldessarini RJ, Conwell Y, Fawcett JA,
   Horton L, Meltzer H, Pfeffer CR, Simon RI. Assessment
   and treatment of patients with suicidal behaviors. APA
   Pract Guidel. 2010:1–183
7. Cerel J, Currier GW, Conwell Y. Consumer and family experiences in the emergency department following a suicide attempt. J Psychiatr Pract. 2006;12(6):
   341–7.
8. Oldham JM. Borderline personality disorder and suicidality. Am J Psychiatr. 2006;163:20–6.
9. American Psychiatric Association. Practice guideline
   for the treatment of patients with borderline personality disorder. American Psychiatric Publ. 2001;158(10
   Suppl):1–52.
10. Oumaya M, Friedman S, Pham A, Abou AT, Guelfi
    JD, Rouillon F. Borderline personality disorder, self-
    mutilation and suicide: literature review. L'Encephale.
    2008;34(5):452–8.
11. Zanarini MC, Laudate CS, Frankenburg FR, Wedig
    MM, Fitzmaurice G. Reasons for self-mutilation
    reported by borderline patients over 16 years of pro-
    spective follow-up. J Personal Disord. 2013;27(6).
    https://doi.org/10.1521/pedi_2013_27_115.
12. Black DW, Blum N, Pfohl B, Hale N. Suicidal behav-
    ior in borderline personality disorder: prevalence, risk
    factors, prediction, and prevention. J Personal Disord.
    2004;18(3):226.
13. Zaheer J, Links PS, Liu E. Assessment and emer-
    gency management of suicidality in personality disor-
    ders. Psychiatr Clin N Am. 2008;31(3):527–43.
14. Obegi JH, Rankin JM, Williams Jr JC, Ninivaggio
    G. How to write a suicide risk assessment that's clini-
    cally sound and legally defensible. Curr Psychiatr Ther.
    2015;14(3):50.

15. Bergmans Y, Brown AL, Carruthers AS. Advances in crisis management of the suicidal patient: perspectives from patients. Curr Psychiatry Rep. 2007;9(1):74–80.
16. Owens PL, Mutter R, Stocks C. Mental health and substance abuse-related emergency department visits among adults, 2007. Healthcare cost and utilization project (HCUP) statistical brief #92, July 2010. Agency for Healthcare Research and Quality, Rockville, MD. http://www.hcup-us.ahrq.gov/reports/statbriefs/sb92.pdf. Accessed 25 Sep 2016.
17. Lieb K, Zanarini MC, Schmahl C, Linehan MM, Bohus M. Borderline personality disorder. Lancet. 2004;364(9432):453–61.
18. Linehan M. Cognitive-behavioral treatment of borderline personality disorder. New York: Guilford Press; 1993.
19. Markham D. Attitudes towards patients with a diagnosis of 'borderline personality disorder': social rejection and dangerousness. J Ment Health. 2003;12(6):595–612.
20. McElroy AL, Sheppard G. The assessment and management of self-harming patients in an accident and emergency department: an action research project. J Clin Nurs. 1999;8(1):66–72.
21. Lofchy J, Boyles P, Delwo J. Emergency psychiatry: clinical and training approaches. Can J Psychiatry. 2015;60(6):1–7.
22. Lykouras L, Douzenis A. Do psychiatric departments in general hospitals have an impact on the physical health of mental patients? Curr Opin Psychiatry. 2008;21(4):398–402.
23. Leucht S, Burkard T, Henderson J, Maj M, Sartorius N. Physical illness and schizophrenia: a review of the literature. Acta Psychiatr Scand. 2007;116(5):317–33.
24. Zun LS. Evidence-based evaluation of psychiatric patients. J Emerg Med. 2005;28(1):35–9.
25. Lukens TW, Wolf SJ, Edlow JA, Shahabuddin S, Allen MH, Currier GW, Jagoda AS. Clinical policy: critical issues in the diagnosis and management of the adult psychiatric patient in the emergency department. Ann Emerg Med. 2006;47(1):79–99.
26. Holloman GH, Zeller SL. Overview of project BETA: best practices in evaluation and treatment of agitation. Western Journal of Emergency Medicine. 2012;13(1):1–2.
27. Allen MH, Forster P, Zealberg J, Currier G. Report and recommendations regarding psychiatric emergency and crisis services. A review and model program descriptions. APA Task Force on Psychiatric Emergency Services; 2002.
28. Moscovitch A, Chaimowitz GA, Patterson PG. Trainee safety in psychiatric units and facilities: the position of the Canadian Psychiatric Association. Can J Psychiatry/La Rev Can Psychiatr. 1990. https://ww1.cpa-apc.org/Publications/Position_Papers/Trainee.asp. Accessed 25 Sep 2016.
29. Harris M, Fallot RD. Trauma-informed inpatient services. New Dir Ment Health Serv. 2001;2001(89):33–46.
30. Richmond JS, Berlin JS, Fishkind AB, Holloman GH, Zeller SL, Wilson MP, Rifai MA, Ng AT. Verbal de-escalation of the agitated patient: consensus statement of the American Association for Emergency Psychiatry Project BETA De-escalation Workgroup. West J Emerg Med. 2012;13(1):17–25.
31. Poole N. In: Greaves L, editor. Becoming trauma informed. Toronto, ON: Centre for Addiction and Mental Health; 2012.
32. Yeager K, Cutler D, Svendsen D, Sills GM, editors. Modern community mental health: an interdisciplinary approach. New York: Oxford University Press; 2013.

A Complex Case of Binge Eating Disorder (BED)

18

Kuppuswami Shivakumar, Shabbir Amanullah and Nicolas Rouleau

18.1 Case Example of Binge Eating Disorder (BED)

This is the case of a 35-year-old married female, mother of three school-going kids. She has been treated for depression for the last 5 years with poor response and weight gain. Over the last 2 years, she noticed increased levels of fatigue, poor concentration, and irritability, prompting her husband to request "a change in medication." Despite three different antidepressants, the patient continued to report fatigue and weight gain. When seen in clinic, she presented on her own with concerns about fatigue and her mood. Her low libido was contributing to some of their marital difficulties.

She is 5′3″, 230 lbs., yielding a body mass index of 39.5 (morbidly obese). Any discussions around her eating habits seem to trigger anger and a response

K. Shivakumar, MD, MPH, MRCPsych(UK), FRCPC (✉)
Associate Professor, Department of Psychiatry,
Northern Ontario School of Medicine (NOSM),
Sudbury, ON, Canada
e-mail: kshivakumar@hsnsudbury.ca

S. Amanullah, MD, DPM, FRCPsych(UK), CCT,FRCPC
Department of Psychiatry,
Woodstock General Hospital, Woodstock, ON, Canada
e-mail: samanullah@wgh.on.ca

N. Rouleau, PhD
Department of Biomedical Engineering, Initiative for Neural Science, Disease and Engineering (INScide) at Tufts University, Science and Engineering Complex (SEC), 200 College Ave., Medford, MA 02155, Canada
e-mail: nicolas.rouleau@tufts.edu

"I'm doing my best." On careful probing, she finally admitted to eating fairly large quantities of food that included three bags of chips, a number of candy bars, a tub of ice cream, and a large amount of popcorn with two cans of pop. She claims that she finds it hard to stop and feels intensely guilty about this behavior and has tried to stop many times only to succumb to temptation. She tends to eat in the above manner at least three times per week when the children have gone to school and her husband is out at work, as she has no control during the episode. She eats until she is uncomfortably full and states clearly that she is not eating because she is hungry. She strongly denies any purging behavior, excessive exercising, or any restrictive or compensatory behaviors.

She also goes on to talk about her poor educational performance and difficulty with teachers in school because she did not like to be told what to do. Although she had friends, they were few and far between. She grew up in a critical environment with little emotional support. There was also some remote history of sexual abuse by a cousin when she was growing up.

18.2 Epidemiology

The prevalence of BED in the USA varies from 1.6% to 0.8% based on gender, with females having 1.6% prevalence over a 12-month period. Prevalence rates across racial and ethnic groups seem to be similar. Lifetime prevalence is 3.5%

for females and 2.0% for males in the general population, making it the most common eating disorder [13]. For comparison, anorexia nervosa is associated with a lifetime prevalence of 0.9% in females and 0.3% in males. Similarly less prevalent, bulimia nervosa is associated with rates of 1.5% in females and 0.5% in males. BED is associated with a late mean age of onset (25.4 years) relative to bulimia nervosa (19.7 years) and anorexia nervosa (18.9 years). This condition is considered to have significant morbidity including impaired health-related quality of life, increased medical morbidity and mortality, higher risk of weight gain, and potential obesity. Early intervention is key in achieving full recovery, and various treatment approaches are used lately. The onset of BED is associated with a late mean age of onset (25.4 years) compared with bulimia nervosa (19.7 years) and anorexia nervosa (18.9 years). Although BED can be associated with increased weight, it can occur in normal weight or obese adults [9]. Compared to individuals who are not obese and who report no binge eating, individuals affected with BED can experience impairments with work productivity [21]. It is also known that daily stressful life events, such as death of spouse or close family member, divorce, separation, prolonged illness, or job loss, can contribute to the development of BED. A study by Wolff et al. [22] suggests that stress and negative mood (depression, anger, excessive guilt, self-blame) are likely antecedents to binge eating disorder.

18.3 Etiology

Etiology of binge eating disorder is complex and multifactorial. Twin studies have suggested that genetic factors are responsible for 40–60% of liability for binge eating disorder. Neurochemical studies have shown that the reward mechanism has been implicated in the development of the disorder, including activation of opiate or cannabinoid receptors. Other stresses such as physical, emotional, and sexual abuse, significant early trauma, life events, and daily stresses have been strongly implicated with the development of BED. It is also important to understand the family environment;

the family's attitude to eating, weight, and shape; and the emotional support that they receive from the family which could be an important factor in the development of BED [8].

18.4 BED Is a Distinct Diagnosis Entity in the DSM-5

The term binge eating disorder was classified under the category of eating disorders not otherwise specified in DSM-IV, and recently in DSM-5 it was considered as a specific psychiatric disorder [12].

Summary of the current DSM-5 criteria for a diagnosis of BED:

- Recurrent episodes of binge eating behavior (eating in a discrete period and a sense of lack of control over eating).
- Binge eating episodes are usually associated with eating rapidly or eating until feeling uncontrollable or eating large amounts even when not hungry or eating alone or having emotional consequences after eating large amount of food.
- Significant distress after binge eating, which should occur frequently (once a week for 3 months) and not associated with any other inappropriate compensatory behaviors.
- Binge eating does not occur during the course of bulimia or anorexia nervosa.

Although current studies have shown an increased prevalence of BED, symptoms are underreported especially around mood and binging secondary to shame and denial. Multiple factors (Table 18.1) have been identified in underreporting of symptoms and a lower treatment rates.

Table 18.1 Possible reasons for low detection rates of BED

Patient related factors	Physician related factors
Feelings of shame and guilt	Poor knowledge of BED
Fear of accepting a diagnosis	Low comfort levels in asking appropriate questions to diagnose BED
Unawareness of a diagnosable disorder	Lack of familiarity in using appropriate screening tools
Stigma	Negative feelings toward a diagnosis of BED

Table 18.2 Comorbidities and prevalence in BED

Comorbidities	Prevalence
Specific phobia[1]	37%
Social phobia[1]	32%
Alcohol abuse or dependence[1]	21%
Unipolar major depression[1]	32%
Post-traumatic stress disorder[1]	26%
Any personality disorder[2]	29%
Avoidant personality disorder[2]	12%
Borderline personality disorder[2]	10%
Obsessive-compulsive personality disorder[2]	10%
Three or more conditions[3]	49%

[a]Kessler et al. [14]
[b]Friborg et al. [3]
[c]Hudson et al. [9]

18.4.1 Psychiatric Comorbidity in Binge Eating Disorder

Binge eating disorder (BED) is associated with significant comorbid psychiatric conditions including specific phobia, social phobia, unipolar major depression, post-traumatic stress disorder, and alcohol use or dependence. In general, according to a survey completed in the USA, 79% of BED population had a lifetime history of at least one other psychotic disorder, and 49% had a lifetime history of three or more comorbid disorders (Table 18.2).

18.4.1.1 Medical Comorbidity in Binge Eating Disorder

Medical comorbidities associated with BED (Fig. 18.1) which may be related to obesity include type 2 diabetes (mellitus), hypertension, sleep/pain conditions, and dyslipidemia, whereas those which present independent of obesity can include asthma, gastrointestinal symptoms, intracranial hypertension, polycystic ovarian syndrome, and menstrual dysfunction [15]. The history and physical examination should focus on medical comorbidities which are commonly observed in binge eating disorder.

18.5   Assessment

The assessment of binge eating disorder relies quite heavily on good rapport and a thorough history. Childhood experiences, trauma, genetic factors, and seeking weight-loss treatment have been linked to the above conditions and, hence, play a critical role in management. A variety of questionnaires have been used to assess binge eating including the 9-item Binge Scale, [16] the 16-item Binge Eating Scale (BES) [17], and the Eating Disorder Inventory – a 64-item multi-scale inventory [18]. SCOFF questionnaire (which is not a specific questionnaire to BED) has been shown to be an effective and quick screening tool that can be easily administered [20].

The 16-item Binge Eating Scale (BES) can be used to assess the presence of binge eating behaviors. The scale is not required for diagnosis but represents a useful screening tool. Scoring involves assigning a numerical value where scores <17 represent non-binging, 18–26 represent moderate binging, and >26 represent severe binging [17]. The 7-item BED screener is an easy tool which can be administered rapidly in outpatient settings (Fig. 18.2).

A thorough assessment will include a history of the patient's comorbidities with the view to predicting outcomes. Patients with BED who had a lifetime history of depression seemed less likely to receive full remission. Patients with poor self-esteem also fared worse with behavioral weight-loss treatment than interventions like cognitive behavioral therapy. Medical comorbidity is also an important area, but except for obesity, there is poor evidence base on specific medical conditions.

18.6   Treatment

Treatment options vary for binge eating disorder (BED), and include psychological, pharmacological [19], and dietary interventions. Psychological treatments include individual or group therapy, CBT, interpersonal therapy (IPT), dialectical behavior therapy (DBT) [24], behavioral weight-loss treatment (BWLT), guided self-help therapy (GSHT), and combination therapy (COMB) (Fig. 18.3). Close to a half of patients with BED do not seem to benefit from psychological and behavioral interventions, and hence pharmacotherapy with either behavioral or

Fig. 18.1 Visual representation of medical issues associated with BED

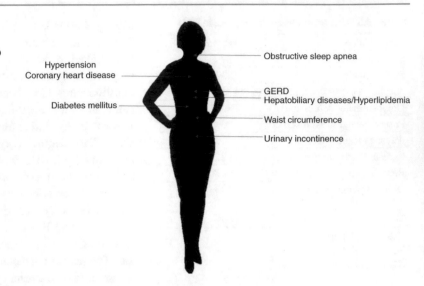

Hypertension
Coronary heart disease

Diabetes mellitus

Obstructive sleep apnea

GERD
Hepatobiliary diseases/Hyperlipidemia

Waist circumference

Urinary incontinence

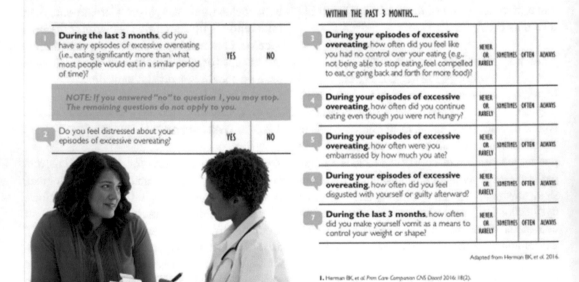

7-Item Binge-Eating Disorder Screener (BEDS-7)

These questions may help you identify adults with Binge Eating Disorder in your practice[1]

1 During the last 3 months, did you have any episodes of excessive overeating (i.e., eating significantly more than what most people would eat in a similar period of time)?	YES	NO

NOTE: If you answered "no" to question 1, you may stop. The remaining questions do not apply to you.

2 Do you feel distressed about your episodes of excessive overeating?	YES	NO

WITHIN THE PAST 3 MONTHS...

	NEVER OR RARELY	SOMETIMES	OFTEN	ALWAYS
3 During your episodes of excessive overeating, how often did you feel like you had no control over your eating (e.g., not being able to stop eating, feel compelled to eat, or going back and forth for more food)?				
4 During your episodes of excessive overeating, how often did you continue eating even though you were not hungry?				
5 During your episodes of excessive overeating, how often were you embarrassed by how much you ate?				
6 During your episodes of excessive overeating, how often did you feel disgusted with yourself or guilty afterward?				
7 During the last 3 months, how often did you make yourself vomit as a means to control your weight or shape?				

Adapted from Herman BK, et al. 2016.

1. Herman BK, et al. Prim Care Companion CNS Disord 2016; 18(2).

Fig. 18.2 BEDS-7 tool (Herman et al. [10]. Used with permission ©2014 Shire US Inc., Lexington, MA 02421)

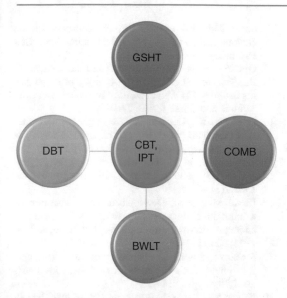

Fig. 18.3 Therapeutic options associated with BED. Cognitive behavioral therapy (CBT), interpersonal therapy (IPT), dialectical behavior therapy (DBT), behavioral weight-loss treatment (BWLT), guided self-help therapy (GSHT), and combination therapy (COMB)

Table 18.3 Drugs used to treat BED

Centrally acting sympathomimetics – Approved	Substance abuse treatment agents – Out of license
Lisdexamfetamine[a(starting at 30mg per day)] [a]Only one approved drug by the US Food and Drug Administration for the treatment of BED	Naltrexone Baclofen ALKS-33 Acamprosate
Antidepressants – Out of license	Anti-seizure medication – Out of license
SSRIs (e.g., Citalopram, Sertraline, Fluvoxamine) SNRIs (e.g., Venlafaxine, Duloxetine) NRIs (e.g., Reboxetine) NDRIs (e.g., Bupropion)	Topiramate Zonizamide Lamotrigine
Anti-obesity medication – Not licensed	
Orlistat Fenfluramine Sibutramine[a]	

Adapted from Goracci et al. [4] and Parker et al. [20]
[a]This medication is no longer used due to side effects such as headache, dry mouth, insomnia, constipation, dizziness, non-fatal myocardial infarction, and non-fatal stroke

psychological interventions may have better outcomes. However, a recent article shows that this clinical strategy has generally failed [5]. Only one study supported the benefits of combining the two. The addition of topiramate, however, has shown some promising results when added to CBT. CBT and IPT have the most evidence for effectiveness [1, 11].

Treatment should also focus on providing nutritional counseling, normalizing portion sizes/regularizing food intake [2], addressing eating behavior, and dealing with excessive concerns with body image. Psychiatric comorbid conditions should be treated with antidepressants, anticonvulsants, centrally acting sympathomimetics, and psychostimulants. IPT is an effective treatment for binge eating disorder (BED). A follow-up study performed by Wilson et al. [23] comparing IPT and CBT showed that both therapies were significantly more effective than behavioral weight-loss treatment in eliminating binge eating after 2 years [6]. In common clinical practice, the combination of pharmacological and psychological treatments such as CBT or behavioral weight loss are widely used which seems to be superior to medication management or psychological treatment alone [7].

Table 18.3 describes some commonly used medications in BED.

Response to treatment is found to in some cases predict eventual remission posttreatment. Some studies pointed out to a rapid response to treatment, and this seems to be a positive predictive factor. In patients receiving pharmacotherapy, the absence of a rapid response indicated no further improvement which should lead the clinician to consider alternative pharmacotherapy.

References

1. Ansell EB, Grilo CM, White MA. Examining the interpersonal model of binge eating and loss of control over eating in women. Int J Eat Disord. 2012;45(1):43–50.
2. Brownell KD. LEARN program for weight management 2000. American Health; 2000.
3. Friborg O, Martinussen M, Kaiser S, Øvergård KT, Martinsen EW, Schmierer P, Rosenvinge JH. Personality disorders in eating disorder not otherwise specified and binge eating disorder: a meta-analysis of comorbidity studies. J Nerv Ment Dis. 2014; 202(2):119–25.

4. Goracci A, di Volo S, Casamassima F, Bolognesi S, Benbow J, Fagiolini A. Pharmacotherapy of binge-eating disorder: a review. J Addict Med. 2015;9(1):1–19.
5. Grilo CM. Psychological and behavioural treatments for binge-eating disorder. J Clin Psychiatry. 2017; 78:20–4.
6. Grilo CM, Masheb RM, Wilson GT, Gueorguieva R, White MA. Cognitive–behavioral therapy, behavioral weight loss, and sequential treatment for obese patients with binge-eating disorder: a randomized controlled trial. J Consult Clin Psychol. 2011;79(5):675.
7. Grilo CM, Reas DL, Mitchell JE. Combining pharmacological and psychological treatments for binge eating disorder: current status, limitations, and future directions. Curr Psychiatry Rep. 2016;18(6):55.
8. Grilo CM, White MA, Gueorguieva R, Wilson GT, Masheb RM. Predictive significance of the overvaluation of shape/weight in obese patients with binge eating disorder: findings from a randomized controlled trial with 12-month follow-up. Psychol Med. 2013;43(6):1335–44.
9. Hudson JI, Hiripi E, Pope HG, Kessler RC. The prevalence and correlates of eating disorders in the National Comorbidity Survey Replication. Biol Psychiatry. 2007;61(3):348–58.
10. Herman BK, et al. The primary care companion for CNS Disorders. J Clin Psychiatry. 2016;18(2):82–8.
11. Iacovino JM, Gredysa DM, Altman M, Wilfley DE. Psychological treatments for binge eating disorder. Curr Psychiatry Rep. 2012;14(4):432–46.
12. DSM 5 American Psychiatric Association. Diagnostic and statistical manual of mental disorders. 5th ed. Arlington, VA: American Psychiatric Association; 2013.
13. Hudson. The prevalence and correlates of eating disorders in the National Comorbidity Survey Replication (vol 61, pg 348, 2007). Biol Psychiatry. 2012;72(2):164.
14. Kessler RC, Berglund P, Demler O, Jin R, Merikangas KR, Walters EE. Lifetime prevalence and age-of-onset distributions of DSM-IV disorders in the National Comorbidity Survey Replication. Arch Gen Psychiatry. 2005;62(6):593–602.
15. Olguin P, Fuentes M, Gabler G, Guerdjikova AI, Keck PE, McElroy SL. Medical comorbidity of binge eating disorder. Eat Weight Disord-Studies on Anorexia, Bulimia and Obesity. 2016;22:1–14.
16. Hawkins RC, Clement PF. Development and construct validation of a self-report measure of binge eating tendencies. Addict Behav. 1980;5(3):219–26.
17. Gormally J, et al. The assessment of binge eating severity among obese persons. Addict Behav. 1982;7(1):47–55.
18. David MG, et al, Development amd validation of a multidimensional eating disorders inventoryfor anorexia nervosa and bulimia. Eating disorders. 1983;2(2):15–34.
19. McElroy Susan L. Pharmacological treatments for binge eating disorder. J Clin Psychiatry. 2017;78(Suppl 1):14–9.
20. Parker SC, Lyons J, Bonner J. Eating disorders in graduate students: exploring the SCOFF questionnaire as a simple screening tool. J Am Coll Heal. 2005;54(2):103–7.
21. Striegel RH, Bedrosian R, Wang C, Schwartz S.Why men should be included in research on binge eating: results from a comparison of psychosocial impairment in men and women. Int J Eat Disord. 2012;45(2):233–40. doi: 10.1002/eat.20962. Epub 2011 Oct 26.
22. Gretchen E., Wolff, Ross D. Crosby, Jennifer A. Roberts, David A. Wittrock Differences in daily stress, mood, coping, and eating behavior in binge eating and non binge eating college women, 2000;25(2):205–16.
23. Wilson GT, Wilfley DE, Agras WS, Bryson SW. Psychological treatments of binge eating disorder. Arch Gen Psychiatry. 2010;67(1):94–101.
24. Wiser S, Telch CF. Dialectical behavior therapy for binge-eating disorder. J Clin Psychol. 1999;55(6): 755–68.

A Complex Case of 'Speaking in Tongues'

19

Oyedeji Ayonrinde
and Sanjeevan Somasunderam

19.1 Case Presentation: Part I

A 23-year-old man of West African heritage is brought to the emergency room by the police following concerns raised by members of the public at a train station. He had been observed outside the station, pacing up and down, waving his arms in gesticulation, speaking in a loud tone, and intermittently shouting incoherently while shaking his head. His mood was elated and he said he had the gift of 'speaking in tongues'. Alarm was raised when he held onto strangers insisting that they listen to him as he felt they were possessed by the devil. He demanded they showed repentance for their sins in prayer or deed. During the police safety search, a packet of cannabis seeds, pieces of paper and a bible were found in his pocket.

While in the emergency room, he insisted he was the 'Son of God' and that no one should speak to him. He was observed looking around as if perplexed and muttering incoherently. As he was approached by clinical staff, he shouted 'back off you sinners!'

O. Ayonrinde, FRCPsych, MBA (✉)
Queen's University, Kingston, ON, Canada

Kingston Health Sciences Centre,
Hotel Dieu Hospital, Kingston, ON, Canada
e-mail: oyedeji.ayonrinde@queensu.ca

S. Somasunderam, MBBS, MRCPsych
Maudsley Hospital, Denmark Hill, London, AZ, UK
e-mail: sanj34@me.com

19.2 Questions

1. What differential diagnoses would you consider at this stage?
2. What features of the presentation would support or refute each differential diagnosis?
   (Discussion on differentials below)
3. How would you establish rapport with this man during this state of agitation?
4. What would be the most appropriate initial investigations at this stage?

19.3 Case Presentation: Part II

The man's parents attend the emergency room relieved to have located him and expressed concern about his wellbeing. They are seen separately in a quiet room and you ascertain the following:

His father is a faith leader in a West African Pentecostal church. The family migrated from West Africa about 5 years ago. They felt integrated into the new society and belong to a large supportive faith group network. He reported that his son was an outstanding postgraduate university student and an emerging church leader. He was proud of his son's faith outreach and leadership of an antidrug campaign. Over the past two nights, while preparing for exams, their son had been overheard praying loudly and continuously in his room until the early hours of the morning.

This was unlike him. Devoted members of the congregation were said to be blessed with the ability to 'speak in tongues', while senior clergy were also able to 'see visions' and carry out 'divine healing'.

His mother had additional concerns when he informed her he was receiving spiritual messages from the microwave when turned on, which she found quite odd.

Although they referred to him as their son, he had been adopted in infancy and had only realised this a few weeks ago. His biological mother had been a member of the congregation and died during his birth. Little was known of his estranged biological father, other than that he had died of a sleep medication and pain medication overdose 10 years ago. Their son never knew either of his biological parents.

In the emergency room, both parents expressed the belief that the current presentation was a 'spiritual and demonic attack' on their son.

19.4   The Relationships Between Spirituality and Mental Health

19.4.1 Religion and Spirituality in Psychiatric Diagnosis

Religion and spirituality are addressed in the American Psychiatric Association's handbook of diagnostic classification (DSM-5*) [1] in the chapter on 'Other Conditions That May Be a Focus of Clinical Attention'. These conditions, which are not mental disorders, may affect the diagnosis, course, prognosis or treatment of a patient's mental disorder and as such deserve attention in the course of treatment (see Tables 19.1 and 19.2). From *DSM-5: Religious or Spiritual Problem This category can be used when the focus of clinical attention is a religious or spiritual problem. Examples include distressing experiences that involve loss or questioning of faith, problems associated with conversion to a new faith, or questioning of spiritual values that may not necessarily be related to an organized church or religious* institution. *Diagnostic and Statistical Manual of Mental Disorders, Fifth Edition* [1].

Table 19.1 Relationship between culture, faith and health

Relationship between culture, faith and health
Distinguishing between 'normality' and 'abnormality'
Aetiological influence on some disorders
Influencing clinical presentation
Influencing interpretation of behaviours
Influencing rates and distribution of illness
Determining the recognition of disorders
Generating labels for disorders
Explanatory models of disorders
Determining treatment options
Determining care pathways
Influencing the outcome of treatment interventions

Table 19.2 Brief assessment of spirituality and faith issues

Assessment and therapeutic awareness of faith issues (reference)
Are religious or spiritual beliefs an important part of your life?
How do these beliefs influence the way you take care of yourself?
Do you rely on your faith beliefs to help you cope with health problems?
Do you belong to a faith community?
Are there specific faith issues that need addressing?
Who would you like to address these issues?
How would you like the issues addressed by others?

19.4.2 A Role for Spirituality

Some studies show that people involved in a religious, faith or spiritual group may have a lower risk of premature death or illness than those not involved. The reasons for this apparent benefit are not well understood. But the fellowship, goodwill and emotional support offered by religious or spiritual groups may also promote healthy living and mental health. Some faith communities offer pastoral counselling services, which can be an additional support to therapy and/or medication and may help people cope with mental health challenges (Mental Health: a guide for faith leaders, APA 2016).

19.4.3 The Cultural Formulation Interview (CFI), DSM-5 [1]

The core features of the Cultural Formulation Interview are as follows:

1. Cultural definition of the problem
2. Cultural perception of the cause
3. Cultural perception of the context
4. Cultural perception of support

19.4.4 Cultural Formulation Interview (CFI), Adapted from DSM-5 [1]

Guide to interview	Questions
The following questions aim to clarify key aspects of the presenting clinical problem from the point of view of the individual and other members of the individual's social network (i.e. family, friends or others involved in the current problem). This includes the problem's meaning, potential sources of help and expectations for services	*Introduction* I would like to understand the problems that bring you here so that I can help you more effectively. I want to know about *your* experience and ideas. I will ask some questions about what is going on and how you are dealing with it. Please remember there are no right or wrong answers
Cultural definition of the problem (Explanatory model, level of functioning)	
Elicit the individual's view of core problems and key concerns *Focus on the individual's own way of understanding the problem* *Use the term, expression or brief description elicited to identify the problem in subsequent questions (e.g. 'your conflict with your son')*	1. What brings you here today? People often understand their problems in their own way, which may be similar to or different from how doctors describe the problem. How would *you* describe your problem?
Ask how the individual frames the problem for members of the social network	2. Sometimes people have different ways of describing their problem to their family, friends or others in their community. How would you describe your problem to them?
Focus on the aspects of the problem that matter most to the individual	3. What troubles you most about your problem?

Guide to interview	Questions
Cultural perceptions of cause, context and support	
Causes (Explanatory model, social network, older adults)	
This question indicates the meaning of the condition for the individual, which may be relevant for clinical care	4. Why do you think this is happening to you? What do you think are the causes of your [*problem*]?
Note that individuals may identify multiple causes, depending on the facet of the problem they are considering	Prompt further if: Some people may explain their problem as the result of bad things that happen in their life, problems with others, a physical illness, a spiritual reason or many other causes
Focus on the views of members of the individual's social network. These may be diverse and vary from the individual's	5. What do others in your family, your friends or others in your community think is causing your [*problem*]?

19.4.5 The Traditional Psychiatric Formulation Versus the Cultural Formulation

There are a number of differences between the traditionally used psychiatric formulation and the Cultural Formulation (see Table 19. 3 below)

Table 19.3 Key components of the Psychiatric Formulation and Cultural Formulation

Traditional psychiatric formulation	Cultural formulation
Predisposing factors	Cultural definition of the problem
Precipitating factors	Cultural perception of the cause
Presenting factors	Cultural perception of the context
Perpetuating factors	Cultural perception of support
Protective factors	

19.5 Case Presentation: Part III

19.5.1 Further Information

A urine drug screen was negative for any psychoactive substances, and the breath alcohol reading was zero. This was consistent with both patient and family emphasis that he neither used alcohol nor drugs. It transpired that a member of the public had handed over the cannabis seeds to him in response to his demands to repent and change his ways.

The man's father reported that he had a similar though less severe episode, around 3 years ago while studying for his undergraduate university exams. The family felt his behaviour at the time was related to a desire to succeed and poor sleep during exam preparation. They had not brought it to the attention of health services.

19.6   Questions

1. Do you think this is a culture-specific mental disorder, cultural concept of distress or culture-bound syndrome?
2. If so what disorder or syndrome?
3. What are the contemporary distinctions between culture-bound syndromes and cultural concepts of distress?

In the DSM-IV-TR (2000) [2], the term culture-bound syndrome 'denotes recurrent, locality-specific patterns of aberrant behaviour and troubling experience that may or may not be linked to a particular DSM-IV diagnostic category'.

Characteristics of Culture-Bound Syndromes

(a) Indigenously   considered   illness   or afflictions
(b) Local names – often in the indigenous language and may be part of folk diagnostic categories
(c) Symptoms, course and social response often influenced by local cultural factors
(d) Limited to specific societies or cultural areas
(e) Localised – therefore experiences that are not globally recognised

In the *DSM-5 (2013)* [1], the concept of culture-bound syndromes was discarded with a preference for the term *cultural concepts of distress* defined as 'ways cultural groups experience, understand, and communicate suffering, behavioural problems, or troubling thoughts and emotions'.

The three cultural concepts of distress are:

Syndromes – clusters of symptoms and attributions occurring among individuals in specific cultures
Idioms of distress – shared ways of communicating, expressing or sharing distress
Explanations – labels and attributions suggesting causation of symptoms or distress

The DSM-5 contends that the terminology culture-bound syndromes insufficiently appreciates the influence of culture on the range of expression of distress, stressing all mental distress is culturally framed, and different populations have culturally determined ways of communicating their distress, explanations of causality, coping and help-seeking behaviour.

Both the World Health Organisation [3] and American Psychiatric Association diagnostic classificatory systems continue to incorporate social, cultural and anthropological research findings in the understanding of mental distress in different populations.

19.6.1 Culture-Bound Syndrome: Brain Fag Syndrome

In 1960 Raymond Prince a Canadian psychiatrist working in Nigeria described a cluster of symptoms among students, associated with intensive study and examinations. Their reference to mental exhaustion ('brain fag') led to him terming the symptom cluster - 'brain fag syndrome' [4].

Distinctive symptoms of the syndrome were described as:

• Intellectual impairment
• Sensory impairment (chiefly visual)
• Somatic complaints, most commonly of pain or burning in the head and neck
• Other complaints affecting the student's ability to study
• An unhappy, tense facial expression
• A characteristic gesture of passing the hand over the surface of the scalp or rubbing the vertex of the skull

This clinical presentation of distress was initially felt to be a culture-bound syndrome localised to southern Nigeria. However, subsequent reports in other African regions have brought this into question. There has been considerable debate as to whether this actually constitutes a unique nosological entity, cultural expression or mixed presentation of mental disorders with local idioms of distress [4].

It may be attractive to consider the case above as a West African cultural presentation of affective, psychotic and anxiety disorders. After all, the man is a student of West African heritage presenting with emotional distress while preparing for exams. However, such a consideration would be simplistic and ignores the presentation and phenomena.

19.7   Learning Points

1. *Psychoactive substance issues:* where possible, objective testing or clinical evidence of substance use should be made before making a definitive diagnosis. In this case the presence of cannabis seeds did not indicate use.
2. *Spirituality and mental health:* in the Pentecostal Christian faith, speaking in tongues is part of the spiritual experience and generally acceptable. Collateral information and faith considerations are relevant to diagnostic clarification (see Table 19.4).
3. *Cultural concepts of distress:* unfamiliar disturbing experiences in this West African student preparing for examinations is not a 'culture-bound' brain fag syndrome.

It is important to objectively verify the use of psychoactive substances where possible. While tempting to assume the cannabis seeds found on the patient were for his consumption, they had actually been handed over to him by a stranger during his crusade outside the station. The patient did not drink alcohol and had never used a psychoactive substance before.

Speaking in tongues is not uncommon in a number of Christian Pentecostal faith groups and actually an encouraged practice during prayers. While the unfamiliar phenomena may be considered as *glossolalia* or *neologisms* with different associations, within the faith subculture, this is normal.

There may be additional clinical challenges if the patient also speaks an unfamiliar language or with a different accent.

19.8   Outpatient Clinic Review 2 Weeks Later

The patient presents low in mood with reduced eye contact, psychomotor retardation and anxious. He said he recently found out that his biological father had been a violent man and drank heavily. He died following an alcohol, sleep medication and pain tablet overdose.

The man is worried about the risk of being like his biological father and asks for advice to reduce risk and promote his positive mental wellbeing.

19.8.1 Question

1. What advice would you give him?

Suggestions for Advice

1. Exploratory discussion about his concerns and perceptions
2. To consider alternate explanatory models for his distress
3. Sleep hygiene advice – particularly at certain times of heightened stress (i.e. exams)
4. Consider the potential for future dependence on opioid analgesics due to family hisvtory
5. To explore the idea of accessing psychological therapies (such as cognitive behaviour therapy)
6. Involvement of the family in discussions with patients consent – family work

---

Table 19.4 Relationship between faith and mental wellbeing

Some reported benefits of faith to mental wellbeing
Wellbeing, happiness and life satisfaction
Hope and optimism
Purpose and meaning to life
Self-esteem
Social support and less loneliness
Lower levels of depression, anxiety
Lower levels of substance misuse
Greater relationship stability
Adjustment to loss and bereavement

Adapted from Royal College of Psychiatrists – Spirituality and Mental Wellbeing

Conclusion

This conundrum involves a 23-year-old man of West African heritage who came to the attention of mental health services following a behavioural disturbance in a public place. He was brought to the emergency room by the police for a psychiatric assessment. He had no previous contact with mental health services. Presentation was characterised by an elated mood, and he was perceived to make expansive comments of a religious nature. In addition, cannabis seeds were found in his pocket. Investigations did not identify an organic cause. The potential predisposing factors were initially unknown; however it subsequently came to attention that he was adopted in infancy and previously had a similar episode in the context of studying for another exam. In addition, he was going through some acculturisation to the new country. A recent systematic review and meta-analysis (Mindlis and Boffetta, 2017) [5] observed a relative risk of 1.25 and 1.16 of mood disorders among first- and second-generation immigrants, respectively. Men were found to be at higher risk. The precipitating factors include sleep deprivation in the context of exam preparation against a backdrop of being told he was an adopted child. Initially, the question of whether cannabis use was related to his presentation was raised; however, it was realised that in fact he did not use cannabis, was a staunch leader of the antidrug campaign in his local church community and also had negative urine drug screens. The perpetuating factors appear to be unresolved issues regarding his identity and his attempts to cope with this. The potential protective factors include his close supportive family and faith group. The young man also had positive health attitudes regarding reducing the risk of harm from psychoactive substance misuse.

It is important to be mindful that predisposing, precipitating, perpetuating and protective factors are dynamic in nature and may change. This case highlights a number of complex issues further conceptualised through the use of a cultural formulation and the inherent risk of early assumptions when faced with unfamiliar clinical presentations. With a sensitive and considered use of formulations, a clearer understanding of this man's distress became apparent while sustaining an important therapeutic relationship.

Disclosure Statement "The authors have nothing to disclose."

References

1. Diagnostic and Statistical Manual of the American Psychiatric Association (Fifth edition) DSM 5 (2013).
2. Diagnostic and Statistical Manual of the American Psychiatric Association (Fourth edition) DSM IV -TR (2000).
3. International Classification of Diseases Tenth Edition (ICD 10) – World Health Organisation (WHO) (1992).
4. Ayonrinde OA, Obuaya C, Adeyemi SO. Brain fag syndrome: a culture-bound syndrome that may be approaching extinction. Br J Psychiatry Bull. 2015; 39(4):156–61.
5. Mindlis I, Boffetta P. Mood disorders in first-and second-generation immigrants: systematic review and meta-analysis. Br J Psychiatry. 2017;210:182–9.

Other Useful Resources

https://www.psychiatry.org/File%20Library/Psychiatrists/Cultural-Competency/faith-mentalhealth-guide.pdf. (American Psychiatrists Association advice for faith healers).

Mental Health: A Guide for Faith Leaders: American Psychiatric Association Foundation and the Mental Health and Faith Community Partnership Steering Committee, 2016 American Psychiatric Association Foundation.

http://www.rcpsych.ac.uk/healthadvice/treatmentswellbeing/spirituality.aspx.

Complex Cases of Social Anxiety Disorder (SAD)

20

Akiko Kawaguchi and Norio Watanabe

20.1 A Complicated Case of Social Anxiety Disorder

A 25-year-old man

Although nothing particular in mental state was pointed out at early childhood examinations, after starting his elementary school, he was often teased or left out by his classmates.

In his adolescence, some symptoms started to appear. He was concerned about blushing, and he felt that his voice and hands trembled while speaking in front of the classmates. He also felt his hands shaking while having a meal with others, so he started avoiding having meals with peers. Despite these concerns, he still had a few friends he could get along with through his hobbies such as playing video games.

He did not particularly have a problem in his academic performance and went to university to study engineering. There, he was interested in research and continued his study up to a postgraduate master's course.

He thought of continuing his study to a doctoral course. However, since his parents recommended that he should work after graduation, he started job hunting. He felt nervous and often could not talk well at job interviews. It was a struggle until he got a job offer. Eventually, he joined a major manufacturing company as a technical engineer.

After his job training was over and he actually started his work, he began to feel strongly nervous and distressed in speaking at the morning group meeting or communicating with his boss and colleagues. Moreover, his self-esteem decreased since his boss pointed out that he was slow in learning his job in comparison with his colleagues. Gradually, he started feeling reluctant to go to work. He felt strong fatigue after going back home and could not even play his favorite games on holidays. His appetite and weight reduced. He started having trouble falling asleep, and even when he managed to fall asleep, he woke up in the middle of night thinking about his work.

20.2 What Is Social Anxiety Disorder (SAD)?

Social anxiety disorder (SAD) is characterized by the excessive fear and avoidance for several social situations, according to Diagnostic and Statistical Manual-5 (DSM-5).

Clark and Wells suggested the psychological model of SAD [1]. In this model, patients with

A. Kawaguchi, MD, PhD (✉)
Department of Psychiatry and Cognitive-Behavioral Medicine, Nagoya City University Graduate School of Medical Sciences, Nagoya, Japan

N. Watanabe, MD, PhD
Department of Health Promotion and Human Behavior, Department of Clinical Epidemiology, Graduate School of Public Health, Kyoto University, Kyoto, Japan

© Springer International Publishing AG, part of Springer Nature 2018
K. Shivakumar, S. Amanullah (eds.), *Complex Clinical Conundrums in Psychiatry*,
https://doi.org/10.1007/978-3-319-70311-4_20

SAD quite often ruminate on themselves with negative cognition when they are exposed to social situations where they feel fear. They nearly always expect negative evaluation by others in such situations, too. Their attention tends to be self-focusing, and they easily lose chances to observe responses from others. They use several types of "safety behaviors" (e.g., a patient wears heavy makeup because he/she fears blush) so that they decrease their embarrassment although those efforts often end up with enhancing their self-focusing attention and making their symptom worse. Furthermore, misinterpretation of internal information (e.g., heartbeat, shake) is another aspect of SAD. Cognitive behavioral therapy (CBT) which is the most effective psychotherapy for SAD [2] has been conducted based on this model.

Its lifetime and 12-month prevalence is estimated at 13.0 and 7.4% [3], although the prevalence rates vary by country or culture [4]. SAD is the fourth most frequent psychiatric disorder [5]. SAD usually develops from adolescence and often persists unless it is treated [6]. Because of its chronicity, it contributes serious social dysfunction such as unemployment or the loss of the marriage opportunity [7, 8].

Not only psychological studies but also a large number of biological studies have been conducted on SAD. Among those studies, genetical studies and neurobiological studies have the majority.

Genetical studies have accumulated possibly responsible genes. However, among psychiatric disorders, genetical studies usually focus on "endophenotypes" which mediate gene and disease [9]. As endophenotypes, neurobiological studies are gathering attention. There have been functional magnetic resonance imaging (fMRI) studies and structural MRI studies. Most of the fMRI studies of SAD have focused on the limbic (hippocampal/amygdala) hyperactivity with unpleasant (angry or disgust) facial expressions [10, 11]. Those areas have been also highlighted by the volumetric studies [12–14]. Similar to other anxiety disorders [15, 16], it has been reported that hippocampal/amygdala volume was reduced in patients with SAD. Although it was a small sample study, we also reported insula volume reduction [17]. Hyperactivity and volume reduction is also mentioned in insula. Insula hyperactivity causes altered interoception in patients with SAD.

Furthermore, SAD has been known as a psychiatric disease with a high probability of other comorbid psychiatric problems. In this chapter, we focused on SAD as complex cases of anxiety disorder.

20.2.1 Psychiatric Assessments

Several tools are used for psychiatric assessment of SAD. Liebowitz Social Anxiety Scale (LSAS) [18] is the most popular one which estimates the social anxiety with 24 performance or social interaction situations. Each situation is separately scored for both fear (0–3 indicate none, mild, moderate, and severe, respectively) and avoidance (0–3 indicate never, occasionally, often, and usually, respectively). LSAS was originally developed as a rater-administered assessment tool; however, self-reported version has also been developed and validated. Apart from LSAS, Social Interaction Anxiety Scale/Social Phobia Scale (SIAS/SPS) [19] is also used for measurements of social anxiety. The SPS provides the fear of being observed, whereas the SIAS measures fear of social interaction. Both SPS and SIAS are 20-item self-report questionnaires with ratings on a 4-point scale from 0 (not at all characteristic or true of me) to 4 (extremely characteristic or true of me). Otherwise, the Fear of Negative Evaluation (FNE) Scale or its brief version, the Brief version of the Fear of Negative Evaluation Scale (BFNE), can be used for assessment of SAD symptoms.

20.2.2 Treatment

Some patients cannot reach treatment or go treatment after long time of nontreatment [20, 21] because they believe that their concern is just within their characters. Once they can access psychiatric medical care, selective serotonin reuptake inhibitors (SSRI) or CBT has been frequently used for SAD. More recently, Mayo-Wilson et al. conducted network meta-analysis which included both psychological and pharmacological interventions for SAD [2]. According to this study, interventions which showed high effect sizes compared with waitlist were mono-amine oxidase inhibitors(SMD −1.01, 95% credible interval (CI) −1.56 to −0.45), benzo-diazepines (−0.96, −1.56 to −0.36), SSRIs and serotonin-norepinephrine reuptake inhibitors (SNRIs) (−0.91, −1.23 to −0.60), individual CBT (−1.19, −1.56 to −0.81), and group CBT (−0.92, −1.33 to−0.51).

In the aspect of pharmacotherapy for SAD, there have been a number of randomized control trials [22–25] and some meta-analytic studies. For example, Blanco et al. conducted a meta-analysis of pharmacotherapy for SAD [26]. Although they reported that some medications such as phenelzine, clonazepam, and gabapentin have showed larger effect sizes rather than SSRIs, they recommended SSRIs as the first-line treatment in regard to the safety, tolerability, and comorbid condition. On the other hand, in the previously mentioned network meta-analysis, the efficacy of benzodiazepines was also superior to that of SSRIs and SNRIs. However, the number of the included participants is further limited in ben-zodiazepines, and in case of SAD, benzodi-azepine use should be cautious because of its dependency or tolerance. Considering the high rate of depression comorbidity [27], SSRIs may be a good treatment choice except for those with bipolar depression (i.e., concerns for manic switch) or for children or adolescent cases (i.e., agitation or suicidal side effects) [28]. Psychotherapy might be better than phar-macotherapy in those cases.

Similar to pharmacotherapy, positive effects of CBT have been repeatedly reported [2, 29].

The following is a brief introduction of CBT program for SAD of the authors [30]. We have developed our manual based on the one written by Andrews et al. [31] and then modified the pro-gram according to Clark and Wells' model [1]. A group is composed by three patients with one principal therapist and one co-therapist. One ses-sion lasts for 120 min once a week, and the total number of the session is 12–16 depending on patients' needs. We also assign homework every session.

Session 1	Psychoeducation about SAD
Session 2	Introduction about the individual cognitive behavioral model of SAD
Session 3	Cognitive restructuring
Session 4–5	Attention training to shift focus away from themselves to the task or the external social situation
Session 6–7	Video feedback of role-playing in anxious situations to modify their self-image
Session 8 to last	Experiments to drop safety behavior and self-focused attention In vivo exposure using behavioral experiments to test the patient's catastrophic predictions Cognitive restructuring

Our single-arm, naturalistic, follow-up study included 113 patients with SAD (of those, 70 patients finished 1-year follow-up). The effect sizes of SPS/SIAS at the posttreatment were 0.64 (95% confidence interval 0.37–0.90)/0.76 (0.49–1.03), in the intention-to-treat group and 0.81 (0.46 1.15)/0.76 (0.49–1.10) in completers, respectively. The effect sizes of SPS/SIAS at the 1-year follow-up were 0.68 (0.41–0.95)/0.76 (0.49–1.03) in the intention-to-treat group and 0.77 (0.42–1.10)/0.84 (0.49–1.18) in completers. Older age at baseline, late onset, and lower sever-ity of SAD were predictors for a good outcome [30]. From what is known to date, individual CBT was superior to group 1 [2], but we con-ducted group CBT because of its cost-effectiveness [32].

Network meta-analysis of Mayo-Wilson et al. [2] also revealed that combined treatment (phar-macotherapy and psychological therapy) was superior to either approach alone. Actually, in the clinical practice, combined treatment can be helpful. For example, at our clinic, patients with severe symptom might be able to join group CBT sessions under the medication.

As mentioned regarding the pharmacotherapy, concurrent psychiatric problems make treatment of SAD complicating. Patients with SAD often suffer from comorbid depression, other anxiety disorders, and substance dependence disorders [27] which lead to social dysfunction. More recently SAD is paid attention to as the major comorbid psychiatric problems of neurodevelopmental disorders such as autism spectrum disorder (ASD) or attention deficit hyperactivity disorder (ADHD) even in adult cases. In this chapter, we focused on those comorbidities as complex cases of SAD, and we also introduced a tip for psychological treatment for taijin-kyofu-sho syndrome (TKS) which has been known as a cultural variation of SAD.

20.3 SAD with Autism Spectrum Disorder (ASD)

Autism spectrum disorder (ASD) is characterized by the persistent deficits in social communication and social interaction (DSM-5). Patients with ASD are at increased risk of anxiety disorders. Among those anxiety disorders, SAD is no exception. Especially for patients with high-functioning ASD, their comorbidity rate of SAD is estimated at 21–57% [33–36]. Comorbid SAD with ASD makes their social adaptation difficult [37]. They sometimes also accompany social skill deficits [38]. Some previous studies have reported that SAD with ASD tends to occur later than pure SAD [36] because SAD with ASD develops as a result of repeated failure communication. In those cases, some studies have showed that the level of social anxiety was milder than that of pure SAD, and the others have showed that there was no difference. [36, 39].

20.3.1 Psychiatric Assessments

Because there are some symptom overlaps (e.g., avoidance of social situation, hypersensitivity for internal sense) between ASD and SAD, the diagnosis of ASD tends to be delayed under the preceding SAD diagnosis [36].

It is very difficult to detect ASD with comorbid SAD during the clinical course. In case it is suspected, several tools for ASD such as Autism Diagnostic Observation Schedule (ADOS) [40] and Autism Diagnostic Interview-Revised (ADI-R) [41] are used for diagnosis. Furthermore, as a screening tool for ASD, Autism-Spectrum Quotient (AQ) [42] is broadly used in general psychiatric clinical practice. However, in patients referred to a specialist clinic for suspected ASD, sensitivity and specificity of AQ to detect clinical diagnosis of ASD among those with SAD were calculated at 0.81 and 0.25, respectively [43]. Positive and negative predictive values were calculated at 76% and 31%, respectively [44]. Thus, the AQ may not be able to adequately find those with clinically diagnosed ASD among SAD patients. Eriksson et al. argued that two questions were useful to discriminate ASD from SAD: 1) "It is very difficult for me to work and function in groups" and 2) "How to make friends and socialize is a mystery to me," both of which were derived from the brief version of Ritvo Autism and Asperger Diagnostic Scale-Revised (RAADS-R) [45]. Apart from this, Kreiser et al. have developed an assessment tool which is named Social Anxiety Scale for People with ASD (SASPA) [46, 47]. Those attempts are still in the process of research. An effective way to diagnose SAD with comorbid ASD or discriminate SAD and ASD is expected in the future study.

20.3.2 Treatment

For patients with SAD and comorbid ASD, typical CBT for SAD might be insufficient. Some attempts using modified manual of CBT have been conducted for children or adolescent cases [48–50]. Such modified manual included additional treatment components such as the use of visual aids, parents' education, and group social skill training. Although modified CBT program for adult with both SAD and ASD is still developing, small group style or social skill training might be helpful for adult cases [51].

20.4 SAD with Comorbid Attention Deficit Hyperactivity Disorder (ADHD)

Attention deficit hyperactivity disorder (ADHD) is one of the most prevalent neuropsychiatric disorders in childhood. These days, ADHD is known to be highly likely to persist until adulthood. ADHD is defined by the inattention, hyperactivity, and impulsivity. Patients with ADHD have much difficulty in school, work, and their personal life, so that it has a significant impact on the quality of life of sufferers.

The prevalence rate of adult ADHD is estimated at 4.4% [52]. Among those patients, comorbid anxiety disorder is common. Especially, SAD is the most prevalent anxiety disorder in ADHD. Its 12-month prevalence rate is nearly 30%. Moreover, 14% of patients with SAD are suffering from ADHD [52]. According to Koyuncu et al. [53], SAD coexistence with ADHD was more frequent in inattentive type of ADHD. Children with inattentive type ADHD have difficulty in participating social interaction due to their shyness. Those tendencies lead to late social anxiety. Even grown-ups with combined type ADHD (both of inattentive and hyperactivity/impulsivity symptom) feel anxiety as a result of gradually reducing hyperactivity symptom. Inattentive symptom seems to contribute SAD in ADHD.

> Koyuncu et al. also reported that, among patients with SAD and comorbid ADHD, SAD symptoms were more severe, and depression symptoms were more frequently observed than those with SAD alone. They also mentioned high probability of bipolar depression among patients with SAD with comorbid ADHD.

20.4.1 Psychiatric Assessments

In adult cases, a generally used diagnostic measurement is the Conners Adult ADHD Rating Scales (CAARS) [54]. For screening the general population, the World Health Organization Adult ADHD Self-Report Scale (ASRS) is frequently used [55]. However, to date, any specific tools for SAD with ADHD has not been developed.

20.4.2 Treatment

> Little has been known with regard to treatment of comorbid SAD and ADHD, especially in adult cases. Comorbid anxiety with ADHD can be moderated by the treatment outcome [56]. It is reported that behavioral treatment can be better than pharmacological treatment or combined treatment [56].

Regarding pharmacotherapy, a RCT was conducted to determine the efficacy of atomoxetine for patients with SAD and comorbid ADHD [57]. It reported that atomoxetine improved both ADHD and SAD symptoms. On the other hand, Lakshmi et al. failed to show the efficacy of atomoxetine for the SAD in the absence of the ADHD [58]. Thus, for the patients with SAD, atomoxetine is one of the useful treatment options in case of the comorbid ADHD. In our clinical practice, sometimes it is difficult to diagnose ADHD at the first examination. When we find ADHD during the course of the SAD treatment, atomoxetine can be an additional treatment.

20.5 Taijin-Kyofu-Sho Syndrome as a Cultural Variation of SAD

Taijin-kyofu-sho syndrome (TKS) is thought to be a cultural variation of SAD in East Asia, especially Japan and Korea [59, 60]. Using the diagnosis criteria of Western countries, the prevalence rate of SAD is lower in East Asia than that in Western countries, which may imply that symptom difference between Western countries and East Asian countries exists [4]. TKS has become known after stated in the appendix of the Diagnostic and Statistical Manual of Mental Disorders (DSM-IV). Its prevalence rate is estimated as 8% [61].

In East Asian countries, TKS has been well known for its specific therapy such as Morita therapy [62]. Morita therapy was developed by Shoma Morita in the early 1990s. Its treatment components include isolation from others, bed rest, diary writing, and some routine works. The idea of Morita therapy has often been related to the third-wave CBT such as mindfulness-based stress reduction.

Most symptoms of TKS overlap with those of SAD; however, "offensive symptom" might be specific [59, 63]. Patients with SAD tend to ruminate negative evaluation from others; in contrast, patients with offensive-type TKS fear that they have offended others. In other words, SAD is self-oriented and TKS is other-oriented [64]. More detail, this offensive symptom means that the patients with TKS fear to make someone raise an unpleasant feeling by their gaze or their behavior. Although it is limited, TKS has been studied in English-speaking countries such as the USA or Australia [59, 63, 65] in last two decades. Those attempts made DSM-5 criteria include the offensive symptom as SAD symptom (DSM-5 SAD criteria B). After this, TKS might be combined to SAD than before; however, the effective treatment of TKS symptom or offensive symptom should be further studied.

20.5.1 Treatment

With regard to pharmacotherapy of TKS, the efficacy of SSRI or SNRI has been reported [66–68] similar to SAD.

In case of psychotherapy, there has not been any consensus for TKS. Although it is just our clinical CBT experience, we suggest a tip for the offensive type symptoms. We often conduct group experiments for the patients who believe their gaze makes someone unconfutable. In those experiments, patients made a role-play about certain situation (e.g., conversation with the colleagues at lunch), and we took video from the direction which the patient fears. If the patient fears more than two directions, we used two video cameras. Then all of the experiment participants watched the video together and discussed about how it was. Through this experiment, patients easily accept the idea that their gaze might not be offensive for surrounding people rather than cognitive reconstruction on the paper.

Disclosure Statement "The authors have nothing to disclose."

References

1. Clark D, Wells A. A cognitive model of social phobia. In: Heimberg RG, Liebowitz M, Hope DA, Schneier FR, editors. Social phobia: diagnosis, assessment and treatment. Guilford press, New York. 1995.
2. Mayo-Wilson E, Dias S, Mavranezouli I, Kew K, Clark DM, Ades AE, et al. Psychological and pharmacological interventions for social anxiety disorder in adults: a systematic review and network meta-analysis. Lancet Psychiatry. 2014;1(5):368–76.
3. Kessler RC, Petukhova M, Sampson NA, Zaslavsky AM, Wittchen HU. Twelve-month and lifetime prevalence and lifetime morbid risk of anxiety and mood disorders in the United States. Int J Methods Psychiatr Res. 2012;21(3):169–84.
4. Weissman MM, Bland RC, Canino GJ, Greenwald S, Lee CK, Newman SC, et al. The cross-national epidemiology of social phobia: a preliminary report. Int Clin Psychopharmacol. 1996;11(Suppl 3):9–14.
5. Kessler RC, Berglund P, Demler O, Jin R, Merikangas KR, Walters EE. Lifetime prevalence and age-of-onset distributions of DSM-IV disorders in the national comorbidity survey replication. Arch Gen Psychiatry. 2005;62(6):593–602.
6. Keller MB. The lifelong course of social anxiety disorder: a clinical perspective. Acta Psychiatr Scand Suppl. 2003;417:85–94.
7. Katzelnick DJ, Kobak KA, DeLeire T, Henk HJ, Greist JH, Davidson JR, et al. Impact of generalized social anxiety disorder in managed care. Am J Psychiatry. 2001;158(12):1999–2007.
8. Stein MB, Roy-Byrne PP, Craske MG, Bystritsky A, Sullivan G, Pyne JM, et al. Functional impact and health utility of anxiety disorders in primary care outpatients. Med Care. 2005;43(12):1164–70.
9. Bas-Hoogendam JM, Blackford JU, Bruhl AB, Blair KS, van der Wee NJ, Westenberg PM. Neurobiological candidate endophenotypes of social anxiety disorder. Neurosci Biobehav Rev. 2016;71:362–78.
10. Etkin A, Wager TD. Functional neuroimaging of anxiety: a meta-analysis of emotional processing in PTSD, social anxiety disorder, and specific phobia. A J Psychiatry. 2007;164(10):1476–88.
11. Hattingh CJ, Ipser J, Tromp SA, Syal S, Lochner C, Brooks SJ, et al. Functional magnetic resonance imaging during emotion recognition in social anxiety disorder: an activation likelihood meta-analysis. Front Hum Neurosci. 2012;6:347.
12. Irle E, Ruhleder M, Lange C, Seidler-Brandler U, Salzer S, Dechent P, et al. Reduced amygdalar and hippocampal size in adults with generalized social phobia. J Psychiatry Neurosci. 2010;35(2):126–31.
13. Liao W, Xu Q, Mantini D, Ding J, Machado-de-Sousa JP, Hallak JE, et al. Altered gray matter morphometry and resting-state functional and structural connectivity in social anxiety disorder. Brain Res. 2011;1388:167–77.

14. Meng Y, Lui S, Qiu C, Qiu L, Lama S, Huang X, et al. Neuroanatomical deficits in drug-naive adult patients with generalized social anxiety disorder: a voxel-based morphometry study. Psychiatry Res. 2013;214(1):9–15.

15. Morey RA, Gold AL, LaBar KS, Beall SK, Brown VM, Haswell CC, et al. Amygdala volume changes in post-traumatic stress disorder in a large case-controlled veterans group. Arch Gen Psychiatry. 2012;69(11):1169–78.

16. Hayano F, Nakamura M, Asami T, Uehara K, Yoshida T, Roppongi T, et al. Smaller amygdala is associated with anxiety in patients with panic disorder. Psychiatry Clin Neurosci. 2009;63(3):266–76.

17. Kawaguchi A, Nemoto K, Nakaaki S, Kawaguchi T, Kan H, Arai N, et al. Insular volume reduction in patients with social anxiety disorder. Front Psych. 2016;7:3.

18. Liebowitz MR. Social phobia. Mod Probl Pharmacopsychiatry. 1987;22:141–73.

19. Mattick RP, Clarke JC. Development and validation of measures of social phobia scrutiny fear and social interaction anxiety. Behav Res Ther. 1998;36(4):455–70.

20. Schneier FR. Clinical practice. Social anxiety disorder. N Engl J Med. 2006;355(10):1029–36.

21. Gross R, Olfson M, Gameroff MJ, Shea S, Feder A, Lantigua R, et al. Social anxiety disorder in primary care. Gen Hosp Psychiatry. 2005;27(3):161–8.

22. Liebowitz MR, Gelenberg AJ, Munjack D. Venlafaxine extended release vs placebo and paroxetine in social anxiety disorder. Arch Gen Psychiatry. 2005; 62(2):190–8.

23. Liebowitz MR, DeMartinis NA, Weihs K, Londborg PD, Smith WT, Chung H, et al. Efficacy of sertraline in severe generalized social anxiety disorder: results of a double-blind, placebo-controlled study. J Clin Psychiatry. 2003;64(7):785–92.

24. Stein DJ, Stein MB, Pitts CD, Kumar R, Hunter B. Predictors of response to pharmacotherapy in social anxiety disorder: an analysis of 3 placebo-controlled paroxetine trials. J Clin Psychiatry. 2002;63(2): 152–5.

25. Stein MB, Fyer AJ, Davidson JR, Pollack MH, Wiita B. Fluvoxamine treatment of social phobia (social anxiety disorder): a double-blind, placebo-controlled study. Am J Psychiatry. 1999;156(5):756–60.

26. Blanco C, Schneier FR, Schmidt A, Blanco-Jerez CR, Marshall RD, Sanchez-Lacay A, et al. Pharmacological treatment of social anxiety disorder: a meta-analysis. Depress Anxiety. 2003;18(1):29–40.

27. Schneier FR, Johnson J, Hornig CD, Liebowitz MR, Weissman MM. Social phobia. Comorbidity and morbidity in an epidemiologic sample. Arch Gen Psychiatry. 1992;49(4):282–8.

28. Hammad TA, Laughren T, Racoosin J. Suicidality in pediatric patients treated with antidepressant drugs. Arch Gen Psychiatry. 2006;63(3):332–9.

29. Liebowitz MR, Heimberg RG, Schneier FR, Hope DA, Davies S, Holt CS, et al. Cognitive-behavioral group therapy versus phenelzine in social phobia: long-term outcome. Depress Anxiety. 1999;10(3):89–98.

30. Kawaguchi A, Watanabe N, Nakano Y, Ogawa S, Suzuki M, Kondo M, et al. Group cognitive behavioral therapy for patients with generalized social anxiety disorder in Japan: outcomes at 1-year follow up and outcome predictors. Neuropsychiatr Dis Treat. 2013;9:267–75.

31. Andrews G, Creamer M, Crino R, Hunt C, Lampe L, Page A. The treatment of anxiety disorders clinician guides and patient manuals. Cambridge University Press, Cambridge. 2002.

32. Gould RA, Buckminster S, Pollack MH, Otto MW, Massachusetts LY. Cognitive-behavioral and pharmacological treatment for social phobia:a meta-analysis. Clin Psychol Sci Pract. 1997;4(4):291–306.

33. Kuusikko S, Pollock-Wurman R, Jussila K, Carter AS, Mattila ML, Ebeling H, et al. Social anxiety in high-functioning children and adolescents with autism and asperger syndrome. J Autism Dev Disord. 2008;38(9):1697–709.

34. Bellini S. Social skill deficits and anxiety in high-functioning adolescents with autism spectrum disorders. Focus Autism Other Dev Disabl. 2004;19(2):78–86.

35. Lugnegard T, Hallerback MU, Gillberg C. Psychiatric comorbidity in young adults with a clinical diagnosis of Asperger syndrome. Res Dev Disabil. 2011;32(5):1910–7.

36. Bejerot S, Eriksson JM, Mortberg E. Social anxiety in adult autism spectrum disorder. Psychiatry Res. 2014;220(1–2):705–7.

37. White SW, Kreiser NL, Pugliese C, Scarpa A. Social anxiety mediates the effect of autism spectrum disorder characteristics on hostility in young adults. Autism : Int J Res Pract. 2012;16(5):453–64.

38. White SW, Albano AM, Johnson CR, Kasari C, Ollendick T, Klin A, et al. Development of a cognitive-behavioral intervention program to treat anxiety and social deficits in teens with high-functioning autism. Clin Child Fam Psychol Rev. 2010;13(1):77–90.

39. Cath DC, Ran N, Smit JH, van Balkom AJ, Comijs HC. Symptom overlap between autism spectrum disorder, generalized social anxiety disorder and obsessive-compulsive disorder in adults: a preliminary case-controlled study. Psychopathology. 2008; 41(2):101–10.

40. Lord C, Rutter M, Goode S, Heemsbergen J, Jordan H, Mawhood L, et al. Autism diagnostic observation schedule: a standardized observation of communicative and social behavior. J Autism Dev Disord. 1989; 19(2):185–212.

41. Lord C, Rutter M, Le Couteur A. Autism diagnostic interview-revised: a revised version of a diagnostic interview for caregivers of individuals with possible pervasive developmental disorders. J Autism Dev Disord. 1994;24(5):659–85.

42. Baron-Cohen S, Wheelwright S, Skinner R, Martin J, Clubley E. The autism-spectrum quotient (AQ): evidence from Asperger syndrome/high-functioning autism, males and females, scientists and mathematicians. J Autism Dev Disord. 2001;31(1):5–17.

43. Ashwood KL, Gillan N, Horder J, Hayward H, Woodhouse E, McEwen FS, et al. Predicting the diagnosis of autism in adults using the Autism-Spectrum Quotient (AQ) questionnaire. Psychol Med. 2016;46(12):2595–604.

44. Freeth M, Bullock T, Milne E. The distribution of and relationship between autistic traits and social anxiety in a UK student population. Autism : Int J Res Pract. 2013;17(5):571–81.

45. Eriksson JM, Andersen LM, Bejerot S. RAADS-14 screen: validity of a screening tool for autism spectrum disorder in an adult psychiatric population. Molecular Autism. 2013;4(1):49.

46. Kreiser NL, White SW. Measuring social anxiety in adolescents and adults with high functioning autism: the development of a screening instrument. In: Kreiser NL, Pugliese C, editors. Co-occurring psychological and behavioral problems in adolescents and adults with features of autism spectrum disorder: assessment and characteristics. Toronto: Symposium conducted at the meeting of the Association for Behavioral and Cognitive Therapies; 2011.

47. Kreiser NL, White SW. Assessment of social anxiety in children and adolescents with autism spectrum disorder. Clin Psychol Sci Pract. 2014;21:18–31.

48. White SW, Ollendick T, Scahill L, Oswald D, Albano AM. Preliminary efficacy of a cognitive-behavioral treatment program for anxious youth with autism spectrum disorders. J Autism Dev Disord. 2009;39(12):1652–62.

49. Wood JJ, Ehrenreich-May J, Alessandri M, Fujii C, Renno P, Laugeson E, et al. Cognitive behavioral therapy for early adolescents with autism spectrum disorders and clinical anxiety: a randomized, controlled trial. Behav Ther. 2015;46(1):7–19.

50. Wood JJ, Drahota A, Sze K, Har K, Chiu A, Langer DA. Cognitive behavioral therapy for anxiety in children with autism spectrum disorders: a randomized, controlled trial. J Child Psychol Psychiatry. 2009;50(3):224–34.

51. Kuroda M, Kawakubo Y, Kuwabara H, Yokoyama K, Kano Y, Kamio YA. Cognitive-behavioral intervention for emotion regulation in adults with high-functioning autism spectrum disorders: study protocol for a randomized controlled trial. Trials. 2013;14:231.

52. Kessler RC, Adler L, Barkley R, Biederman J, Conners CK, Demler O, et al. The prevalence and correlates of adult ADHD in the United States: results from the National Comorbidity Survey Replication. Am J Psychiatry. 2006;163(4):716–23.

53. Koyuncu A, Ertekin E, Yuksel C, Aslantas Ertekin B, Celebi F, Binbay Z, et al. Predominantly inattentive type of ADHD is associated with social anxiety disorder. J Atten Disord. 2015;19(10):856–64.

54. Conners DE, Sparrow MA. Conners' Adult ADHD Rating Scales (CAARS). New York: Multihealth Systems, Inc.; 1999.

55. Kessler RC, Adler L, Ames M, Demler O, Faraone S, Hiripi E, et al. The World Health Organization Adult ADHD Self-Report Scale (ASRS): a short screening scale for use in the general population. Psychol Med. 2005;35(2):245–56.

56. Moderators and mediators of treatment response for children with attention-deficit/hyperactivity disorder: the Multimodal Treatment Study of children with Attention-deficit/hyperactivity disorder. Arch Gen Psychiatry. 1999;56(12):1088–96.

57. Adler LA, Liebowitz M, Kronenberger W, Qiao M, Rubin R, Hollandbeck M, et al. Atomoxetine treatment in adults with attention-deficit/hyperactivity disorder and comorbid social anxiety disorder. Depress Anxiety. 2009;26(3):212–21.

58. Ravindran LN, Kim DS, Letamendi AM, Stein MB. A randomized controlled trial of atomoxetine in generalized social anxiety disorder. J Clin Psychopharmacol. 2009;29(6):561–4.

59. Choy Y, Schneier FR, Heimberg RG, KS O, Liebowitz MR. Features of the offensive subtype of Taijin-Kyofu-Sho in US and Korean patients with DSM-IV social anxiety disorder. Depress Anxiety. 2008;25(3):230–40.

60. Heimberg RG, Makris GS, Juster HR, Ost LG, Rapee RM. Social phobia: a preliminary cross-national comparison. Depress Anxiety. 1997;5(3):130–3.

61. Kleinknecht RA, Dinnel DL, Kleinknecht EE, Hiruma N, Harada N. Cultural factors in social anxiety: a comparison of social phobia symptoms and Taijin kyofusho. J Anxiety Disord. 1997;11(2):157–77.

62. Wu H, Yu D, He Y, Wang J, Xiao Z, Li C. Morita therapy for anxiety disorders in adults. Cochrane Database Syst Rev. 2015(2):CD008619.

63. Clarvit SR, Schneier FR, Liebowitz MR. The offensive subtype of Taijin-kyofu-sho in New York City: the phenomenology and treatment of a social anxiety disorder. J Clin Psychiatry. 1996;57(11):523–7.

64. Chang SC. Social anxiety (phobia) and east Asian culture. Depress Anxiety. 1997;5(3):115–20.

65. Kim J, Rapee RM, Gaston JE. Symptoms of offensive type Taijin-Kyofusho among Australian social phobics. Depress Anxiety. 2008;25(7):601–8.

66. Matsunaga H, Kiriike N, Matsui T, Iwasaki Y, Stein DJ. Taijin kyofusho: a form of social anxiety disorder that responds to serotonin reuptake inhibitors? Int J Neuropsychopharmacol. 2001;4(3):231–7.

67. Nagata T, van Vliet I, Yamada H, Kataoka K, Iketani T, Kiriike N. An open trial of paroxetine for the "offensive subtype" of Taijin kyofusho and social anxiety disorder. Depress Anxiety. 2006;23(3):168–74.

68. Nagata T, Wada A, Yamada H, Iketani T, Kiriike O. Effect of milnacipran on insight and stress coping strategy in patients with Taijin Kyofusho. Int J Psychiatry Clin Pract. 2005;9(3):193–8.

A Complex Case of Anorexia Nervosa Associated with Pediatric Acute-Onset Neuropsychiatric Disorder Associated with Streptococcal Infection (PANDAS)

21

Peter Ajueze, Kuppuswami Shivakumar, and Kevin Saroka

21.1 Case Study

AB is an 11-year-old young girl living with her parents. She was attending a local elementary school and was referred to the eating disorder clinic due to concerns about her significant weight loss which was precipitated by a period of food restriction. She was reported to be eating the exact same food every day in small quantities. She also had been showing a significant fear of gaining weight, and as a result, she started to count calories, skip meals, and avoid fatty foods. She continued to worry about her body weight and she had an intense fear of gaining weight despite having a current weight that is low for her age and height. Her parents were concerned that she was showing physical symptoms associated with undernourishment (recurring dizziness, recurring headache, light-headedness, amenorrhea).

AB also presented with low-mood, anhedonia, sleep difficulties, loss of interest in previously enjoyable activities, and fleeting suicidal thoughts. She also reported experiencing irritability, anxiety, and frustration, especially around mealtimes. She was compulsively exercising in an effort to lose weight.

Prior to the onset of the above symptoms, she had a bout of severe pharyngitis. At that time there was a positive throat swab for group A streptococcal infection. The initial impres-

P. Ajueze, MD, MRCPsych(UK), FRCPC (✉)
K. Shivakumar, MD, MPH, MRCPsych(UK), FRCPC
Department of Psychiatry, Northern Ontario School
of Medicine (NOSM), Sudbury, ON, Canada
e-mail: pajueze@hsnsudbury.ca

K. Saroka, BSc, MA, PhD
Department of Psychiatry, Health Sciences North,
Sudbury, ON, Canada

© Springer International Publishing AG, part of Springer Nature 2018
K. Shivakumar, S. Amanullah (eds.), *Complex Clinical Conundrums in Psychiatry*,
https://doi.org/10.1007/978-3-319-70311-4_21

sion at the time was that of Kawasaki's or scarlet fever because she had a persistent fever and rash. At the time AB developed other symptoms following this bout of infection including sudden onset of OCD symptoms, recurrent motor and vocal tics, anxiety, irritability, and severe oppositional behavior. AB presents with exacerbation of these symptoms following subsequent streptococcal infections.

It was noted that while some of these symptoms subsided after treatment of the infection, symptoms of her eating disorder, OCD, and tics persisted regardless of treatment. As a result of AB's symptoms, she started avoiding school, her grades declined, she became more defiant toward her parents, and she continued to socially isolate herself due to low self-esteem.

21.2　What Is the Clinical Definition of PANDAS/PANS and How Is It Diagnosed

1. Pediatric Acute-Onset Neuropsychiatric Disorder Associated with Streptococcal Infection (PANDAS) was first described in the early 1900s in a subset of children or adolescents who had obsessive-compulsive disorder and/or tic disorders that followed streptococcal infection such as scarlet fever or strep throat. There is now evidence that symptoms originating from group A streptococcal infection may initiate neuropsychiatric disorders besides OCD and tics, such as anorexia nervosa.

2. PANS is a newer term that describes Pediatric Acute-Onset Neuropsychiatric Syndrome and includes all cases of abrupt onset of psychiatric symptoms, not just those associated with streptococcal infection, for example, mycoplasma, influenza A, chicken pox, Lyme disease, and other known infectious diseases. As reported by Chang et al. (2013), the most common antecedent infection seems to be upper respiratory infection including rhinosinusitis, pharyngitis, or bronchitis.

21.2.1　Key Differences Between PANS and PANDAS

Pediatric Acute-Onset Neuropsychiatric Syndrome (PANS)	Pediatric Acute-Onset Neuropsychiatric Disorder Associated with Streptococcal Infection (PANDAS)
Abrupt, dramatic onset of obsessive-compulsive disorder or severely restricted food intake (anorexia)	1. Presence of obsessive-compulsive disorder and/or a tic disorder
Presence of additional neuropsychiatric symptoms, with similarly severe and acute onset, from at least two of the following seven categories	2. Pediatric onset of symptoms (age 3 years to puberty)
Anxiety	3. Episodic course of symptom severity
Emotional lability and/or depression	4. Association with group A beta-emolytic streptococcal infection (a positive throat culture for strep or history of scarlet fever)
Irritability, aggression, and/or severely oppositional behaviors	5. Association with neurological abnormalities (motoric hyperactivity or adventitious movements, such as choreiform movements) [3]
Behavioral (developmental) regression	*1,2,3,4,5 Working diagnostic criteria for PANDAS
Deterioration in public performance	
Sensory or motor abnormalities	
Somatic signs and symptoms, including sleep disturbances, enuresis, or urinary frequency	
Symptoms are not better explained by a known neurologic or medical disorder, such as Sydenham chorea, systemic lupus erythematosus, Tourette syndrome, or others [1, 2]	

Table modified from Thienemann et al. [4]

21.3　Epidemiology of PANDAS

In contrast to the prevalence rates of anorexia nervosa, the epidemiology of PANDAS/PANS in relation to anorexia nervosa appears to be inexistent at this time. The average age of onset of symptoms for tics is 6.3+/−2.7 years and 7.4+/−2.7 years of age for OCD (in PANDAS). Some estimates have suggested that the onset of PANDAS occurs in 10% of those children with the childhood-onset obsessive-compulsive disorder and tic disorder.

21.4 Etiology of PANDAS

The exact pathogenic mechanisms are unknown; however, it is considered to have an autoimmune etiology. Evidence for an autoimmune etiology has been supported by the presence of serum antibodies that cross-react with neurons of the caudate, putamen, and globus pallidus [5, 6]:

- MRI shows enlargement of caudate, putamen, and globus pallidus, which suggest regional inflammation.
- Presence of antineuronal antibodies in majority of patients.

21.5 Assessment and Evaluation of PANDAS

Once there a suspicion of PANDAS/PANS, it is important to get comprehensive medical and psychiatric history and subsequently perform a full examination.

Diagnosis of PANDAS requires a temporal relation between GAS infection and the onset and/or exacerbation of neuropsychiatric abnormalities [4].

In 2013, the PANS Consensus Conference, Chang et al. (2013) are recommended the following for PANS evaluation or diagnosis:

- Family history
- Medical history and physical examination
- Psychiatric evaluation
- Infectious disease evaluation
- Assessment of symptoms and history that points for further evaluation of immune dysregulation (autoimmune disease, inflammatory disease, immunodeficiency)
- Neurological assessment

- Assessment of somatic symptoms, including possible sleep evaluation
- Genetic evaluation

21.6 Laboratory Features

Laboratory features of PANDAS include positive throat or skin ulcer or rapid antigen detection test for GAS as well as a clinically significant rise in antistreptococcal antibody between the onset of symptoms and 4–6 weeks later. These are associated with anti-DNase B titers and are elevated in approximately 80% of PANDAS cases [3].

21.7 Differential Diagnosis

As this condition coexists with several other disorders, the following requirements should be considered as differential diagnosis: (1) obsessive-compulsive disorder, (2) tic disorder, (3) Sydenham chorea, and (4) gastrointestinal disorder, e.g., inflammatory bowel disease and superior mesenteric artery syndrome.

21.8 Management of the Case Study

The initial goal for managing AB is weight restoration by refeeding. Hospitalization may be indicated for the following:

1. Medical stabilization as weight may be markedly low which subsequently may lead to an unstable physical health e.g bradycardia, hypotension and hypothermia.
2. Ensure the patient's safety (from psychological and physical risk).

Fluid and electrolyte levels may need to be restored after refeeding, the emphasis should be on maintaining a healthy weight. The choice of treatment depends on various factors including age and/or living circumstances of the patient. For youths and adolescents, the family-based treatment approach, otherwise known as the Maudsley Approach, is recommended which is a highly structured manual-based approach that requires a therapeutic staff who is highly skilled in this treatment. For older individuals or young adults not living with their parents, other approaches include cognitive behavior therapy (CBT) and cognitive remediation therapy etc. Studies have shown that CBT is superior to simple nutritional counseling alone [7]. With regard to treatment of PANDAS, antibiotics such as penicillin are recommended along with specific targeted treatment for OCD and tic disorders.

Conclusion

In addition to the well-known biopsychosocial factors implicated in the etiology of anorexia nervosa, it is important to consider evaluating for PANDAS/PANS, as this can potentially present as anorexia nervosa, obsessive-compulsive disorder, and tic disorder.

Failure to consider PANDAS/PANS in cases of anorexia nervosa may lead to treatment strategies that are ineffective.

References

1. Swedo SE, Leckman JF, Rose NR. From research subgroup to clinical syndrome: modifying the PANDAS criteria to describe PANS (pediatric acute-onset neuropsychiatric syndrome). Pediatr Therapeut. 2012;2(2):113.
2. Chang K, Frankovich J, Cooperstock M, Cunningham MW, Latimer ME, Murphy TK, Pasternack M, Thienemann M, Williams K, Walter J, Swedo SE. Clinical evaluation of youth with pediatric acute-onset neuropsychiatric syndrome (PANS): recommendations from the 2013 PANS consensus conference. J Child Adolesc Psychopharmacol. 2015;25(1):3–13.
3. Garvey MA, Giedd J, Swedo SE. Topical review: PANDAS: the search for environmental triggers of pediatric neuropsychiatric disorders. Lessons from rheumatic fever. J Child Neurol. 1998;13(9):413–23.
4. Thienemann M, Fewster D, Mazur A, Tona J, Hoppin KM, Stein K, Pohlman D. PANDAS and PANS in school settings: a handbook for educators. Philadelphia: Jessica Kingsley Publishers; 2016.
5. Leonard HL, Ale CM, Freeman JB, Garcia AM, Ng JS. Obsessive-compulsive disorder. Child Adolesc Psychiatr Clin N Am. 2005;14(4):727–43.
6. Snider LA, Swedo SE. PANDAS: current status and directions for research. Mol Psychiatry. 2004;9(10):900–7.
7. Pike KM, Carter JC, Olmsted MP. Cognitive behavioral therapy for anorexia nervosa. In: Grilo CM, Mitchell JE, editors. The treatment of eating disorders: a clinical handbook. New York: Guilford; 2010. p. 83–107.

Index

Printed in the United States
By Bookmasters